SECOND EDITION

PATHOLOGIC BASIS *of* DISEASE

SELF-ASSESSMENT AND REVIEW

CAROLYN C. COMPTON, M.D., Ph.D.

Assistant Professor, Department of Pathology
Massachusetts General Hospital
Harvard Medical School
Boston, Massachusetts

W. B. Saunders Company   **1986**

PHILADELPHIA LONDON TORONTO MEXICO CITY RIO DE JANEIRO SYDNEY TOKYO

W. B. Saunders Company: West Washington Square
Philadelphia, PA   19105

Library of Congress Cataloging-in-Publication Data

Compton, Carolyn C.

Pathologic basis of disease.

1. Pathology—Examinations, questions, etc.   I. Title.
   [DNLM: 1. Pathology—examination questions. QZ 18 C738p]

RB111.C65 1986   616.07   86–3986

ISBN 0–7216–2112–0

Editor: Dana Dreibelbis
Designer: Karen O'Keefe
Production Manager: Bill Preston
Manuscript Editor: Betty Gittens

Pathologic Basis of Disease: Self-Assessment and Review   ISBN   0–7216–2112–0

Last digit is the print number: 9   8   7   6   5   4   3

Our delight in any particular study . . . improves in proportion to the application which we bestow upon it. Thus, what was at first an exercise becomes at length an entertainment.

Addison

PREFACE

This book was conceived and written for students of pathology. In writing it, I really had two purposes in mind. I intended this book (1) to serve as an aid to the comprehension and synthesis of information contained in the companion textbook, *Pathologic Basis of Disease*, and (2) to help make studying pathology a little more sportful and a little less laborious. The questions cover major issues, but some *relevant* trivia is sprinkled in for the challenge and the purpose of specific illustration (*not* to make you throw up your hands in disgust). There are no trick questions; my motives were pure.

The short explanations at the end of each chapter give concise answers to each question and expand on each answer choice. For more information about the topic of the question, consult the referenced pages of the textbook.

The goal in using this book is to strengthen your understanding of the mechanisms and manifestations of disease, a worthy pursuit. In addition, however, it is my hope that you will enjoy the process as much as the product (i.e., knowledge). Learning is, after all, intrinsically entertaining. As Aristotle put it in his *Metaphysics*, "All humans by nature desire to know."

ACKNOWLEDGMENTS

The author thanks:

1. Ms. Jane Frabotta, who cheerfully typed every word of this book (several times)

2. My friends, who provided both moral and editorial support

3. My students and residents, from whom I am always learning

4. Dr. Stan Robbins and Dr. Ramzi Cotran, my much admired mentors

Answer: All of the Above

CONTENTS

1

GENERAL PATHOLOGY

DIRECTIONS: For Questions 1 to 15, choose the ONE BEST answer to each question.

1. Generalized edema results from all of the following disorders EXCEPT:

    A. Systemic hypertension
    B. Congestive heart failure
    C. Cirrhosis
    D. Nephrotic syndrome
    E. Hyperaldosteronism

2. Disorders that predispose to thrombosis include all of the following EXCEPT:

    A. Pancreatic carcinoma
    B. Pregnancy
    C. Vitamin K deficiency
    D. Sickle cell anemia
    E. Diabetes mellitus

3. Chemical agents known to be carcinogenic in human beings include all of the following EXCEPT:

    A. Chemotherapeutic alkylating agents
    B. Asbestos
    C. Arsenic
    D. Saccharin
    E. Vinyl chloride

4. Markedly increased susceptibility to pyogenic infections occurs in all of the following conditions EXCEPT:

    A. Deficiency of the third component of complement (C3)
    B. Common variable immunodeficiency
    C. Chronic granulomatous disease of childhood
    D. DiGeorge's syndrome
    E. Chédiak-Higashi syndrome

5. The feature most important in differentiating a malignant from a benign tumor is:

    A. Lack of encapsulation
    B. High mitotic rate
    C. Presence of necrosis and hemorrhage
    D. Presence of metastases
    E. Nuclear pleomorphism (anaplasia)

6. In hypoxic cell injury, swelling of the cells occurs because:

    A. Intracytoplasmic lipids accumulate
    B. Intracytoplasmic proteins accumulate
    C. Intracytoplasmic glycogen increases
    D. Pinocytotic fluid uptake greatly increases
    E. None of these

7. Cell injury from chemically unstable molecules known as "free radicals" is a major feature of each of the following pathologic processes EXCEPT:

    A. Mercuric chloride poisoning
    B. Irradiation damage
    C. Oxygen toxicity
    D. Carbon tetrachloride poisoning
    E. Bacterial infection

8. In an inflammatory response, neutrophils release molecules that have all of the following effects EXCEPT:

    A. Chemotaxis of monocytes
    B. Chemotaxis of lymphocytes
    C. Degranulation of mast cells
    D. Increased vascular permeability independent of histamine release
    E. Connective tissue digestion

9. In immunologic reactions, lymphocytes make substances (lymphokines) that are chemotactic for all of the following cells EXCEPT:

    A. Neutrophils
    B. Platelets
    C. Eosinophils
    D. Macrophages
    E. Basophils

10. Mediators of increased vascular permeability in acute inflammatory responses include all of the following EXCEPT:

    A. Leukotriene E_4
    B. Complement complex C5b67
    C. Leukotriene C_4
    D. Bradykinin
    E. Platelet activating factor (PAF)

11. The most reliable evidence of chronicity in an inflammatory process in the liver (hepatitis) is the presence of:

  A. Lymphocytes
  B. Bile duct destruction
  C. Councilman bodies
  D. Fibrosis
  E. Plasmacytic infiltrates

12. A large aggregate of epithelioid histiocytes is seen in a microscopic section of an ovary removed at surgery. Your diagnosis is:

  A. Granulation tissue
  B. Granular cell tumor
  C. Granulosa cell tumor
  D. Granuloma
  E. Granulocytosis

13. All of the following neoplasms are malignant EXCEPT:

  A. Glomus tumor
  B. Ewing's tumor
  C. Wilms' tumor
  D. Seminoma
  E. Histiocytosis X

14. Hereditary conditions that are associated with a high risk of malignancy include all of the following EXCEPT:

  A. Von Hippel–Lindau disease
  B. Turcot syndrome
  C. Patau's syndrome
  D. Fanconi's anemia
  E. Ataxia-telangiectasia

15. The diagnosis on a cervical cytology specimen is "Class II." You would tell the patient that:

  A. Her Pap smear was perfectly normal
  B. Atypical cells were found, and the examination will need to be repeated
  C. A high grade cervical dysplasia is present, and biopsy confirmation will be required
  D. Carcinoma *in situ* was found, and surgical excision of the lesion will be necessary
  E. Invasive carcinoma is present, and hysterectomy will be required

DIRECTIONS: For Questions 16 to 41, ONE or MORE of the completions given correctly finishes the incomplete statement. Choose:
  A—if only *1,2, and 3* are correct
  B—if only *1 and 3* are correct
  C—if only *2 and 4* are correct
  D—if only *4* is correct
  E—if all are correct

16. In myocardial ischemia, *irreversibly* injured myofibers are distinguishable by which of the following light microscopic features?

  1. Cytoplasmic fatty change
  2. Cytoplasmic eosinophilia
  3. Cellular swelling
  4. Nuclear shrinkage

   A. 1,2,3   B. 1,3   C. 2,4   D. 4 Only   E. All

17. Generation of free radicals is the *major* mechanism of cell injury in:

  1. Oxygen toxicity
  2. Radiation injury
  3. Carbon tetrachloride poisoning
  4. Ischemia

   A. 1,2,3   B. 1,3   C. 2,4   D. 4 Only   E. All

18. Which of the following conditions are usually associated with delayed wound healing?

  1. Severe granulocytopenia
  2. Cushing's syndrome
  3. Severe thrombocytopenia
  4. Scurvy

   A. 1,2,3   B. 1,3   C. 2,4   D. 4 Only   E. All

19. Cytotoxic lymphocytes are the major mediators in the pathogenesis of:

  1. Renal transplant rejection
  2. Arthus reaction
  3. Graft-versus-host disease
  4. Tuberculin reaction

   A. 1,2,3   B. 1,3   C. 2,4   D. 4 Only   E. All

20. Secondary amyloidosis is associated with:

  1. Ulcerative colitis
  2. Rheumatoid arthritis
  3. Renal cell carcinoma
  4. Waldenström's macroglobulinemia

   A. 1,2,3   B. 1,3   C. 2,4   D. 4 Only   E. All

21. Amyloid is:

  1. Digested by amylase
  2. Stained by Oil Red O

3. Sometimes generated from immunoglobulin heavy chains
4. Sometimes generated from prealbumin

A. 1,2,3   B. 1,3   C. 2,4   D. 4 Only   E. All

22. Hageman factor activates the:

1. Complement system
2. Kinin system
3. Fibrinolytic system
4. Coagulation system

A. 1,2,3   B. 1,3   C. 2,4   D. 4 Only   E. All

23. Red infarctions are usually encountered in:

1. Pulmonary embolism
2. Torsion of the testis
3. Superior mesenteric artery atheroembolism
4. Coronary artery thrombosis

A. 1,2,3   B. 1,3   C. 2,4   D. 4 Only   E. All

24. Shock is commonly associated with which of the following conditions?

1. *E. coli* sepsis
2. Myocardial infarction
3. Cholera
4. Acute pancreatitis

A. 1,2,3   B. 1,3   C. 2,4   D. 4 Only   E. All

25. Human malignancies known to be caused by exposure to radiation include:

1. Acute leukemia
2. Thyroid carcinoma
3. Lung cancer
4. Osteosarcoma

A. 1,2,3   B. 1,3   C. 2,4   D. 4 Only   E. All

26. Neoplasms that are known to be associated with a defect of chromosome 22 include:

1. Adenocarcinoma of the colon
2. Meningioma
3. Malignant melanoma
4. Chronic myelogenous leukemia

A. 1,2,3   B. 1,3   C. 2,4   D. 4 Only   E. All

27. Factors that are assessed in the grading of a malignant tumor include:

1. Numbers of lymph nodes containing metastases
2. Size of the primary lesion
3. Degree of local invasion of the primary tumor
4. Number of mitoses in the primary tumor

A. 1,2,3   B. 1,3   C. 2,4   D. 4 Only   E. All

28. Shock is a frequent complication of large burn injuries that is commonly produced by:

1. Disseminated intravascular coagulation
2. Pseudomonas endotoxemia
3. Transudation of fluid from the wound
4. Anaphylaxis from smoke inhalation

A. 1,2,3   B. 1,3   C. 2,4   D. 4 only   E. All

29. In a myocardial biopsy taken two hours after coronary occlusion and reperfusion, which of the following ultrastructural features would indicate that the myocytes had sustained irreversible ischemic injury?

1. Ribosomal detachment from the rough endoplasmic reticulum
2. Appearance of dense deposits in the mitochondria
3. Loss of intracellular glycogen
4. Loss of intracellular RNA

A. 1,2,3   B. 1,3   C. 2,4   D. 4 only   E. All

30. An immunoperoxidase stain of an anaplastic tumor demonstrates the presence of desmin in the tumor cell cytoplasm. This finding is compatible with a diagnosis of:

1. Fibrosarcoma
2. Squamous cell carcinoma
3. Rhabdosarcoma
4. Lymphoma

A. 1,2,3   B. 1,3   C. 2,4   D. 4 only   E. All

31. Contractile and cytoskeletal elements common to all cells include:

1. Spectrin
2. Actin
3. Myosin
4. Tubulin

A. 1,2,3   B. 1,3   C. 2,4   D. 4 only   E. All

32. Pathologic forms of hyperplasia that are associated with an increased risk of malignancy in the tissue of origin and are therefore considered to be premalignant conditions include:

1. Adenomatous hyperplasia of endometrium
2. Follicular hyperplasia of lymph nodes
3. Hyperplasia of gastric surface mucous glands (Ménétrier's disease)
4. Prostatic gland hyperplasia

A. 1,2,3   B. 1,3   C. 2,4   D. 4 only   E. All

33. Cancers that commonly occur in tissues that have first undergone metaplasia, then become dysplastic, and finally become malignant include:

1. Squamous cell carcinoma of the endocervix
2. Squamous cell carcinoma of the bladder
3. Bronchogenic squamous cell carcinoma
4. Adenocarcinoma of the esophagus

A. 1,2,3   B. 1,3   C. 2,4   D. 4 only   E. All

34. In which of the following diseases do calcium deposits commonly occur in normal tissues?

1. Wilson's disease
2. Multiple myeloma
3. Papillary carcinoma of the thyroid
4. Parathyroid carcinoma

   A. 1,2,3   B. 1,3   C. 2,4   D. 4 only   E. All

35. Factors that promote neutrophil adherence to the endothelium of blood vessels (a prerequisite for leukocyte emigration into tissues in an acute inflammatory response) include:

1. Divalent calcium ions
2. Leukotriene B$_4$
3. The C5a component of the complement system
4. Decreased negative cell surface charges on neutrophils

   A. 1,2,3   B. 1,3   C. 2,4   D. 4 only   E. All

36. Predisposition to bacterial infection in diabetes mellitus is caused by basic defects in leukocyte function that include:

1. Reduced ability of leukocytes to stick to vascular endothelium
2. Reduced numbers of circulating white cells
3. Defective phagocytic function
4. Deficiency of leukocyte glucose-6-phosphate dehydrogenase (G-6-PD)

   A. 1,2,3   B. 1,3   C. 2,4   D. 4 only   E. All

37. Factors that are important in protecting normal cells from potential injury from free radicals generated in the course of an inflammatory response include:

1. Glutathione peroxidase
2. Serum ceruloplasmin
3. Catalase
4. Alpha-2-macroglobulin

   A. 1,2,3   B. 1,3   C. 2,4   D. 4 only   E. All

38. Pathologic lesions produced by vascular congestion include:

1. Nutmeg liver
2. Brown induration of the lung
3. Splenic Gandy-Gamna bodies
4. Koilonychia

   A. 1,2,3   B. 1,3   C. 2,4   D. 4 only   E. All

39. Amyloid of the AA type, in which the fibrils are composed mostly of amyloid-associated (AA) protein, occurs in association with which of the following conditions?

1. Senile cardiac amyloidosis
2. Hereditary neuropathic amyloidosis
3. Medullary carcinoma of the thyroid
4. Ulcerative colitis

   A. 1,2,3   B. 1,3   C. 2,4   D. 4 only   E. All

40. Tumors that tend to spread over the surfaces of viscera or body cavities rather than metastasizing via blood vessels or lymphatics include:

1. Colon carcinoma
2. Ovarian carcinoma
3. Renal cell carcinoma
4. Mesothelioma

   A. 1,2,3   B. 1,3   C. 2,4   D. 4 only   E. All

41. In the United States, which of the following tumors occur(s) with greater frequency in males than in females?

1. Pancreatic carcinoma
2. Colon carcinoma
3. Bladder carcinoma
4. Hepatocellular carcinoma (hepatoma)

   A. 1,2,3   B. 1,3   C. 2,4   D. 4 only   E. All

DIRECTIONS: For Questions 42 to 67, you are to decide whether EACH choice is TRUE or FALSE.

For each of the following statements about histocompatibility antigens, decide whether it is TRUE or FALSE.

42. Histocompatibility antigens are the antigens that evoke graft vs. host disease
43. HLA-DR antigens are found on the cell surface of all normal nucleated cells

44. HLA-DR antigens evoke the formation of humoral antibody in genetically incompatible transplant recipients
45. The chance that two siblings will be HLA-identical is 50%
46. The genes that determine patterns of immune responses are located within the HLA gene complex
47. Recognition of a virally infected cell by a T lymphocyte is dependent on the presence of HLA-D antigens on the infected cells

48. Individuals who posses HLA-B27 antigen are nearly 100 times as likely to get ankylosing spondylitis as those who don't

For each of the following statements about tissue atrophy, decide whether it is TRUE or FALSE

49. Atrophic cells contain fewer than normal numbers of cytoplasmic organelles (mitochondria, endoplasmic reticulum, etc.)
50. Atrophy occurs in otherwise normal tissues if their workload is decreased
51. Atrophy begins to occur in most tissues immediately after death of the individual
52. Atrophy occurs in otherwise normal tissues in which the blood supply has decreased
53. The appearance of autophagic vacuoles in cells undergoing atrophy signals irreversible cell injury and impending cell death

For each of the following statements about the acquired immune deficiency syndrome (AIDS), decide whether it is TRUE or FALSE.

54. The disease is caused by a retrovirus infection
55. The disease is caused by an Epstein-Barr virus infection

56. The number of helper T cells in the peripheral blood is characteristically increased
57. Immunoglobulin levels are characteristically normal or elevated
58. Death from this disease is usually caused by metastatic Kaposi's sarcoma
59. Diffuse undifferentiated (Burkitt-like) lymphoma is a feature of the AIDS syndrome
60. Hemophiliacs are at high risk of developing AIDS

For each of the following statements about malignant cells, decide whether it is TRUE or FALSE

61. Malignant cells require greater amounts of serum factors in the medium for optimal *in vitro* growth than their normal counterparts
62. Malignant cells enter the G_0 stage of the cell cycle at high density in cell culture
63. The cells of most virally induced tumors possess tumor specific transplantation antigens (TSTAs) on their cell surface
64. A syngeneic host can be immunized against transplanted malignant cells bearing TSTAs
65. A syngeneic host can be immunized against transplanted malignant cells bearing tumor-associated antigens (TAAs) on their cell surface
66. Malignant cells are deficient in desmosomes compared with their normal counterparts
67. Malignant cells secrete enzymes that can digest normal tissues

DIRECTIONS: For Questions 68 to 105, the set of lettered headings is followed by a list of numbered words or phrases. For each numbered word or phrase choose:

A—if the item is associated with (A) only
B—if the item is associated with (B) only
C—if the item is associated with *both* (A) and (B)
D—if the item is associated with neither (A) nor (B)

For each process or lesion listed below, choose whether it is primarily characterized by an inflammatory response, an immunologic response, both, or neither.

A. Inflammatory response
B. Immunologic response
C. Both
D. Neither

68. Suture granuloma
69. Marantic endocarditis
70. Streptococcal pneumonia
71. Sunburn
72. Hashimoto's thyroiditis
73. Lead poisoning

For each of the biologic properties listed below, choose whether it is characteristic of interleukin-1, interleukin-2, both, or neither.

A. Interleukin-1
B. Interleukin-2
C. Both
D. Neither

74. Made by macrophages
75. Made by neutrophils
76. Made by lymphocytes
77. Produces fever
78. Stimulates lymphocytes
79. Stimulates fibroblasts
80. Stimulates liver cells

81. Inhibits viral replication
82. Activates complement
83. Activates plasminogen

For each of the biologic properties described below, decide whether it is characteristic of epidermal cells, fibroblasts, both, or neither.

   A. Epidermal cells (keratinocytes)
   B. Fibroblasts
   C. Both
   D. Neither

84. Under physiologic conditions, undergo continuous proliferation throughout life
85. Respond so rapidly to surgical skin incisions that migration across the wound is complete within 24 to 48 hours
86. Produce type IV collagen
87. Produce type II collagen
88. Synthesize fibronectin
89. Are induced to migrate by fibronectin
90. Are induced to divide by a factor secreted by activated macrophages
91. Are induced to divide by urogastrone

92. Are induced to divide by platelet-derived growth factor (PDGF)
93. Produce interleukin-1

For each of the conditions listed below, decide whether it is causally related to cigarette smoking, alcohol abuse, both, or neither.

   A. Cigarette smoking
   B. Alcohol abuse
   C. Both
   D. Neither

94. Esophageal carcinoma
95. Acute esophagitis
96. Pancreatic carcinoma
97. Acute pancreatitis
98. Gastric carcinoma
99. Acute gastritis
100. Renal cell carcinoma
101. Bladder carcinoma
102. Pharyngeal carcinoma
103. Hodgkin's disease
104. Breast carcinoma
105. Ovarian carcinoma

DIRECTIONS: Questions 106 to 266 are matching questions. For each numbered item, choose the most likely associated lettered item from those provided. Each numbered item has ONLY ONE answer. Within each group, each lettered item may be the answer to one, more than one, or none of the numbered items.

For each of the causes of fatty liver listed below, decide whether it increases free fatty acid entry into liver cells, decreases fatty acid oxidation, increases triglyceride formation, decreases apoprotein synthesis, or does all of these.

   A. Increases free fatty acid entry into liver cells
   B. Decreases fatty acid oxidation
   C. Increases triglyceride formation
   D. Decreases apoprotein synthesis
   E. All of these

106. Alcohol ingestion
107. Phosphorus poisoning
108. Carbon tetrachloride poisoning
109. Corticosteroid therapy
110. Starvation

For each of the descriptions of intracellular pigment accumulation listed below, decide whether it refers to lipofuscin, melanin, hemosiderin, or none of these.

   A. Lipofuscin
   B. Melanin
   C. Hemosiderin
   D. None of these

111. Accumulates in cartilage of patients with ochronosis
112. Accumulates in lungs of patients with mitral stenosis
113. Accumulates in lungs of coal miners
114. Accumulates in synovium of patients with pigmented villonodular synovitis
115. Accumulates in colonic mucosa of some laxative abusers

For each of the situations listed below, decide whether the cellular response it typically engenders is hypertrophy, hyperplasia, metaplasia, dysplasia, or none of these.

   A. Hypertrophy
   B. Hyperplasia
   C. Metaplasia
   D. Dysplasia
   E. None of these

116. Response of cardiac muscle to systemic hypertension
117. Response of bronchiolar epithelium in chronic bronchitis

118. Response of adrenocortical cells to a pituitary adenoma producing ACTH
119. Response of prostatic stroma in benign prostatic hypertrophy (BPH)
120. Response of colonic epithelium in long-standing ulcerative colitis

For each of the characteristics of autoimmune disease listed below, decide whether it describes systemic lupus erythematosus (SLE), Sjögren's syndrome, scleroderma, all of these, or none of these.

    A. Systemic lupus erythematosus (SLE)
    B. Sjögren's syndrome
    C. Scleroderma
    D. All of these
    E. None of these

121. The disease occurs with increased incidence in hereditary deficiency of the second component of complement (C2)
122. A 40-fold increased risk of lymphoid malignancy is incurred
123. An underlying epithelial malignancy is found in 10% of patients
124. Dermatomyositis is an associated disorder
125. Articular (joint) pain is a common symptom
126. Anticentromere antibodies are characteristic
127. Glomerular lesions are extremely rare
128. The most common cause of death is renal failure
129. Immunoglobulin deposition is found in normal-appearing skin
130. Response to corticosteroids is excellent

For each of the characteristics of immunodeficiency disease listed below, decide whether it describes X-linked agammaglobulinemia of Bruton, common variable immunodeficiency, DiGeorge's syndrome, or none of these.

    A. X-linked agammaglobulinemia of Bruton
    B. Common variable immunodeficiency
    C. DiGeorge's syndrome
    D. None of these

131. Characterized by a failure of pre-B cells to mature into B cells
132. Caused by a defect in lymphoid stem cells
133. Associated with tetany
134. Associated with a high incidence of systemic lupus erythematosus
135. Often accompanied by nontropical sprue (gluten-sensitive enteropathy)
136. Associated with an increased incidence of lymphoid malignancy
137. Associated with noncaseating granulomas in the liver

For each of the conditions listed below, decide whether the major pathogenetic mechanism of the associated tissue edema and/or ascites is related to:

    A. Decreased plasma oncotic pressure
    B. Increased hydrostatic pressure
    C. Increased endothelial permeability
    D. Lymphatic obstruction
    E. None of these

138. Nephrotic syndrome
139. Congestive heart failure
140. Cirrhosis
141. Thermal burn
142. Kwashiorkor
143. Bee sting
144. Pregnancy
145. Excessive salt intake
146. Hydrops fetalis
147. Constrictive pericarditis
148. Metastatic carcinoma
149. Ménétrier's disease

For each of the conditions listed below, decide whether it most commonly produces coagulation necrosis, liquefaction necrosis, enzymatic fat necrosis, caseous necrosis, or none of these.

    A. Coagulation necrosis
    B. Liquefaction necrosis
    C. Enzymatic fat necrosis
    D. Caseous necrosis
    E. None of these

150. Pulmonary nocardiosis
151. Myocardial infarction
152. Pott's disease
153. Tuberculoid leprosy of skin
154. Acute pancreatitis
155. Wet gangrene of the great toe
156. Giardiasis (small bowel)
157. Cerebral infarction
158. Acute tubular necrosis (kidney)

For each of the conditions listed below, decide whether it is an example of an immunologically mediated disorder of the anaphylactic type (Type I), cytotoxic type (Type II), immune complex type (Type III), cell-mediated type (Type IV), or whether it is not an immunologically mediated disorder at all.

    A. Type I, anaphylactic type immune response
    B. Type II, cytotoxic type immune response
    C. Type III, immune complex disorder
    D. Type IV, cell-mediated hypersensitivity response
    E. Not an immunologically mediated disord

159. Erythroblastosis fetalis
160. Poison ivy dermatitis
161. Hay fever
162. Polyarteritis nodosa
163. Serum sickness
164. Graft vs. host disease
165. Dopamine-induced hemolytic anemia
166. Penicillin-induced urticaria
167. Amphotericin-induced renal injury
168. Chlorpromazine-induced cholestatic jaundice
169. Pulmonar asbestosis
170. Chronic berylliosis

For each of the biologic characteristics listed below, decide whether it describes B cells, T cells, macrophages/monocytes, all of these cell types, or none of these.

    A. T cells
    B. B cells
    C. Macrophages/monocytes
    D. All of the above
    E. None of the above

171. Found in the circulating blood
172. Found in the cortex of lymph nodes
173. Display IgG on their cell surface
174. Do not display HLA-DR antigens on their cell surface
175. Do not have cell surface receptors for complement
176. Are able to lyse antibody-coated target cells by means of a nonphagocytic mechanism
177. Function in the negative regulation (turning off) of the immune response
178. Are capable of lysing tumor cells without previous sensitization
179. Initiate delayed-type cell-mediated hypersensitivity responses
180. Produce leukotriene mediators of anaphylaxis
181. Respond chemotactically to leukotriene B_4
182. Form spontaneous rosettes with sheep erythrocytes (E rosettes)

For each of the situations listed below, decide whether bilirubin, hematin, ceroid, lipofuscin, or none of these pigmentations would be expected to be seen.

    A. Bilirubin
    B. Hematin
    C. Ceroid
    D. Lipofuscin
    E. None of these

183. Myocytes of an elderly, malnourished individual
184. Hepatocytes in an elderly, malnourished individual

185. Kupffer cells in a patient recovering from hepatitis
186. Sinus histiocytes in the peribronchial lymph nodes of a smoker
187. Skin keratinocytes in Addison's disease
188. Kupffer's cells in an individual with hereditary spherocytosis
189. Kupffer's cells in large bile duct obstruction
190. Splenic phagocytes in malaria
191. Splenic phagocytes after a hemolytic transfusion reaction
192. Dermal macrophages of tatooed skin

For each of the conditions listed below, decide whether the associated inflammatory cell infiltrate is composed predominantly of neutrophils, monocytes, eosinophils, plasma cells, or lymphocytes.

    A. Neutrophils
    B. Monocytes/macrophages
    C. Eosinophils
    D. Plasma cells
    E. Lymphocytes

193. Acute myocardial infarction (2 to 3 days in age)
194. Acute B viral hepatitis
195. Sarcoidosis
196. Liver transplant rejection
197. Polyarteritis nodosa
198. Chronic endometritis
199. Primary syphilis
200. Löffler's syndrome
201. Paragonimiasis
202. Bronchial asthma

For each of the elements listed below, decide whether it is chemotactic for neutrophils only, monocytes only, eosinophils only, both neutrophils and monocytes, both monocytes and eosinophils, or all of these cell types.

    A. Neutrophils
    B. Monocytes
    C. Eosinophils
    D. Neutrophils and monocytes
    E. Monocytes and eosinophils
    F. All of these cells

203. The C5a component of the complement system
204. Products of the lipoxygenase pathway of arachidonic acid metabolism
205. Products of the cycloxygenase pathway of arachidonic acid metabolism
206. Bacterial products
207. Histamine
208. Factors liberated by activated lymphocytes
209. Fibronectin fragments

For each of the biologic effects listed below, decide whether it is produced by one or none of the following lymphokines:

  A. Transfer factor
  B. Interferon
  C. Interleukin-2
  D. Lymphotoxin
  E. None of the above

210. Increases macrophage bactericidal activity
211. Increases proliferation of other T cells
212. Directly kills bacteria
213. Inhibits macrophage migration
214. Inhibits intracellular viral replication

For each of the properties listed below, decide whether it is characteristic of killer (K) cells, natural killer (NK) cells, cytotoxic lymphocytes (CTL), all of these, or none of these.

  A. Killer (K) cells
  B. Natural killer (NK) cells
  C. Cytotoxic lymphocytes (CT)
  D. All of the above
  E. None of the above

215. Have the ability to destroy tumor cells
216. Are not phagocytic
217. Contain granules in their cytoplasm
218. Are capable of lysing only antibody-coated cells
219. Do *not* possess cell surface receptors for the Fc fragment of IgG
220. Recognize virally infected cells only by means of altered cell-surface HLA antigens

For each of the conditions listed below, decide whether it is characterized by inflammation of the serous, fibrinous, suppurative, granulomatous, or lymphoplasmacytic type.

  A. Serous inflammation
  B. Fibrinous inflammation
  C. Suppurative inflammation
  D. Granulomatous inflammation
  E. Mononuclear cell inflammation

221. Cat scratch lymphadenitis
222. Acute viral pneumonia
223. Acute appendicitis
224. Rheumatic pericarditis
225. Chronic brucellosis
226. Adult hyaline membrane disease (diffuse alveolar damage)
227. Second degree thermal burns
228. Friction blisters
229. Acute viral hepatitis

230. Acute ascending cholangitis
231. Initial stage of primary biliary cirrhosis
232. Uremic pericarditis

For each of the chemical carcinogens listed below, decide whether it is primarily associated with cancer of the lung, skin, stomach, bladder, or none of these malignancies.

  A. Lung cancer
  B. Skin cancer
  C. Stomach cancer
  D. Bladder cancer
  E. None of the above

233. Aflatoxin B1
234. Beta-naphthylamine (an azo dye)
235. Busulfan
236. Vinyl chloride
237. Chromium compounds
238. Nitrosamines
239. Benzidine

For each of the tumor types listed below, decide which of the following substances would be expected to be found in the tumor cells by immunohistochemical stains and would help to identify the tumor.

  A. Alpha-fetoprotein
  B. Carcinoembryonic antigen
  C. Desmin
  D. Human chorionic gonadotropin
  E. None of the above

240. Lymphoma
241. Ganglioneuroblastoma
242. Hepatoma
243. Colonic carcinoma
244. Choriocarcinoma
245. Medullary carcinoma of the thyroid
246. Rhabdosarcoma

For each of the neoplasms listed below, decide if Epstein-Barr virus, papilloma virus, herpes simplex type 2, hepatitis B virus, or none of these viruses is thought to be causally related to at least some tumors of that type.

  A. Epstein-Barr virus
  B. Papilloma virus
  C. Adenovirus
  D. Hepatitis B virus
  E. None of these

247. Cervical carcinoma
248. Breast carcinoma
249. Nasopharyngeal carcinoma

250. Burkitt's lymphoma
251. Cutaneous squamous cell carcinoma
252. Adult T-cell leukemia
253. Fibrosarcoma
254. Cholangiocarcinoma
255. Hepatoma
256. Angiosarcoma of the liver

C. Renal cell carcinoma
D. Prostatic carcinoma
E. None of these

For each of the paraneoplastic syndromes listed below, decide whether bronchogenic carcinoma, pancreatic carcinoma, renal cell carcinoma, prostatic carcinoma, or none of these is a very strongly associated underlying malignancy.

A. Bronchogenic carcinoma
B. Pancreatic carcinoma

257. Malignant form of acanthosis nigricans
258. Hypercalcemia
259. Cancer-associated dermatomyositis
260. Hypertrophic osteoarthropathy
261. Hyponatremia
262. Polycythemia
263. Nephrotic syndrome
264. Anemia (nonmyelophthisic)
265. Malignancy-associated myasthenia gravis
266. Peripheral neuropathy

1

GENERAL PATHOLOGY

ANSWERS

1. (A) Generalized noninflammatory edema results from any disorder that causes an imbalance in the factors that determine fluid compartmentalization and tips the balance toward the extravascular compartment. Thus, the common primary etiologies include increased hydrostatic pressure (congestive heart failure) or reduced plasma oncotic pressure resulting either from inadequate synthesis (cirrhosis) or increased loss (nephrotic syndrome) of albumin. Increased osmotic tension in the interstitial fluid related to sodium retention is another primary cause of generalized noninflammatory edema, which occurs in the presence of increased circulating levels of aldosterone.

Generalized edema occurs only in the presence of increased hydrostatic pressure in the venous or lymphatic systems, the sites of resorption of extravascular interstitial fluid. Systemic hypertension in the arterial system does not produce this effect (*pp. 85–87*).

2. (C) A number of clinical states are associated with an increased incidence of thrombosis. Included among these are pregnancy and pancreatic carcinoma. The mechanisms underlying the thrombotic tendency in pregnancy are poorly understood but in pancreatic carcinoma may be related to the release of tissue thromboplastin and procoagulant factors from the tumor.

Conditions that produce intravascular stasis also predispose to thrombosis. Sickle cell anemia is a prime example (see Chapter 7, Question 13).

Endothelial injury also causes activation of the coagulation system and prediposes to thrombosis. It is well known that thrombi tend to occur on ulcerated atherosclerotic plaques. Thus, diabetes mellitus with its predisposition to severe atherosclerosis and to hyperlipidemia, which potentiates platelet aggregation, is associated with an increased incidence of arterial thrombosis.

Vitamin K deficiency, in contrast, produces a bleeding tendency rather than a predisposition to thrombosis. Since vitamin K is essential to the biosynthesis of prothrombin and clotting factors VII, IX, and X, vitamin K deficiency produces a coagulopathy on the basis of the depletion of these factors (see Chapter 3, Question 14 and *pp. 97–98*).

3. (D) It is now clear from both epidemiologic and experimental studies that a large number of chemical agents are capable of causing neoplastic transformation of cells, either by direct action or after metabolic transformation into a carcinogenic metabolite. Among the best studied chemical carcinogens are alkylating agents, many of which are used for cancer chemotherapy and have resulted in the iatrogenic induction of second malignancies (particularly lymphoid neoplasms and leukemia). Asbestos is a well-known cause of mesothelioma, a tumor that rarely occurs in other than asbestos-exposed individuals. Arsenic exposure is a well-documented cause of cutaneous squamous cell carcinomas, and vinyl chloride is known to cause the otherwise rare hemangiosarcoma of liver. Saccharin, in contrast, has only been shown to promote bladder cancer in rats previously given marginal doses of carcinogens. There is no epidemiologic evidence that saccharin is carcinogenic in human beings (*pp. 237–238*).

4. (D) The most important defense mechanisms against pyogenic infections are humoral immune responses and inflammatory reactions with neutrophilic phagocytosis. Thus, disorders that affect either of these processes are associated with increased susceptibility to pyogenic infection.

Since the third component of complement plays a critical role as an opsonin in inflammatory responses to pyogenic bacteria, C3 deficiencies increase susceptibility to infection by these agents. Common variable immunodeficiency is associated with a defect in humoral immunity and is also associated with increased susceptibility to pyogenic infection. Chronic granulomatous disease of childhood and the Chédiak-Higashi syndrome are disorders in which the function of phagocytes is deranged. In chronic granulomatous disease of childhood, the myeloperoxidase-dependent bactericidal mechanism of phagocytes is deficient. In the Chédiak-Higashi syndrome, a number of defects in phagocyte function are present, including impaired chemotactic responses and deficient degranulation. Thus, with defective neutrophilic function in these two disorders, pyogenic infection is common.

DiGeorge's syndrome, however, is a disorder of the cellular immune system only. Inflamma' mechanisms and humoral immunity are unimpaired in patients with DiGeorge's syndrome, and susceptibility to pyogenic infection is not increased (*pp. 50–51, 205–207*).

5. (D) Although a number of pathologic features, including anaplasia with nuclear pleomorphism, high mitotic rate, lack of encapsulation, and presence of necrosis and hemorrhage, are typically associated with malignant tumors, benign tumors may occasionally display one or more of these features as well. Therefore, the only feature that is absolutely diagnostic of malignancy is the presence of metastases. Although so-called "benign" tumors are capable of producing considerable morbidity and even mortality through local compressive effects or secretion of systemically active substances such as hormones, benign tumors never metastasize (*p. 229*).

6. (E) Hypoxia is the most common cause of cell injury. It is usually caused by ischemia (decreased blood flow) to the tissue, but depletion of the oxygen-carrying capacity of the blood or toxic injury to the oxidative enzymes within the cells can also cause hypoxic injury. One of the most common histologic hallmarks of hypoxic cell injury, especially in cells with a high rate of aerobic metabolism, is acute cellular swelling (cellular edema). It occurs as a result of an influx of sodium and an iso-osmotic quantity of water into the cell. Since the cell membrane pumps that normally keep the concentration of sodium inside the cell low compared with the extracellular fluid require ATP as their energy source, they will cease to function as oxygen tension within the cell decreases, in turn decreasing oxidative phosphorylation by mitochondria and generation of ATP. Glycogen supplies within the cell cytoplasm can serve as a temporary source of ATP generated from anaerobic glycolysis, but glycogen stores are quickly depleted. Very simply, loss of the biochemical means to produce ATP, the energy source that fuels the active transport enzyme systems of the cell membrane, leads to failure of these pumps to move ions (and fluid) out of the cell.

Although intracytoplasmic accumulations of abnormal amounts of lipid, protein, or glycogen do characterize some forms of cell injury, these do not usually occur with hypoxia. Moreover, although accumulation of any of these substances could indeed cause affected cells to increase in size, the process would not be known as cellular swelling. This term applies exclusively to intracellular edema (*pp. 6–8*).

7. (A) Free radicals are chemically unstable, highly reactive molecules that are generated in many types of chemical and toxic pathologic processes. They are capable of profound cellular injury, chiefly through their ability to damage the unsaturated fatty acids in cell membranes. The initiation of free radicals in biologic materials requires either a powerful outside energy source (ionizing radiation, for example) or an oxidation-reduction reaction that leads to the addition of an extra electron to oxygen or other molecule that can accept electrons in transit from one valency state to another. Thus, atoms or molecules having an odd number of electrons are formed. The unpaired electron of these radicals is free to participate in chemical bond formation, such as lipid peroxidation (e.g., in cell membrane damage). Alternatively, they may donate their extra electrons to yet another molecule that, in turn, becomes a free radical.

In irradiation damage, free radical formation is usually mediated through the radiolysis of water, leading to the formation of hydroxyl radicals that are highly injurious to the cell. In oxygen toxicity, oxygen acts as an electron acceptor to form the highly reactive free radical superoxide. In carbon tetrachloride (CCl_4) poisoning, CCl_4 itself acts as an electron acceptor and becomes a free radical. In bacterial infection, reactive oxygen metabolites (superoxides) are elaborated within the lysosomes of neutrophils and macrophages following phagocytosis of bacterial organisms. Although these free radicals constitute one of the major bactericidal mechanisms of phagocytes, they can unfortunately be released extracellularly and cause damage to the surrounding tissues.

Unlike the above forms of injury mediated by free radical formation, mercuric chloride poisoning is the result of the direct toxic effects of mercury on cell proteins. Mercury binds to the sulfhydryl groups of cell membrane and other proteins, causing increased membrane permeability and inhibition of ATPase-dependent membrane transport. Its biologic activity is not dependent on metabolic conversion or free radical formation (*pp. 10–13, 51, 57*).

8. (B) The azurophilic granules found in the cytoplasm of neutrophils are specialized lysosomes that contain myeloperoxidase, acid hydrolases, neutral proteases, and cationic proteins. The latter include a chemotactic factor for monocytes, a factor that increases vascular permeability by releasing histamine from mast cells, and factors that increase vascular permeability independently of histamine release. Among the neutral proteases are enzymes capable of digesting collagen, elastin, cartilage, and basement membrane material, resulting in connective tissue destruction.

Although activated lymphocytes release molecules (lymphokines) that are chemotactic for neutrophils, the reverse is not true. Neutrophils do not produce chemoattractants for lymphocytes (*pp. 55–56*).

9. (B) Besides being able to initiate, carry out, and terminate immune responses, lymphocytes can also produce acute inflammatory responses through their ability to recruit a variety of inflammatory cell types. Activated T cells manufacture and release a variety of biologically active molecules called lymphokines. A number of lymphokines are chemotactic agents for neutrophils, eosinophils, macrophages, and basophils as well as other lymphocytes.

Platelets do not respond with chemotactic movement to any known substance. In fact, like the erythrocyte, the other blood-borne cell lacking a nucleus, the platelet appears incapable of directed cell movement toward a chemoattractant. Platelets can, however, be *activated* by molecules produced by other cells such as the platelet activating factors (PAFs) derived from basophils and macrophages. "Activation" of platelets causes their aggregation and subsequent release of active constituents such as histamine and serotonin but does not involve chemotaxis (*pp. 57, 170*).

10. (B) Increased permeability leading to tissue edema is one of the hallmarks of acute inflammation. Vascular leakiness is produced by a number of chemical mediators that act directly on blood vessels to increase permeability. Perhaps the best known among these mediators is histamine, an amine released from mast cells and sometimes platelets in response to various forms of tissue injury. Platelet activating factor (PAF), a mediator derived from basophils, can indirectly increase vascular permeability by causing platelets to release their cytoplasmic stores of histamine. In addition, PAF itself is a potent, direct mediator of vascular permeability. In extremely low concentrations, PAF induces vasodilatation and increases vascular permeability with a potency of 100 to 10,000 times greater than that of histamine.

Bradykinin, a potent vasoactive peptide generated during activation of the kinin system following tissue injury, not only increases vascular permeability but causes contraction of smooth muscle, blood vessel dilatation, and pain. Bradykinin is produced when the inactive factor XII of the coagulation system (Hageman factor) is activated through contact with collagen, basement membrane material, cartilage, or endotoxin. Activated factor XII converts the blood-borne factor prekallikrein to kallikrein, which, in turn, enzymatically mediates the conversion of kininogen to bradykinin.

The leukotrienes are arachidonic acid metabolites produced by leukocytes via the cyclooxygenase pathway. Leukotrienes C_4, D_4, and E_4 all cause intense vasoconstriction and bronchospasm and are at least 1000 times as potent as histamine in increasing vascular permeability.

The complement system consists of 18 component plasma proteases (together with their cleavage products) that are activated in inflammatory and immune responses. The end result of complement activation is production of the C5b–9 complex, which produces membrane lysis (hopefully of a microbial agent, although parenchymal cells may be injured). During activation of the cascade, cleavage products are produced that have numerous biologic activities. Among those that produce increased vascular permeability are C3A and C5A, the latter being more potent in this respect than the former. The C5b67 complex has no permeability effect but is a chemotactic agent (*pp. 53–57*).

11. (D) In general, tissue infiltration by mononuclear cells, principally lymphocytes, plasma cells, and macrophages, is considered one of the histologic hallmarks of chronic inflammation. However, in immunologically mediated forms of inflammation such as acute viral hepatitis, inflammatory infiltrates consist primarily of mononuclear cells regardless of the stage of the disease and thus are not reliable indicators of the chronicity of the process. Bile duct destruction and Councilman body formation (representing coagulative hepatocellular necrosis) can both be seen in either acute or chronic phases of numerous inflammatory conditions of the liver. Bile duct proliferation or hepatocellular regeneration accompanied by ceroid pigment in Kupffer's cells (a sign of past hepatocellular destruction) would be more indicative of an inflammatory process of longer duration.

Fibrosis is by far the most reliable indicator of chronicity in any inflammatory process, including that of the liver. Thus, a special stain for collagen is often routinely performed on liver biopsies to estimate the duration, degree of destruction, and subsequent scarring (indicative of irreversible damage) produced by inflammatory processes in the liver (*pp. 51–53, 907–910*).

12. (D) An aggregate of epithelioid histiocytes, no matter where it is found, is known as a granuloma. Granulomas are indicative of inflammatory responses to foreign bodies or type IV (cell-mediated) hypersensitivity responses initiated by specifically sensitized T lymphocytes. Immunologic responses to a variety of microorganisms including mycobacteria, viruses, fungi, protozoa, and parasites are often of the delayed hypersensitivity type and involve granuloma formation.

Granulation tissue is newly forming connective tissue consisting of fibroblasts and new blood vessels found at sites of tissue repair. Granular cell tumors are histologically distinctive (usually benign) neoplasms of Schwann cell origin that may occur in almost any site in the body although rarely in the ovary. Granulosa cell tumors, on the other hand, arise exclusively in the ovary and are derived from the granulosa cells of the ovarian follicle. Granulocytosis refers to the increased numbers of circulating neutrophils, a hallmark of acute inflammatory conditions such as infection. Although the names of these entities may bear certain etymologic similarities, they share no biologic similarities and are in no way related to granuloma (*pp. 64–65, 71–72, 169–170, 655, 1153, 1316*).

13. (A) Unfortunately for oncologists, oncologic surgeons, and students of pathology alike, names of tumors do not always correspond to the simple rules of nomenclature that usually help to indicate if the tumor is benign or malignant. For example, a tumor name composed of the word root for the tissue of origin plus the suffix "oma" denotes a benign neoplasm of that tissue. Designations for malignant tumors are usually compound names: the tissue of origin plus "sarcoma" (if mesenchymal in origin) or "carcinoma" (if epithelial in origin). However, according to accepted nomenclature, it is impossible to know from the names of certain tumors whether they are benign or malignant. In these cases the information must simply be memorized (as unpalatable a suggestion as this may be).

Glomus tumors are completely benign tumors that arise from the modified smooth muscle cells of the glomus body found in arterioles with arteriovenous anastomoses. They usually occur in the distal portions of the fingers and toes where glomus bodies are most commonly found. Simple surgical excision is completely curative (both for the tumor and for the pain they produce).

Ewing's tumor, Wilms' tumor, seminoma, and histiocytosis X are all examples of malignant neoplasms. Ewing's tumor, more correctly called Ewing's sarcoma, is a highly malignant type of primary bone tumor composed entirely of primitive mesenchymal cells. These tumors occur primarily in children and young adults, and when treated by the combined use of surgery, radiation, and chemotherapy, have a five-year survival of 70 to 75%.

Wilms' tumor, another tumor that occurs predominantly in the pediatric age group, is a malignant neoplasm of renal origin. It is composed of a number of different cell types, all derived from the mesonephric mesoderm. Like Ewing's sarcoma, the vastly improved long-term survival now associated with these neoplasms represents a triumph of aggressive combined modality oncologic therapy. When treated with chemotherapy, radiation, and surgery, 90% of patients with Wilms' tumors survive at least five years.

Although they vary in their biologic behavior, all germ cell tumors of the testis are malignant neoplasms. Seminoma, the most common testicular germ cell tumor, is composed of uniform, undifferentiated cells thought to be derived from primary germ cells. Seminomas are extremely radiosensitive and tend to remain localized for long periods of time. Thus they have the best prognosis among the testicular germ cell neoplasms. More than 90% of seminomas that are confined to the testis (Stage I) or that have spread only to the lymph nodes below the diaphragm (Stage II) can be cured.

Histiocytosis X is a proliferative disorder of Langerhans' cells or their bone marrow precursors. In its generalized form histiocytosis X behaves like a malignant tumor. The focal form of this disease is a benign process, perhaps even non-neoplastic, known as eosinophilic granuloma. Diffuse histiocytosis, also known as the Letterer-Siwe disease, usually occurs in infants and children and is a rapidly progressive,

lethal disease unless treated with intensive chemotherapy (this remarkably improves survival, at least in infants under the age of two years) (*pp. 217, 541, 694, 1156–1157, 1092–1093, 1343–1345*).

14. (C). For many types of cancer, it is now well established that heredity plays a role, be it major or minor, in predisposing an individual to the development of malignancy. Some of the most striking and obvious associations between heredity and tumor risk are exemplified by hereditary disorders.

Von Hippel–Lindau disease is a fortunately rare autosomal dominant disorder that is characterized by a strong predisposition to the development of a variety of benign and malignant tumors throughout the body. Among these, the most common and characteristic are retinal hemangioblastoma and hemangioblastoma of the cerebellum (*pp. 139, 264*).

Turcot syndrome is an autosomal recessive disorder in which affected individuals develop brain tumors and polyps of the colon. These individuals are also at increased risk of colon carcinoma, but the magnitude of the risk is still uncertain and is not as great as that in other familial intestinal polyposis syndromes (*p. 868*).

Fanconi's anemia is an autosomal recessive form of aplastic anemia. In addition to profound marrow hypofunction, affected individuals are at increased risk of developing leukemia or lymphoma (*pp. 264, 639*).

Patau's syndrome is a cytogenetic disorder caused by trisomy of chromosome 13. The most severe malformations among all the chromosomal abnormalities occur in this syndrome, and few affected infants live longer than one year, most dying soon after birth. Neoplasms, however, are not a feature of this syndrome, perhaps because death occurs so prematurely (*p. 129*).

15. (B) Next to the biopsy, cytologic diagnosis of cancer is the best histologic method. It is usually cheaper, quicker, and less traumatic for the patient, since the specimen sample required is so small. Cytologic diagnosis has become the most widely used method of screening for carcinoma of the cervix and/or endometrium and is becoming more and more widely used in the diagnosis of cancers of the breast, GI tract, tracheobronchial tree, and urinary tract.

At the present time, however, the most common cytologic examination performed is that on scrapings from the uterine cervical os, known as the Pap smear. With this reliable and simple screening technique, preneoplastic and early, noninvasive lesions can be detected in time for curative therapy to be performed. By long-standing convention, the cytologic findings of Pap smear examinations are divided into five diagnostic categories or classes. A normal cytology is designated Class I. Cervical dysplasia is designated as Class III, carcinoma *in situ* as Class IV, and invasive cancer as Class V. Class II cytology is an indeterminant category and refers to the presence of few atypical cells in the smear. Atypical cells may occur in inflammatory and reparative processes in the cervix, but they may represent true dysplasia that cannot be definitively diagnosed from the cells present. A repeat cytologic examination is recommended when Class II cytology is obtained (*pp. 265–266*).

16. (C) The morphologic changes associated with nonlethal (reversible) ischemic injury to cells typically include cellular swelling and cytoplasmic fatty change. Cellular swelling is the result of the loss of oxidative phosphorylation and generation of ATP in the hypoxic cell. Without ATP, membrane sodium pumps cannot be maintained, intracellular sodium accumulates, and water is osmotically drawn into the cell, causing the cell to swell. (See Question 6.) Fatty change results from metabolic alterations in the injured cell that render it incapable of metabolizing lipids, which thus accumulate in the cytoplasm.

In contrast to reversible injury, irreversible damage can be recognized only after it has produced the death of the cell and the morphologic features of necrosis develop, usually hours after the biologic death of the tissue. Cytoplasmic eosinophilia and nuclear shrinkage are two of the light microscopic hallmarks of necrosis. The former is a result of depletion of basophilic ribonucleic protein in the cytoplasm; the latter is the result of nuclear degeneration (*pp. 7, 14–15*).

17. (A) Free radicals are chemically unstable, highly reactive molecules that are capable of profound biologic injury, often through lipid peroxidation and consequent cell membrane damage. Generation of free radicals in cells is usually the result of oxidation-reduction reactions yielding a free electron. Molecules that absorb the free electron become unstable free radicals. (See Question 7.) Oxygen frequently acts as an acceptor of free electrons yielding the highly reactive free radical superoxide; thus, free radical generation is a major pathogenetic mechanism in oxygen toxicity. Exogenous drugs or chemicals such as carbon tetrachloride can also act as electron-absorbing molecules productive of injurious free radicals.

Less commonly, ionizing radiation initiates free radical formation, usually through the radiolysis of water and the production of hydroxyl radicals, which are particularly damaging to cells.

In contrast to chemical and toxic types of cell injury, which often involve free radical formation, ischemic and hypoxic injuries have a different pathogenetic basis: namely, termination of aerobic metabolism. Loss of oxidative phosphorylation leads to depletion of cellular ATP. Concomitantly, lactic acid accumulates from anaerobic glycolysis, and cellular pH decreases. Depletion of ATP produces mitochondrial dysfunction, and oxygen deprivation with cel-

lular acidosis produces both lysosomal and plasmalemmal membrane injury (*pp. 6–8, 10–12*).

18. (E) Repair of an injury is a complex process involving cell growth and collagen synthesis and remodeling. Numerous factors contribute to the well-orchestrated biologic events in wound healing, and the process may be delayed if any of these critical factors is altered. Since granulocyte collagenase is critical to degrading collagen in the remodeling of connective tissue essential to the repair process, granulocytopenia may be expected to delay wound healing. Granulocytopenia also predisposes to wound infection, which greatly slows the entire reparative process. Cushing's syndrome is the disease process caused by increased systemic levels of corticosteroids. It has long been known that corticosteroids have an inhibitory effect on the wound healing process, probably the result of their anti-inflammatory action and their ability to directly suppress collagen synthesis. Thrombocytopenia may also be expected to interfere with wound healing because (1) excessive amounts of extravasated blood tend to accumulate in the wound site and serve as a medium for bacterial growth; and (2) platelets are the source of a mitogen for fibroblasts and smooth muscle cells called platelet-derived growth factor (PDGF), which is believed to be important in the normal progression of fibroplasia at wound sites. Since vitamin C is critical to the hydroxylation of proline in the biosynthesis of collagen, deficiency of this vitamin, known as scurvy, produces profound defects in wound healing (*pp. 73, 78, 80*).

19. (B) Renal transplant rejection and graft-versus-host disease are processes in which immunologically mediated cellular cytotoxicity plays a major role. In renal transplant rejection, cytotoxic lymphocytes of the host react against incompatible HLA antigens on the surface of the cells of the transplanted tissue. In graft-versus-host disease, in contrast, it is the immunocompetent lymphocytes of the transplanted tissue that react against the tissue antigens of the host.

The Arthus reaction is a localized immune complex–induced vasculitis resulting from the intracutaneous injection of antigen in a previously sensitized individual having circulating antibodies against that antigen. The immunologic process is humoral rather than cellular, and cytotoxic lymphocytes do not participate. Although a tuberculin reaction is a classic example of a delayed hypersensitivity response mediated by the cellular immune system, the reaction is not cytotoxic. Rather, memory T cells previously sensitized to the tuberculin antigen of *Mycobacterium tuberculosis* are stimulated to divide and secrete lymphokines on re-exposure to the antigen. The lymphokines recruit inflammatory cells, especially monocytes and macrophages, to the site of antigen deposition. Cell-mediated cytotoxicity plays little if any role in this reaction (*pp. 169, 171–172, 175*).

20. (E) Amyloidosis occurring in association with an underlying predisposing condition is known as secondary amyloidosis. When occurring as a consequence of a chronic inflammatory condition, it is known as "reactive systemic amyloidosis." Ulcerative colitis and rheumatoid arthritis are among the most frequent causes of this form of the disease. Reactive systemic amyloidosis may also occur in association with nonlymphoid tumors such as renal cell carcinoma. If the underlying disease is a plasma cell dyscrasia or B lymphocyte malignancy, such as Waldenström's macroglobulinemia, the secondary amyloidosis is categorized as "immunocyte-derived" (p. 199).

21. (D) Despite its name, amyloid is not biochemically related to starch and is not digested by amylase. Rather, amyloid is a protein with a complex substructure and is commonly identified in histologic section by the Congo Red stain. Oil Red O is a stain used for neutral lipid. In immunocyte-derived amyloidosis, amyloid is generated from immunoglobulin light chains. In senile cardiac and senile cerebral amyloidosis, as well as in Portuguese and Swedish polyneuropathic forms of familial amyloidosis, the normal plasma protein prealbumin appears to be the major protein constituent of the amyloid (pp. 197–200).

22. (E) Hageman factor is a critical agent in the complex series of events that follow vascular injury and are critical to hemostasis. The activated Hageman factor (factor XII), which is generated through the contact of serum with collagen or injured endothelium following vascular disruption, in turn activates several enzymatic cascades with diverse biologic effects. Hageman factor can activate the complement system, potentiating complement-mediated inflammatory responses. It also activates the kinin system, leading to the generation of the vasoactive inflammatory mediator bradykinin. Perhaps most importantly, Hageman factor plays the schizophrenic role of activating both the thrombogenic and anticlotting mechanisms. Plasminogen is proteolytically converted to plasmin by activated factor XII, which simultaneously initiates thrombosis through the intrinsic coagulation pathway (pp. 53–54).

23. (A) Red infarctions are named for their hemorrhagic appearance. They are usually encountered in tissues with a double circulation such as the lung and liver, in loose tissues, or in tissues previously congested. In most other tissues, they commonly occur with venous occlusion. Classic examples of red infarctions include pulmonary infarctions from pulmonary embolism and torsion of the testis, which causes venous occlusion and intense congestion before the development of infarction. Infarction of the small intestine with its submucosal loose connective tissue is typically hemorrhagic whether caused by arterial occlusion or venous thrombosis. Coronary artery thrombosis, in contrast, is an example of arterial occlusion in a solid tissue and typically produces a white infarct (p. 108).

24. (E) Shock is a state of inadequate perfusion of all body tissues. It first produces reversible hypoxic injury to cells but if sufficiently prolonged may cause irreversible organ damage or even death. A number of categories of disorders may produce hemodynamic or vascular collapse and shock (see Question 24). Among the most common are bacterial infections producing so-called "septic shock," the result of pooling of blood in the peripheral circulation. Cardiogenic shock, the result of reduced cardiac output, is most commonly caused by myocardial infarction. The watery diarrhea of cholera leads to massive fluid losses and a reduction of the effective circulating blood volume causing hypovolemic shock. Hypovolemic shock may also occur in acute pancreatitis, which causes excessive transudation and exudation of fluid from the site of inflammation into the peritoneal cavity (p. 113).

25. (E) Radiant energy in the form of ultraviolet light, electromagnetic radiation (e.g., x-rays), or particulate radiation (e.g., alpha particles or beta particles of radioisotopes) is carcinogenic. Even therapeutic irradiation has been responsible for the induction of malignancies, especially leukemia. Head and neck irradiation in infants and children has resulted in the development of thyroid cancer later in life in 9% of those exposed. Osteogenic sarcoma has been a common consequence of exposure to radium among watch dial painters. Lung cancer occurs with a 10-fold increased frequency among miners of ores containing radioactive elements (p. 242).

26. (C) Although chromosomal changes are present in the cells of many types of human neoplasms, specific and consistent chromosomal defects have been identified only in about 20 different tumors. In about 90% of meningiomas, a partial deletion or monosomy of chromosome 22 is present. Similarly, 90% of adults with chronic myelogenous leukemia have myeloid cells that contain a specific chromosomal translocation, the distal segment of the long arm of chromosome 22 to chromosome 9 (the Philadelphia chromosome). To date, however, no nonrandom karyotypic changes have been discovered in many of the more common solid tumors such as adenocarcinoma of the colon or malignant melanoma (pp. 231–232).

27. (D) The grading of a malignant neoplasm is based on the degree of cytologic differentiation of tumor cells and the number of mitoses. In general, there is a positive correlation between the degree of anaplasia and the biologic aggressiveness of the tumor. In contrast to grading, staging of a tumor involves assessment of the size of the primary lesion, the extent of local infiltration, spread to regional lymph nodes, and the presence or absence of blood-borne metastases. Staging often affects the therapeutic approach to the tumor and almost always affects survival (statistically). In general, the greater the stage of the tumor, the worse the prognosis. (p. 229).

28. (A) Hemodynamic or vascular collapse causing inadequate perfusion of tissues is known as shock. (See Question 24.) Shock may be induced by a number of mechanisms and is a common clinical problem. The major categories of shock are delineated by hemodynamic mechanism rather than by specific etiology and include (1) cardiogenic shock, encompassing all causes of reduced cardiac output; (2) hypovolemia, caused by hemorrhage or fluid loss of any kind; (3) pooling of blood in the peripheral vasculature, usually associated with neuropathic or infectious causes; (4) anaphylaxis, immunologically mediated systemic circulatory collapse; and (5) disseminated intravascular coagulation. The latter can be either a primary cause of shock or may complicate shock of another etiology.

Patients with severe thermal burns are at high risk of developing shock from at least three major complications of this devastating injury. With massive tissue injury, large amounts of tissue thromboplastin are released into the circulation and precipitate disseminated intravascular coagulation (DIC) by activating the extrinsic pathway of the coagulation system. Widespread vascular injury leads to progressive loss of fluid from burn wounds, producing hypovolemia and reduced circulating blood volume. Another common complication that not only produces shock but is the most common cause of death in severely burned patients is burn wound infection. The gram-negative bacillus *Pseudomonas aeruginosa* is now the most common cause of burn wound sepsis. This organism is the source of many powerful toxins, including endotoxin, which causes pooling of blood in peripheral vessels, producing what is known as "endotoxic shock."

Although smoke inhalation may cause severe pulmonary complications including the acute respiratory distress syndrome, it is not known to cause anaphylaxis or shock (pp. 113, 313, 462, 649–650).

29. (C) The sequence of morphologic events following acute hypoxic cellular injury is now known. The early changes are reversible if oxygen is restored, but if hypoxia continues, morphologic changes that correspond to irreversible cell injury develop. Among the early, reversible changes are ribosomal detachment from rough endoplasmic reticulum and loss of intracellular glycogen as the cell begins to generate ATP through anaerobic glycolysis. These changes are usually accompanied by acute cellular swelling as ATP

concentration is reduced and the sodium ion pumps of the cell membrane cease to function.

Irreversible damage is associated with the appearance of dense deposits in the mitochondria and loss of intracellular RNA. In the heart, these changes can be seen as early as 30 to 40 minutes after ischemia. The loss of cytoplasmic RNA is the result of lysosomal membrane damage and leakage of enzymes into the cytoplasm. As a consequence, RNA, DNA, protein, and other cellular constituents undergo enzymatic digestion. Although this process of autodigestion has been called the "suicide-bag hypothesis" of irreversible cell injury, it is now known that the point of irreversibility has already passed by the time lysosomal rupture occurs (pp. 6–7).

30. (B) The cytoskeletal intermediate filaments of different classes of cells can be separated biochemically and immunochemically into at least five distinctive types: keratin filaments, desmin, vimentin, glial filaments, and neurofilaments. Although vimentin is produced by a wide variety of cells, including all mesenchymal cells and many types of epithelial cells, the other intermediate filaments are more limited and specific in their distribution. Keratins are made only by epithelial cells. Glial filaments and neurofilaments are formed only by glial cells and neurons, respectively. Desmin is produced only by muscle cells and fibroblasts.

Because of their cell-type specificity, intermediate filaments can be helpful in tumor diagnosis. The presence of desmin in an anaplastic tumor, for example, would offer strong evidence that the cell of origin was either a fibroblast or a muscle cell, since desmin is unique to these cell types. Analogously, the intermediate filament that one would expect to find in a squamous cell carcinoma is keratin. Lymphoma, although it may express vimentin, is best identified by markers that are specific for lymphocytes since vimentin is produced by such a wide variety of cells (p. 28).

31. (C) Although the fully differentiated, specialized cell types of the human body possess many unique structural and functional properties, they also share some features common to all human cells. Among these are the cytoplasmic proteins, tubulin and actin. The latter is a ubiquitous contractile protein that plays a role in such cell functions as movement and cell-shape changes. Tubulin is the major structural component of microtubules, which are essential to spindle formation in mitosis, cilia (epithelial cells) and flagellum (sperm) formation, phagocytosis, and intracellular transport of secretions.

Myosin is a contractile protein found in most but not all cells. It is found in higher concentration in cells specialized for contraction, smooth and striated muscle cells. Spectrin is an element of the filamentous meshwork of proteins lining the inner membrane surface of certain cells, particularly erythrocytes, but is not found in all cells (*pp. 28–29*).

32. (B) Hyperplasia refers to an increase in the number of cells in an organ or tissue that is capable of mitotic activity. In some circumstances, hyperplasia represents a normal physiologic response and is beneficial. Compensatory hyperplasia, such as occurs in the remaining kidney after unilateral nephrectomy, and hormonal hyperplasia, such as that which occurs in the endometrium during the proliferative phase of the menstrual cycle, are two common examples.

Postmenopausal endometrial gland hyperplasia, however, is distinctly abnormal and is considered a pathologic form of hyperplasia. It signifies an increase in the absolute or relative amount of estrogen present. When it continues unabated, the hyperplastic changes become excessive (adenomatous hyperplasia) and finally atypical. Both adenomatous hyperplasia and atypical hyperplasia of the endometrium in postmenopausal women are considered premalignant lesions since they go on to develop endometrial carcinoma in 22% and 57%, respectively.

Another form of pathologic hyperplasia that is associated with an increased risk of malignancy is hyperplasia of the gastric surface mucosal glands, a condition known as Ménétrier's disease. The transition from hyperplasia to neoplasia is less common in this setting than in the above-mentioned example of endometrial hyperplasia.

Follicular hyperplasia of lymph nodes and prostatic gland hyperplasia are not premalignant lesions. Follicular hyperplasia of lymph nodes is considered a physiologic form of hyperplasia, since it represents a normal immunologic response to an antigenic challenge. Prostatic gland hyperplasia is so common in elderly men (it occurs in 95% of those over the age of 70) that it can be considered a normal aging process. Because it is extremely common, prostatic gland hyperplasia can often be found in a prostrate carcinoma, but the two conditions are not believed to be causally related (*pp. 32–33, 813, 1102–1104*).

33. (E) Metaplasia is a reversible change in which one adult cell type is replaced by another normal cell type. It usually represents an adaptive change to chronic irritation. Although metaplasia itself is a benign process, the conditions that predispose to metaplastic change, if persistent, may go on to produce malignant change in the metaplastic tissue. Common examples include squamous cell carcinoma of the endocervix and squamous cell carcinoma of the lung. The normal endocervix and lung contain no squamous epithelium, and yet the most common type of carcinoma arising in these tissues is squamous cell carcinoma. These cancers arise from a glandular epithelium that first undergoes squamous metaplasia, becomes progressively more dysplastic, and finally

becomes cancerous. Although less common than the above examples, squamous cell carcinoma of the bladder and adenocarcinoma of the esophagus are also examples of malignant transformation of metaplastic transitional cell epithelium and non-keratinizing squamous cell epithelium, respectively.

Squamous metaplasia is by far the most common type of metaplastic change, whereas adenomatous metaplasia is distinctively unusual. Thus, adenomatous metaplasia of the esophagus (Barrett's esophagus) developing in response to chronic acid reflux from the stomach is the only common example of this type of change (*pp. 33–34, 753, 1075, 1126*).

34. (C) Calcium deposits in tissues are known as "dystrophic" calcifications when they occur in dead or dying tissue and as "metastatic" calcifications when they occur in normal tissue. The cause of metastatic calcification is hypercalcemia. Thus, any disorder that produces increased levels of serum calcium may be associated with metastatic calcification. Multiple myeloma with its characteristic lytic bone lesions commonly produces hypercalcemia. Myeloma cells are known to make an osteoclast activating factor (OAF) that stimulates bone resorption, liberating calcium from the mineralized matrix. Parathyroid carcinoma is a rare cause of primary hyperparathyroidism that tends to cause greater elevation in serum calcium than any other form of hyperparathyroidism. In fact, death from this disease is more often caused by complications of hyperparathyroidism than by the tumor itself. Metastatic calcifications are usually numerous and widespread with this disease. Wilson's disease is a disorder of copper metabolism and does not affect serum calcium levels at all.

Papillary carcinoma of the thyroid often produces dystrophic calcifications within the tumor itself. These laminated concretions of calcium and other mineral salts are known as psammoma bodies. They are thought to represent the tombstones of dead cells that slough off the tips of the papillary fronds formed by the tumor (*pp. 35, 691, 1220, 1229*).

35. (E) One of the hallmarks of an acute inflammatory response is neutrophilic infiltration. Drawn to the site of inflammation by chemotactic substances, migrating neutrophils first marginate to the periphery of vessels in the region of inflammation, stick to the endothelium, and then emigrate through the vessel wall to invade the tissue where their phagocytic talents may be needed. Although under normal circumstances small numbers of neutrophils may transiently marginate and stick to vascular endothelium in some tissues, these processes are markedly amplified in acute inflammation. Several factors are known to promote neutrophil "stickiness." These include (1) reduction of the negative cell surface charges on either the endothelium or the neutrophil, which usually cause them to repel one another; (2) the presence of divalent cations such as CA^{++}, which serve as bridges between the negative charges on endothelium and white cells or as co-factors in other interactions necessary for adhesion; and (3) the presence of chemical mediators such as C5a and lipoxygenase pathway products of arachidonic acid metabolism such as leukotriene B_4 (p. 47).

36. (B) Normal leukocyte function is essential to the body's defense against bacterial organisms. Thus, disorders that are associated with defects in leukocyte function predispose affected individuals to bacterial infection. Diabetes mellitus is an example of a disorder that produces several basic defects in leukocyte function, including defective leukocyte adherence to vessel walls, impaired chemotaxis, and decreased phagocytosis.

The total number of circulating white cells and the leukocyte content of G-6-PD is usually normal in diabetes mellitus (p. 51).

37. (A) To protect themselves from the harmful effects of free radicals generated in inflammatory responses, normal tissues possess several antioxidant protective mechanisms. Serum proteins such as the copper-containing compound ceruloplasmin and the iron-free fraction of serum transferrin are important endogenous antioxidants that serve to inactivate free radicals. Cellular enzymes such as catalase and glutathione peroxidase are capable of detoxifying hydrogen peroxide, and the enzyme superoxide dismutase can inactivate superoxide. Ultimately, the prevention of tissue destruction by an acute inflammatory process depends upon these mechanisms and the balance between production and inactivation of free radicals.

Alpha-2-macroglobulin is an antiprotease found in serum and various secretions. Although it is important in protecting normal tissues from the harmful effects of lysosomal proteases released from leukocytes during inflammatory reactions, it has no effect on free radicals (pp. 10–11, 56–57).

38. (A) Congestion is a general term referring to an increased volume of blood in a tissue caused by reduced venous drainage. Congestion may occur as a systemic phenomenon (e.g., in right- and left-sided congestive heart failure) or may occur as a localized process. Passive congestion of the liver, for example, produces a pattern known as "nutmeg liver" characterized by deeply reddened centrilobular zones surrounded by pale, yellow-brown zones of uncongested liver at the lobular periphery. Chronic passive congestion of the lungs produces a lesion known as "brown induration"—brown owing to hemosiderin deposition and indurated owing to collagen deposition in the chronically edematous alveolar septae. In the spleen; chronic passive congestion produces lesions known as Gandy-Gamna bodies. These are small fibrous nodules with hemosiderin deposition. Gandy-Gamna nodules occur with increased portal pressure

that results in the deposition of collagen in the basement membrane of the splenic sinusoids.

Koilonychia refers to a concave, spoon-shaped deformity of the nails that is characteristic of iron deficiency anemia. It is not a lesion associated with vascular congestion (pp. 89–90, 613, 701).

39. (D) In contrast to amyloid of the AL type in which the fibrils are composed of immunoglobulin light chains, amyloid of the AA type is composed mostly of amyloid-associated (AA) protein. This type of amyloid characteristically occurs in two basic categories of disease: reactive systemic amyloidosis occurring in association with malignant tumors or chronic inflammatory conditions (e.g., ulcerative colitis) and the form of hereditary amyloidosis known as familial Mediterranean fever.

In senile cardiac amyloidosis and the hereditary neuropathic forms of amyloidosis, both Portuguese and Swedish types, the amyloid is derived from prealbumin (see Question 21). In the localized form of amyloidosis that occurs in association with medullary carcinoma of the thyroid, the amyloid is derived from thyrocalcitonin produced by the neoplastic cells (pp. 198–199).

40. (C) Most malignant tumors tend to metastasize via the lymphatic or blood vessels. Only a few tumor types deviate from these patterns and tend to spread over the surfaces of viscera or body cavities. Ovarian carcinomas and mesotheliomas are two such tumors. So characteristic of mesothelioma is this pattern of metastatic spread that this tumor can often be diagnosed radiologically by the thick rind of tumor tissue it produces over the surface of an involved lung. Although usually less confluent than mesothelioma in its spread, ovarian carcinoma characteristically studs the surfaces of the peritoneal cavity and the abdominal viscera, a pattern easily recognized at surgery.

Colon carcinoma is a prime example of a malignant tumor that metastasizes primarily via the lymphatic system. Renal cell carcinoma, on the other hand, is a common example of a tumor that typically spreads by a hematogenous route. Neither of these tumors characteristically spreads over body cavities or organ surfaces (pp. 226–227).

41. (E) In the United States, with the exception of tumors of the female reproductive organ, every major type of malignancy occurs with greater frequency in males than in females. Moreover, the disparity between cancer death rates between men and women appears to be increasing. In the fifteen years between 1953 and 1978, cancer death rates among males increased 25%, whereas those among females decreased by 7%. The steady increase in the death rate among males has been ascribed mainly to lung cancer (pp. 260–263).

42. (True); **43.** (False); **44.** (False); **45.** (False); **46.** (True); **47.** (False); **48.** (True)

(42) Histocompatibility antigens are cell surface antigens encoded by a set of closely linked genes on chromosome 6 that are usually inherited en bloc. They are the antigens that evoke rejection of transplanted organs in an immunocompetent host or immune attack by immunocompetent cells from transplanted tissue on the tissues of an immunoincompetent recipient. Simply put, histocompatibility (HLA) antigens constitute the immunologic basis of "self," since they are the means by which lymphocytes from one individual can recognize "foreign" cells or tissues from a genetically nonidentical individual.

(43 and 44) Two major classes of HLA antigens have been defined. Class I antigens are glycoproteins coded by HLA-A, -B, and -C loci, each representing a separate gene within the major histocompatibility complex on chromosome 6. Class I antigens are present on virtually all nucleated cells and evoke the formation of humoral antibody in genetically nonidentical transplant recipients. Class II antigens are those encoded by the HLA-D and HLA-DR loci of the major histocompatibility complex. Although the term HLA refers to "human leukocyte antigens," it is only the Class II HLA antigens that are distributed almost exclusively on leukocytes—specifically cells of the immune system. In contradistinction to Class I antigens, Class II antigens evoke cellular rather than humoral immune responses to genetically nonidentical cells.

(45) As mentioned above, the genes that code for both classes of HLA antigens are closely linked and inherited as a set that constitutes a haplotype. One set or haplotype is inherited from each parent. According to the laws of Mendelian genetics, siblings can have only four possible combinations of haplotypes. There is only a 25% chance that two siblings will be HLA-identical. The odds are 50% that two siblings will share one haplotype and 25% that they will not share any haplotype. The concept of haplotype sharing becomes important when genetically related or genitically identical organ transplant donors are sought.

(46 and 47) It is now clear that the genes controlling immune responses are intimately linked to the genes of the major histocompatibility complexes. There is considerable evidence in both the mouse and the human that the genes controlling the magnitude of both cellular and humeral immune responses are located within the major histocompatibility complex. In humans, immune response (Ir) genes map within the HLA-D/DR region of the HLA complex, and HLA-D/DR antigens may, in fact, be products of Ir genes. A corollary to this close association between HLA antigens and immune responses is that T cell–mediated cell-to-cell interactions in immune responses are critically dependent on cell surface HLA antigens. For example, recognition of a virally infected cell by a T lymphocyte is dependent on the coincident presence of Class I HLA molecules on the infected cell. In other words, cytotoxic lymphocytes cannot recognize viral antigens independent of the Class I HLA molecules. The Class II HLA antigens, however, do not appear to play a role in this response.

(48) It is also clear that a variety of diseases are strongly associated with certain HLA types. Perhaps the best known and strongest association is that between ankylosing spondylitis and HLA-B27. Individuals who possess the HLA-B27 antigen have a 90-fold greater chance of developing this disease than those who lack this antigen (*pp. 160–162*).

49. (True); **50.** (True); **51.** (False); **52.** (True); **53.** (False)

(49, 50, 52) Atrophy is the term that refers to diminished cell size. This is due to a reduction in the structural components of the cell, including cytoplasmic organelles and cytostructural elements. Atrophy may refer to individual cells of diminished size or to an entire tissue or organ composed of shrunken cells. Although atrophy may be accompanied by decreased cell functon, it does not imply that the cells are dead or moribund. Atrophy may occur in otherwise normal tissues whose workload or blood supply has been decreased. Other causes of atrophy are loss of innervation, inadequate nutrition, and loss of endocrine stimulation.

(51 and 53) Although autophagic vacuoles may be seen in cells undergoing atrophy, this is not a sign of irreversible cell injury. Autophagy is a mechanism by which injured (e.g., from hypoxia) or effete organelles are eliminated from the *living* cell. Autophagy is to be distinguished from autolysis, the process by which *dead* tissues are enzymatically digested by lysosomal enzymes released from necrotic cells (*pp. 15, 26–30*).

54. (True); **55.** (False); **56.** (False); **57.** (True); **58.** (False); **59.** (True); **60.** (True)

(54 and 55) Since the first cases of the acquired immune deficiency syndrome (AIDS) were reported in 1981, this devastating and lethal disease has been the subject of intensive research and enormous public concern. AIDS is an infectious disease transmitted sexually (primarily in homosexual males) or parenterally (e.g., blood transfusions or intravenous drug use) and is now known to be caused by a retrovirus known as HTLV. Although the designation refers to human T-cell leukemia virus, HTLV represents a family of retroviruses only one subtype of which causes T-cell leukemia. Although all of the members of the HTLV family characteristically infect lymphocytes, one subtype may cause uncontrolled proliferation (T-cell leukemia), whereas another subtype apparently causes uncontrolled suppression and destruction of effector T cells (AIDS). Although infection with cytomegalovirus (CMV), herpes simplex virus, or Epstein-Barr virus (EBV) is common in AIDS, these viral infections occur as a result of immunosuppression. They are not causally related to AIDS, however.

(**56 and 57**) Typically, AIDS presents clinically with fever, weight loss, and persistent generalized lymphadenopathy. Affected individuals characteristically have a lymphopenia and a selective impairment of T-cell function. In contrast to the circulating T-cell population of normal individuals in which the ratio of helper to suppressor cells is approximately 2:1, this ratio is inverted in AIDS patients owing to a severe deficiency of helper/inducer cells. Immunoglobulin levels, on the other hand, are often elevated in AIDS patients owing to rising antibody titers to infectious agents such as EBV or CMV.

(**58 and 59**) Although a particularly aggressive form of Kaposi's sarcoma is a common feature of the AIDS syndrome, death from overwhelming infection usually ensues before death from metastatic tumor can occur. Another tumor type occurring with a high rate of frequency in AIDS patients is a diffuse, undifferentiated lymphoma (Burkitt's lymphoma). Burkitt's lymphoma has been causally linked to EBV, and it has been postulated that in the absence of immunologic competence, EBV may initiate oncogenesis more readily than in the presence of a normally functioning immune system.

(**60**) As mentioned above, AIDS can be transmitted by blood transfusion. Thus, hemophiliacs are at especially high risk of developing AIDS. They receive factor VIII concentrates derived from pooling blood obtained from several thousand blood donors (*pp. 208–210, 292, 543–544*).

61. (False); 62. (False); 63. (True); 64. (True); 65. (False); 66. (False); 67. (True)

(**61 and 62**) Many of the altered growth properties of malignant cells can best be studied in cell culture. For example, it appears that malignant cells are less fastidious than normal cells and can grow and divide under conditions that would not support optimal growth of normal cells. Lacking a requirement for attachment to a solid substrate, cancer cells can grow in a fluid or semisolid medium and require lower serum concentrations in the medium for optimal growth than normal cells. In further contrast to normal cells that arrest at the G_0 stage of the cell cycle (i.e., they stop dividing) at high density in cell culture, cancer cells do not exhibit "contact inhibition" or cessation of locomotion and division confluence. They are, therefore, less suceptible to what has been termed "density-dependent inhibition of growth" (*pp. 230–231*).

(**63, 64, 65**) Malignant cells also differ from normal cells in their antigenic properties. Although they may express some of the same antigens found on normal cells, they may also possess "neoantigens" found only in tumor cells. One such example is the tumor-specific transplantation antigens (TSTAs) found on the surface of nearly all neoplastic cells transformed by oncogenic viruses and the cells of many chemically induced tumors. Unlike the TSTAs of a chemically induced cancer, which are immunologically distinct from those of other tumors produced by the same agent, the TSTAs of all tumors induced by a specific virus are identical. A syngeneic host can be immunized against malignant cells bearing TSTAs, hence their designation as "transplantation" antigens. In contrast to TSTAs, however, tumor-associated antigens (TAAs) do not evoke transplantation immunity. TAAs encompass a wide variety of antigens that are not necessarily unique to tumor cells but are often expressed by them (e.g., alpha-fetoprotein and carcinoembryonic antigen). Unfortunately, TSTAs are expressed on only a very few human cancers, whereas TAAs are extremely common (*pp. 233–234*).

(**66 and 67**) Contrary to what might be expected from their property of being less cohesive than normal cells, malignant cells appear to have the same number of desmosomal junctions as their normal counterparts. However, malignant cells do differ from their normal counterparts in their ability to elaborate a number of lytic enzymes. Some of these enzymes, including collagenases and lysosomal hydrolases, are released from the surfaces of malignant cells and are capable of digesting normal host tissues. It is believed that the secretion of such enzymes may contribute to the invasive potential of cancer cells (*pp. 225, 236*).

68. (A); 69. (D); 70. (C); 71. (A); 72. (B); 73. (D)

Inflammation and immunologic responses are complex reactions that have evolved because of their overall benefit to the organism. However, these same reactions can also cause injury to the organism and form the basis of a disease process. In general, inflammation occurs in vascularized living tissue as a response to local injury of almost any cause, whereas immune responses are highly specific reactions directed against specific molecular substances known as antigens.

(**68**) A granulomatous response to an inert foreign body such as surgical suture material is a type of inflammation and, in contrast to type IV hypersensitivity responses with granuloma formation, requires no participation of the immune system (*p. 59*).

(**69**) In contrast to infectious endocarditis, which evokes an inflammatory response in the surrounding valvular tissue, marantic endocarditis is characterized by the formation of bland fibrin thrombi on valve leaflets with no significant accompanying inflammatory reaction. Although its pathogenesis is uncertain, marantic endocarditis is thought to be related to hypercoagulability (*pp. 584–585*).

(**70**) Streptococcal infection produces both an exuberant inflammatory response and an immunologic reaction to the organism. Since both responses are important host-defense mechanisms against pyogenic bacteria, disorders that produce defects in either lead to increased susceptibility to staphylococcal and other pyogenic infections (*p. 306*).

(**71**) Sunburn is a classic example of inflammation induced by cutaneous injury from the radiant energy of ultraviolet light (*p. 46*).

(**72**) Although the name implies an inflammatory response in the thyroid, Hashimoto's thyroiditis is an autoimmune disorder mediated by both cellular and humeral immune responses to thyroidal antigens (*p. 1207*).

(**73**) Lead poisoning is caused by the direct toxic effects of lead on the hematopoietic system, the nervous system, and the kidneys. It evokes neither an inflammatory nor an immunologic response (*pp. 453–455*).

74. (A); 75. (D); 76. (B); 77. (A); 78. (C); 79. (A); 80. (A); 81. (D); 82. (D); 83. (D)

Interleukin-1 and interleukin-2 are leukocyte products that have significant biologic effects in inflammatory responses and immune responses, respectively.

(**74, 77, 79, 80**) Interleukin-1 is a polypeptide made by macrophages that produces a number of pathophysiologic responses including fever production (it has been called "endogenous pyrogen" in the past), lymphocyte activation, and stimulation of specific protein synthesis by other cells (e.g., acute-phase proteins in liver, collagenase in fibroblasts).

(**76 and 78**) Interleukin-2 is a growth factor produced only by activated T cells. Its only known action is promotion of the proliferation of other T cells, specifically those involved in mediating cellular immunity.

(**75, 81, 82, 83**) Neither of these two substances is made by neutrophils or any other granulocyte. Neither do these compounds share any of the biologic activities of other macrophage or lymphocyte products such as interferon (a viral replication inhibitor). Likewise, they do not interact with the complement system, the kinin system, or any of the other serum protease cascades that play roles in inflammatory and/or immune responses (*pp. 60, 68–69, 171*).

84. (A); 85. (A); 86. (A); 87. (D); 88. (C); 89. (C); 90. (B); 91. (C); 92. (B); 93. (A)

During cutaneous wound healing two diverse cell types, keratinocytes and fibroblasts, synchronously proliferate and interact to repair the defect.

(**84, 85, 86, 87**) Unlike fibroblasts that normally undergo proliferation only in response to tissue injury (a "stable" cell type), epidermal cells undergo continuous proliferation throughout life (a "labile" cell type). Following a cutaneous wound such as a clean surgical incision, epidermal cells rapidly migrate across the wound, establishing epithelial continuity with 24 to 48 hours. This speedy response takes place long before the reparative response of the underlying connective tissue has begun to evolve. The basal cells of the newly re-formed epithelium lay down new basement membrane, the primary component of which is type IV collagen. Type IV collagen is the only collagen type presently known to be produced by epidermal cells. Fibroblasts are capable of pro-ducing both type I and type III collagen, but neither keratinocytes nor fibroblasts produce type II collagen, a type found only in cartilage, intervertebral discs, and the vitreous body (*pp. 70, 73, 77*).

(**88, 89, 90**) Fibroblasts are capable of abetting the process of epithelial cell migration referred to above through their production of fibronectin. This large glycoprotein is involved in the process of epithelial cell attachment and spreading upon the collagenous matrix below, although the mechanisms by which this occurs are still unclear. Moreover, there is recent experimental evidence that keratinocytes themselves can synthesize fibronectin.

Fibronectin may also be involved in the induction of connective tissue cell migration across the healing wound, since fibronectin fragments are known to be chemotactic for fibroblasts. In addition fibroblasts are activated and induced to divide by a factor secreted by activated macrophages (usually plentiful in healing wounds) (*p. 79*).

(**91**) Urogastrone is a polypeptide that can be purified from the submaxillary glands of mice or from human urine. Although it is also known as epidermal growth factor (EGF) because of its ability to enhance epidermal proliferation and keratinization, urogastrone is mitogenic for cultured fibroblasts as well. What role, if any, it plays in cutaneous wound healing is unknown (*pp. 75–76*).

(**92 and 93**) Other factors that stimulate fibroblast activity and probably do so during the wound healing process are platelet-derived growth factor (PDGF) and interleukin-1. PDGF is a polypeptide stored in the alpha granules of platelets and released upon platelet activation. It is a powerful mitogen and chemotactic factor for fibroblasts. Interleukin-1 is a polypeptide produced mainly by macrophages that among other activities stimulates collagenase production in fibroblasts. It is now known that epidermal cells produce interleukin-1 or, as it is sometimes called, epidermal thymocyte activating factor (ETAF) (*pp. 60, 76*).

94. (C); 95. (C); 96. (A); 97. (B); 98. (C); 99. (C); 100. (D); 101. (A); 102. (C); 103. (D); 104. (D); 105. (D)

Sadly, a very great number of debilitating inflammatory conditions and human cancers are self-inflicted via the chronic use of two highly injurious substances, cigarettes and alcohol.

(**94, 95, 96, 97, 98, 99, 101, 102**) The esophagus and stomach are both highly susceptible to injury and neoplastic transformation by cigarettes and alcohol. Acute esophagitis, acute gastritis, esophageal carcinoma, and gastric carcinoma are all causally related to both cigarettes and alcohol. Pharyngeal carcinoma is also closely linked with both cigarette smoking and alcohol abuse. The pancreas responds somewhat differently from the esophagus in that acute pancreatitis has been linked only to alcohol abuse, whereas pancreatic carcinoma is associated with cigarette smoking. Cancers of the GI tract are not the only malignancies caused by cigarette smoking, however. Transitional cell carcinoma of the bladder also occurs with significantly greater frequency in cigarette smokers.

(**100, 103, 104, 105**) There is no known association between either cigarette smoking or alcohol abuse and renal cell carcinoma, Hodgkin's disease, breast carcinoma, or ovarian carcinoma, but this is small consolation (*pp. 801, 1143*).

106. (E); 107. (D); 108. (D); 109. (A); 110. (A)

(**106**) Fatty change refers to intracellular accumulation of neutral lipids within parenchymal cells produced by some imbalance in the cellular production, utilization, or mobilization of fat. It is usually the result of some form of nonlethal cell injury. Although it may occur in other organs, fatty change is most frequently seen in the liver, the major site of fat metabolism.

In the United States, alcohol is the most common cause of fatty liver. It has a variety of lipogenic effects, including increased free fatty acid mobilization and entry into liver cells, decreased fatty acid oxidation, increased esterification of fatty acids to triglycerides, and decreased lipoprotein secretion.

(**107 and 108**) Toxic exposure to phosphorus or carbon tetrachloride produces lipid accumulation in liver cells principally by reducing apoprotein synthesis, which consequently decreases secretion of lipoprotein (the export form of lipid).

(**109 and 110**) Increased lipid mobilization from adipose tissue leading to excessive entry of free fatty acids into the liver is the major mechanism of hepatic fatty change caused by corticosteroids or starvation (*pp. 18–19*).

111. (D); 112. (C); 113. (D); 114. (C); 115. (B)

(**111**) Although pigment accumulation is usually not harmful to cells, it can be a reflection of certain distinctive pathologic processes. In patients with alkaptonuria, a rare inherited metabolic disease, accumulation of the brown-black pigment homogentisic acid occurs in the skin, connective tissue, and cartilage where the pigmentation is known as ochronosis.

(**112**) Patients with mitral stenosis classically develop brown, indurated lungs. The brown color is due to hemosiderin accumulation, the result of pulmonary hypertensive vascular changes and chronic leakage of red blood cells.

(**113**) The color of the lungs in coal miners' disease, however, is due to a marked accumulation of an inhaled exogenous pigment, carbon.

(**114**) Pigmented villonodular synovitis is an unusual condition of unknown etiology characterized by dramatic synovial overgrowth (probably neoplastic) usually involving the knee or hip. Typically, the proliferating mass of synovium is variably pigmented by hemosiderin, presumably of traumatic origin.

(**115**) In yet another bizarre condition of unknown etiology called melanosis coli, the colonic mucosa becomes diffusely blackened by deposition of a type of melanin pigment in mucosal macrophages. The origin of the pigment is unknown, but the condition is associated with chronic use of cathartics of the anthracene type (see Chapter 8, Question 18 and *pp. 22–25, 142, 433, 858, 1365*).

116. (A); 117. (C); 118. (B); 119. (B); 120. (D)

Hypertrophy, hyperplasia, and metaplasia are adaptive changes that cells may undergo in response to alterations in their environment. In brief, hypertrophy refers to increase in cell size, hyperplasia to increase in cell numbers, and metaplasia to a change in cell type through altered cellular differentiation. Dysplasia, in contrast, is not considered to be an adaptive response. It refers to some derangement in normal cellular responses producing atypical development. In epithelial tissues, dysplasia is strongly associated with the development of malignancy and often precedes overt cancers.

(**116**) A classic example of *hypertrophy* is the response of cardiac muscle to systemic hypertension. Cardiac muscle cannot proliferate. Therefore, in response to an increased work load, each cell becomes larger by increasing its cytoplasmic content of contractile elements.

(**117**) One of the cardinal histopathologic features of chronic bronchitis is goblet cell *metaplasia* of the bronchiolar epithelium. In contrast to normal bronchioles, which are lined only by ciliated columnar cells and Clara cells, the bronchioles of the chronic bronchitic contain large numbers of mucin-producing goblet cells. They develop from the bronchiolar reserve cells as a result of chronic exposure to cigarette smoke. Early in the course of the disease, the metaplastic change is an adaptive one and appears to be reversible.

(**118**) Prolonged increased stimulation by ACTH typically induces adrenocortical *hyperplasia*. The hyperplasia may be nodular or diffuse, and its extent is a function of the duration and level of the ACTH excess.

(**119**) The "hypertrophy" referred to in the disorder known as "benign prostatic hypertrophy" (BPH) is that of the entire gland, which diffusely enlarges. On microscopic examination, however, it becomes obvious that the glandular enlargement is due to *hyperplasia* of the stromal and glandular elements of this tissue.

(**120**) Perhaps the most important pathologic change associated with long-standing ulcerative colitis is *dysplasia* of the colonic epithelium. It has long been known that patients with ulcerative colitis are at greatly increased risk of developing colonic carcinoma. It is now clear that epithelial dysplasia precedes the development of malignancy in these patients, and is therefore considered a premalignant change (*pp. 31–33*).

121. (A); 122. (B); 123. (E); 124. (D); 125. (A); 126. (C); 127. (B); 128. (A); 129. (A); 130. (E)

As the name. implies, autoimmune diseases are disorders caused by immunologic attack directed against constituents of the body's own tissues ("self-antigens"). Both systemic lupus erythematosus (SLE) and scleroderma are *primary* disease processes involving multiple organ systems. Although Sjögren's syndrome may occur in primary form as an isolated disorder, it occurs more frequently as a *secondary* process in association with other autoimmune diseases.

(**121, 125, 128, 129**) SLE is believed to be caused by a fundamental defect in the immune system producing abnormalities of both B and T cells. The disease clearly has a genetic predisposition and a positive correlation with HLA-DR2 and DR3 antigens. Furthermore, SLE is associated with inherited deficiency of the second component of complement (C2), the genes for which are located within the HLA region. Thus, the association of SLE and hereditary C2 deficiency may reflect genetic derangements in certain chromosomal regions governing the immune response. Although SLE involves virtually every organ system, joint involvement with articular pain is the single most common clinical manifestation and must be differentiated from other forms of arthritis. The most devastating manifestation, however, is kidney involvement with renal failure, the major cause of mortality. As in many other autoimmune disorders, skin involvement is common in SLE. In contrast to the skin involvement in dermatomyositis, scleroderma, and chronic discoid lupus erythematosus, however, immunoglobulin deposition is found along the dermoepidermal junction of *normal*-appearing as well as clinically involved skin in SLE.

(**122 and 127**) Sjögren's syndrome is an uncomfortable disorder characterized by dry eyes and dry mouth resulting from immunologically mediated destruction of lacrimal and salivary glands. It also has the unfortunate distinction of being associated with a 40-fold increased risk of developing a lymphoid malignancy. Another feature of Sjögren's syndrome that distinguishes it from SLE and scleroderma is the rarity of glomerular lesions, which are quite common in the latter two disorders. Instead of glomerular disease, renal involvement in Sjögren's syndrome takes the form of tubulointerstitial nephritis.

(**123**) Epithelial malignancy is most commonly associated with dermatomyositis, in which the incidence of underlying carcinoma is about 10%. SLE, Sjögren's syndrome, and scleroderma do not share this association.

(**124**) However, in another subset of patients without underlying malignancy, dermatomyositis is associated with other autoimmune connective tissue disorders including SLE, Sjögren's syndrome, and scleroderma.

(**126**) Scleroderma, a disorder characterized by altered collagen synthesis with systemic fibrosis, shares a variety of serologic abnormalities with other autoimmune connective tissue disorders. Recently, however, two autoantibodies more or less unique to scleroderma and useful in establishing this diagnosis have been discovered: an anticentromere antibody and antibody against a non-histone nuclear protein called Scl-70.

(**130**) Although immunosuppression with corticosteroids is of variable benefit in controlling the clinical manifestations of most autoimmune connective tissue disorders, a consistently excellent response to this mode of therapy is associated only with mixed connective tissue disease (*pp. 181–195*).

131. (A); 132. (D); 133. (C); 134. (A); 135. (B); 136. (B); 137. (B)

In contrast to immunodeficiencies that arise as a secondary consequence of infection, malnutrition, aging, autoimmune disease, or exposure to immunosuppressive agents, primary immunodeficiency disorders are almost always genetic in origin. Study of the specific defects inherent in each of these disorders has greatly broadened our understanding of the functions of individual components of the immune system.

(**131, 134**) X-linked agammaglobulinemia of Bruton is a disease restricted to males and characterized by the virtual absence of immunoglobulin production. The disorder is a classic example of a primary B cell deficiency in which the underlying defect is a failure in pre-B cell maturation. Although patients with this disorder fail to mount humoral immune responses against infectious organisms, they are paradoxically at greatly increased risk of developing autoimmune diseases such as systemic lupus erythematosus, rheumatoid arthritis, and dermatomyositis. Although a high frequency of rheumatoid arthritis is also associated with common variable immunodeficiency, systemic lupus erythematosus is not particularly common in association with this disease as compared with X-linked agammaglobulinemia of Bruton.

(**132**) As in X-linked agammaglobulinemia of Bruton, common variable immunodeficiency and DiGeorge's syndrome are both characterized by derangements in immunocyte maturation rather than an underlying defect in lymphoid stem cells. Stem cell defects produce a much more serious disease known as severe combined immunodeficiency.

(**133**) DiGeorge's syndrome is a selective T cell deficiency. It is caused by a failure of development of the third and fourth pharyngeal pouches, the embryologic origin of both the thymus and the parathyroids. Thus, the total absence of cell-mediated immunity is accompanied by deranged serum calcium regulation and tetany.

(**135, 136, 137**) Common variable immunodeficiency is the most common form of immunodeficiency with serious clinical impact. As its name implies, it represents a group of syndromes with variable functional defects of either B cells or T cells or both. Disorders falling into this category have several unusual features in common, however. Patients with common variable immunodeficiency are often affected by a gluten-sensitive, spruelike malabsorption syndrome. Furthermore, noncaseating granulomas without any consistent microbial cause are frequently found in the liver, lungs, spleen, and skin. Of graver significance is the association of this disorder with the development of lymphoid malignancy, which sometimes develops late in the course of this disease (*pp. 205–210*).

138. (A); 139. (B); 140. (B); 141. (C); 142. (A); 143. (C); 144. (B); 145. (E); 146. (A); 147. (B); 148. (D); 149. (A)

Edema is the term that refers to the accumulation of an abnormal amount of fluid in the interstitial tissue spaces or body cavities. Ascites is a localized form of edema in which edema fluid collects in the peritoneal cavity. Edema is the result of a disturbance in the forces that normally keep about 75% of all the extracellular fluid in the body within the intravascular compartment. The remaining 25% is interstitial fluid that is separated from the intravascular fluid by a semipermeable endothelial barrier. Maintenance of this balance between the interstitial and intravascular fluid compartments depends upon several factors: (1) the intravascular hydrostatic pressure, (2) the oncotic pressure exerted by the plasma proteins, (3) the hydrostatic pressure of the interstitial fluid, (4) the lymphatic drainage of the interstitial tissue spaces, and (5) the integrity of the vascular endothelium. Disorders that either decrease the plasma oncotic pressure, lymphatic drainage, or endothelial integrity or increase the intravascular hydrostatic pressure or the osmotic tension of the interstitial fluid (usually related to sodium retention) will promote edema.

(**138, 142, 146, 149**) Decreased plasma oncotic pressure is the major cause of edema in the nephrotic syndrome, kwashiorkor, hydrops fetalis, and Ménétrier's disease. In the nephrotic syndrome, excessive glomerular permeability results in the loss of large amounts of protein into the urine. Excessive protein loss is also the underlying problem in Ménétrier's disease, but in this condition, protein is secreted into the gut in the form of mucus produced by hyperplastic gastric mucosal cells. Underproduction (rather than excessive loss) of plasma proteins is the underlying defect in kwashiorkor and hydrops fetalis. In kwashiorkor, profound protein malnutrition produces severe protein deprivation in all tissues of the body, including the liver, severely limiting hepatic plasma protein production. In hydrops fetalis, the result of a hemolytic anemia produced by blood-group incompatibility between mother and child, hypoxic injury to the liver leads to markedly reduced synthesis of albumin and other major plasma proteins.

(**139, 140, 144, 147**) Increased intravascular hydrostatic pressure is the major contributor to the edema associated with congestive heart failure and constrictive pericarditis. In congestive heart failure, the most common cause of edema, the failing heart is unable to generate a normal cardiac output. Consequently, blood is not adequately emptied from the venous system of the lungs (left heart failure) or the systemic venous system (right heart failure), and venous hydrostatic pressure increases, causing edema in the lungs or the periphery, respectively. In pregnancy and constrictive pericarditis, venous return to the heart is restricted by external compression, and hydrostatic pressure in the venous system proximal to the point of compression increases. Thus pregnancy-associated edema is primarily in the lower extremities, whereas the edema associated with constrictive pericarditis is characteristically systemic. In cirrhosis, hepatic scarring and obliteration of portal architecture greatly diminishes portal flow through the liver and increases hydrostatic pressure in the portal system, producing ascites.

(**141 and 143**) Disruption of endothelial integrity with increased vascular permeability produces edema in thermal burns and bee stings. In thermal burns, direct tissue injury as well as mediators of vascular permeability generated in the accompanying inflammatory response lead to a massive outpouring of fluids into injured tissue. Bee stings most commonly produce a mild inflammatory response and localized edema. In sensitized individuals, however, IgE-mediated hypersensitivity responses lead to increased vascular permeability on a wider scale, producing hives or anaphylaxis.

(**148**) Edema associated with metastatic carcinoma is most often the result of lymphatic blockage by tumor. Other mechanisms, such as veous compression by tumor, protein wasting, or hepatic replacement by metastatic tumor, are possible but are less common.

(**145**) Excessive salt intake in normal individuals does not ordinarily cause edema. In those predisposed to sodium retention, however, edema may result from elevated osmotic pressure in interstitial fluid containing increased numbers of sodium ions (*pp. 42–43, 85–88, 400, 487, 813*).

150. (B); 151. (A); 152. (E); 153. (D); 154. (C); 155. (B); 156. (E); 157. (B); 158. (A)

Morphological patterns of tissue necrosis depend on the balance between progressive enzymatic digestion of dead cells and coagulation of denatured proteins in the cytoplasm of dead cells. At least four distinctive morphological patterns of necrosis can be recognized: coagulation necrosis, liquefaction necrosis, enzymatic fat necrosis, and caseous necrosis.

(**151, 158**) Coagulation necrosis is the most common pattern of necrosis and is characterized by preservation of the basic cellular shape, permitting recognition of the cell outlines and tissue architecture despite the loss of nuclei from the dead cells. It is the result of coagulation of denatured proteins in dead cells and delayed proteolysis by lysosomal enzymes. This type of necrosis commonly occurs in myocardial infarction with ischemic necrosis of myocytes. Coagulation necrosis also predominates in acute tubular necrosis resulting from sudden severe ischemia to the kidney or after chemical injury such as mercuric chloride poisoning. In these injuries, entire renal tubules may undergo necrosis but the outlines of the tubular epithelial cells can still be recognized (*pp. 15, 561*).

(150, 155, 157) Liquefaction necrosis is the result of enzymatic digestion of dead cells, resulting in obliteration of tissue architecture. This occurs when lysosomal enzymes within the dead and dying cells are activated (autolysis) or when the powerful hydrostatic enzymes of bacteria or leukocytes contribute to the digestion of dead cells (heterolysis). This pattern of necrosis characteristically occurs in pulmonary nocardiosis and wet gangrene of an extremity. In both these examples the liquefactive action of bacteria and attracted leukocytes largely determines the pattern of necrosis. Liquefaction necrosis is also characteristic of ischemic destruction of brain tissue, but in this case it is primarily autolytic in nature (*pp. 15, 17*).

(154) Enzymatic fat necrosis is highly characteristic of acute pancreatitis. In this condition powerful lipases and proteases are released into the surrounding peripancreatic fat and catalyze the decomposition of triglycerides that leak from the damaged adipose cells, producing free fatty acids. Indistinct outlines of necrotic adipose cells are seen in association with granular, basophilic deposits that represent calcium soaps formed by the reaction of calcium with the released free fatty acids (*p. 965*).

(152) Pott's disease is the term by which tuberculous spondylitis is known. The granulomatous lesions of *Mycobacterium tuberculosis*, wherever they are found in the body, are characterized by a distinctive pattern of necrosis known as caseation. Caseous necrosis represents a combination of coagulative and liquefactive necrosis in which the outlines of the dead cells are neither totally destroyed nor well preserved. Grossly, caseous necrosis resembles clumped cheesy material, and microscopically, distinctive amorphous granular debris is seen. This pattern of necrosis is highly characteristic and virtually diagnostic of mycobacterial infection (*p. 17*).

(153) Although tuberculoid granulomas are characteristic of the vigorous T cell–mediated immune response mounted by individuals infected with *Mycobacterium leprae* in tuberculoid leprosy, the granulomatous lesions do not characteristically undergo necrosis and instead remain as hard tubercles (*pp. 347–349*).

(156) Infection with the intestinal flagellate *Giardia lamblia* usually produces dramatic symptomatology such as copious, watery diarrhea; cramps; and even malabsorption. Ironically, however, the organism induces relatively few morphologic changes in the small bowel. Although the intestinal morphology may range from virtually normal to markedly abnormal with villous flattening, necrosis is virtually never seen (*p. 364*).

159. (B); 160. (D); 161. (A); 162. (C); 163. (C); 164. (D); 165. (B); 166. (A); 167. (E); 168. (E); 169. (E); 170. (D)

Although immune responses are essential for survival in a world filled with microbes, they can also cause debilitating and even fatal diseases. Disorders resulting from tissue-damaging immune reactions can be separated into four major categories based on the immunologic mechanism that mediates the disease.

(161 and 166) In Type I disease, exposure to an antigen leads to the production of cytotropic IgE antibodies that become affixed to mast cells and basophils. On re-exposure, antigen combines with the cell-bound antibody, causing release of vasoactive amines, increased vascular permeability, and edema within a few minues of encountering the antigen. Depending on the allergen and the portal of entry, localized reactions may take the form of cutaneous swellings (hives, or urticaria), nasal and conjunctival discharge, hay fever, bronchial asthma, or allergic gastroenteritis. Systemic reactions, usually developing after an intravenous injection of the offending antigen, can produce a state of shock that is sometimes fatal. Hay fever and penicillin-induced urticaria are examples of localized Type I (anaphylactic type) hypersensitivity response (*pp. 165–166*).

(159 and 165) Type II (cytotoxic type) hypersensitivity responses are caused by the formation of antibodies directed toward antigens present on the surface of cells or other tissue components. The antigen may be one intrinsic to the cell membrane or an adsorbed exogenous antigen. Antibody-coated cells are then susceptible to three separate modes of injury: (1) complement activation and direct complement-mediated membrane damage; (2) phagocytosis promoted by opsinization; or (3) antibody-dependent cell-mediated cytotoxicity by nonsensitized cells that have Fc receptors such as monocytes, neutrophils, eosinophils, and K cells. Erythroblastosis fetalis, a hemolytic anemia in the newborn caused by blood-group incompatibility between mother and child, is a prime example of a Type II hypersensitivity reaction. In this disorder the mother's immune system reacts to blood group antigens expressed by the fetal red blood cells. Another example is the hemolytic anemia induced by the antihypertensive agent alpha-methyldopa (dopamine). The drug initiates (in some unknown manner) the production of antibodies that are directed against intrinsic red blood cell antigens. As in erythroblastosis fetalis, the red cell antigens that are usually the target of the immunologic response in dopamine-induced hemolytic anemia are the Rh blood group antigens (*pp. 166, 629*).

(**162 and 163**) Immune complex disorders (Type III hypersensitivity responses) are caused by antigen-antibody complexes that cause tissue damage through their ability to activate a variety of serum mediators, principally the complement system. Such a reaction usually requires at least two exposures to the antigen: a sensitizing exposure to induce circulating antibody followed by a second exposure sometime later. However, persistence of the antigen through the phase of the primary immune response when circulating antibody is present can also lead to immune complex formation. Polyarteritis nodosa is a necrotizing form of vasculitis thought to be produced by complement-fixing immune complexes that become localized to vessel walls, particularly the small or medium-sized muscular arteries. Although the inciting antigen is not known in most cases, about 30% of patients with polyarteritis nodosa have hepatitis B antigen in their serum and circulating HBsAg–anti-HBs immune complexes. Serum sickness is a systemic immune complex disorder caused by the formation of small, soluble antigen-antibody aggregates within the circulation. The inciting antigen in this disorder is usually a foreign protein contained in some therapeutic antiserum derived from an animal (e.g., horse tetanus antitoxin) or a drug (*pp. 166–169*).

(**160, 164, 170**) Hypersensitivity responses mediated by specifically sensitized T lymphocytes are known as Type IV (cell-mediated) reactions. Poison ivy dermatitis, graft vs. host disease, and chronic berylliosis are all examples of cell-mediated hypersensitivity. Poison ivy is a type of contact dermatitis in which a delayed hypersensitivity response is mounted against the plant-derived antigen affixed to epidermal cells. In graft vs. host disease, the immunocompetent cells in the grafted tissue mount an immune response against the tissue of the immunocompromised recipient. In chronic berylliosis, T cells immunized against beryllium initiate granuloma formation, the hallmark of chronic berylliosis, through their production of lymphokines, which regulate macrophage activity (*pp. 169–171*).

(**167, 168, 169**) In amphotericin-induced renal injury, chlorpromazine-induced cholestatic jaundice, and pulmonary asbestosis, the tissue injury is caused by the direct toxic effects of the causative agent. Immunologic responses are not known to play any direct role in these disorders. Although some alterations in the immune system have been detected in individuals with asbestos-induced disease, such as reduced numbers of circulating T cells, elevated immunoglobulins, and defective cell-mediated immunity, the significance of these is as yet unclear (*pp. 439–441, 445*).

171. (D); 172. (D); 173. (B); 174. (A); 175. (A); 176. (E); 177. (A); 178. (E); 179. (A); 180. (C); 181. (C); 182. (A)

(**171 and 172**) The three major cell types that comprise the immune system are T lymphocytes, B

lymphocytes, and macrophages. In varying proportions, all of these cell types are found in the circulating blood (monocytes are the circulating form of macrophages) and in the peripheral lymphoid tissues. In the cortex of lymph nodes, B cells are found primarily in the germinal centers, whereas T cells and macrophages are found predominantly in the paracortical zones (*pp. 159–160, 653*).

(**174, 175, 177, 179, 182**) T lymphocytes are the major effector cells in cellular immune reactions such as delayed hypersensitivity responses and in the regulation (both initiation and termination) of all immune responses. Unlike B cells and macrophages/monocytes, T lymphocytes do not display HLA-DR antigens on their cell surface, nor do they have cell surface receptors for complement. They are characterized by their distinctive and somewhat peculiar ability to form spontaneous rosettes with sheep red blood cells (E rosettes) (*pp. 158–159*).

(**173**) B lymphocytes are the major effector cells in humoral immune responses. They express cell surface immunoglobulin (IgG) that is thought to be identical in specificity to the immunoglobulin secreted by that cell when it differentiates into a plasma cell (*pp. 158–159*).

(**180 and 181**) Macrophages play several key roles in the immune response. They function as antigen-presenting cells and also act as powerful effector cells in certain cell-mediated immune responses, usually under the direction of lymphokines produced by activated T cells. Along with mast cells and neutrophils, macrophages produce lipoxygenase derivatives of arachidonic acid, known as leukotrienes. Leukotrienes C_4, D_4, and E_4 are powerful mediators of anaphylaxis. In addition, macrophages respond chemotactically to another of these lipoxygenase derivatives, leukotriene B_4, a mediator of acute inflammation (*pp. 55–56, 165*).

(**176 and 178**) Although macrophages are capable of phagocytizing and lysing antibody-coated target cells, only killer (K) cells are capable of lysing antibody-coated target cells by means of a nonphagocytic mechanism. This process is called antibody-dependent cellular cytotoxicity (ADCC). Obviously, however, ADCC requires previous sensitization by the antigen and the production of cytophilic antibody. Cells capable of lysing target cells, such as tumor cells or virus-infected cells, without previous sensitization are called natural killer (NK) cells. Although NK cells share some cell surface properties with T cells, B cells, and macrophages, they are thought to be distinct from any of these cell types. They are considered to be important as the first line of defense against tumors and viral infections (*p. 160*).

183. (D); 184. (D); 185. (C); 186. (E); 187. (E); 188. (E); 189. (A); 190. (B); 191. (B); 192. (E)

Pigment accumulation in cells is most often the result of a pathologic process. Normal examples of pigment accumulation are few and include melanin in melanocytes and neighboring basal keratinocytes of the skin and iron stores in the form of hemosiderin in the bone marrow. Examples of pathologic accumulations of pigment in cells are much more numerous, however, and certain disorders characteristically produce accumulations of a specific pigment type.

(183 and 184) Lipofuscin, an insoluble brown pigment that is the product of cell membrane breakdown—often the result of lipid peroxidation by free radicals—is considered "wear-and-tear" or aging pigment. It is present in abundance in the heart and liver of elderly, malnourished individuals. In severe cases, when lipofuscin deposition is accompanied by organ shrinkage, the condition is known as "brown atrophy." Lipofuscin is not injurious to cells, nor does it interfere with cellular function.

(185) Ceroid pigment is lipofuscin that has been chemically altered, probably by auto-oxidation. It is commonly found in Kupffer's cells in the liver following hepatocellular injury. Lipofuscin is liberated from dying liver cells and taken up by sinusoidal phagocytes that convert it to ceroid pigment.

(189) In liver diseases that disrupt the flow of bile, such as large bile duct obstruction, profound cholestasis ensues, and bile infarcts may occur. In this setting, Kupffer's cells mop up the spilled bile and become laden with bilirubin, the major bile pigment.

(188, 190, 191) Hematin is a hemoglobin-derived pigment whose precise chemical composition is unknown. It is seen most commonly within mononuclear phagocytes following a massive hemolytic crisis such as that which may occur in malaria or a hemolytic transfusion reaction. In conditions characterized by increased destruction of red blood cells such as hereditary spherocytosis (see Chapter 7, Question 1), large deposits of *hemosiderin* are found in mononuclear phagocytes. Hemosiderin pigment represents aggregates of ferritin micelles that accumulate in a local or systemic excess of iron. Iron excess can result from any one of a number of conditions, including increased absorption of dietary iron, impaired utilization of iron, hemolytic anemias, or blood transfusions (an exogenous iron load).

(186, 187, 192) Carbon is the pigment encountered in sinus histiocytes of the lungs and peribronchial lymph nodes of smokers. In tattooed skin, carbon is injected into the dermal tissues and taken up by dermal macrophages. The hyperpigmentation that occurs in Addison's disease, a condition caused by adrenal insufficiency, is seen microscopically as an accumulation of melanin in epidermal keratinocytes. Increased melanocytic production of melanin in Addison's disease is probably the result of increased ACTH released from the pituitary gland. One end of this molecule is homologous to melanocyte stimulating hormone (MSH) *(pp. 23–26).*

193. (A); 194. (E); 195. (B); 196. (E); 197. (A); 198. (D); 199. (D); 200. (C); 201. (C); 202. (C)

The type of inflammatory cell infiltrate found in injured tissues is primarily determined by the nature of the underlying pathologic process, namely, immunologic or inflammatory. There is much overlap in the cellular responses evoked by these two processes, however. On the one hand, although lymphocytes, monocytes, and plasma cells characteristically predominate in most responses that are immunologically mediated, the same cell types predominate in inflammatory responses of a chronic nature. On the other hand, although neutrophilic infiltrates are usually associated with acute inflammatory reactions, neutrophils are also the major cell type present in necrotizing immunologic responses mediated by complement-fixing antibody or immune complexes.

(193 and 197) Neutrophils are the predominant inflammatory cell type seen in infarcted myocardium 48 to 72 hours after injury and represent an acute inflammatory response to the necrotic tissue. Neutrophils are also the predominant cell type present in the early phases of polyarteritis nodosa. In this case they are attracted by chemotactic cleavage products generated from complement activation by the circulating immune complexes believed to cause this disease *(pp. 520, 563).*

(194) Although its name implies that it is an acute inflammatory reaction, acute viral hepatitis B is an immunologically mediated disease. It is caused by a cellular immune response to virally infected hepatocytes. The effector cells in this disease are lymphocytes, and they are the predominant cell type seen in the affected liver *(p. 602).*

(195) Sarcoidosis is a disease of unknown etiology that produces lesions identical to those of a delayed hypersensitivity response. Noncaseating granulomas composed of epithelioid histiocyes (macrophages) occur in virtually any tissue or organ in this disease *(p. 391).*

(196) Liver transplant rejection is most commonly the result of cytotoxic type and delayed hypersensitivity type immunologic reactions to the foreign histocompatability (HLA) antigens of the transplanted tissue. Thus, the predominant cell type seen in transplant rejection reactions is the lymphocyte *(p. 171).*

(198 and 199) Although the causes of chronic endometritis are diverse and include infectious as well as noninfectious etiologies, the histologic hallmark of this inflammatory process is plasma cell infiltration. Conversely, although primary syphilis is an acute disease of singular etiology, namely the spirochete *Treponema pallidum*, the associated inflammatory response is characteristically composed principally of plasma cells *(pp. 336, 1130).*

(200, 201, 202) Eosinophilic inflammation is characteristic of anaphylactic type hypersensitivity responses and parasitic infections. Both Löffler's syndrome and bronchial asthma are examples of Type I allergic reactions in the lung with prominent eosinophilic infiltrates. Paragonimiasis or lung fluke infection is just one of innumerable examples of parasitic infections that induce florid eosinophilic inflammatory infiltrates (*pp. 378, 388, 728, 748*).

203. (F); 204. (D); 205. (C); 206. (D); 207. (C); 208. (F); 209. (B)

Chemotaxis is the directed movement of a cell along a chemical gradient toward a substance to which it is attracted. It is the mechanism by which inflammatory cells and immunocompetent cells are drawn to sites of injury or microbial invasion. The source and composition of many of these chemoattractant substances and their differential effect on various cell types is not known. Of the many chemotactic factors produced during an acute inflammatory response, some affect only the monocyte, and some stimulate migration of all types of leukocytes.

(**203**) During activation of the complement system, biologically active cleavage products are generated that are chemotactic for white cells. The most potent of these is C5a. it is highly chemotactic for neutrophils and monocytes but also attracts eosinophils.

(**204 and 206**) Substances that are known to be chemotactic for both neutrophils and monocytes but not eosinophils are leukotriene B_4 (a product of the lipoxygenase pathway of arachidonic acid metabolism) and bacterial products. HETE, another of the metabolic derivatives of the lipoxygenase pathway, is a potent chemotactic agent for neutrophils only. Both HETE and leukotriene B_4 are produced by leukocytes, and both are chemotactic for leukocytes.

(**205 and 207**) In contrast to products of the lipoxygenase pathway that do not attract eosinophils, some products of the cyclooxygenase pathway of arachidonic acid metabolism (e.g., prostaglandin D_2) are chemotactic *only* for eosinophils. Eosinophils are also uniquely attracted to histamine released from degranulated mast cells or basophils.

(**208**) A variety of substances (lymphokines) with diverse biologic activities are released from activated T cells during an immune response. Among these are chemotactic factors for neutrophils, eosinophils, basophils, monocytes, and other lymphocytes.

(**209**) Although monocytes respond chemotactically to many of the same substances that attract neutrophils (such as C5a, leukotriene B_4, and factors released from neutrophils and lymphocytes), they appear to be uniquely attracted to fibronectin fragments. This characteristic may be important in the wound-healing process (*pp. 48–49, 55–56, 79, 171*).

210. (B); 211. (C); 212. (E); 213. (E); 214. (B)

(**210, 213, 214**) Activated T cells produce a number of lymphokines that affect macrophage activity. Among them are a chemotactic factor for monocytes, a factor that inhibits normal active migration of macrophages (macrophage migration inhibition factor, or MIF), and a gamma-interferon that increases the level of metabolic activity and the bactericidal capacity of macrophages. Until recently, the latter was thought to be an independent lymphokine previously termed "macrophage activating factor" (MAF), but is now known to be an interferon. Interferons were originally discovered for their antiviral activity. Sensitized T cells are induced to produce alpha- and beta-interferon during viral infections. These interferons inhibit intracellular viral replication and therefore constitute an important host defense mechanism in viral infection.

(**211**) Interleukin-2, a lymphokine also known as T-cell growth factor, is produced by activated T cells and in turn causes proliferation of other T cells, principally those involved in cellular immunity.

(**212**) Although a lymphokine known as lymphotoxin will kill tumor cells *in vitro*, lymphocytes do not produce substances that directly kill bacteria. Transfer factor is a lymphokine that has the ability to transfer sensitivity to mycobacterial antigens (tuberculin) to previously unsensitized individuals, but it has no direct effect on the organisms themselves (*pp. 170–171, 278*).

215. (D); 216. (D); 217. (B); 218. (A); 219. (C); 220. (C)

(**215 and 216**) Killer (K) cells, natural killer (NK) cells, and cytotoxic lymphocytes (CTL) are all effector cells of the immune system that are capable of destroying tumor cells. None of these cell types is phagocytic (*pp. 160, 171*).

(**217, 218, 219**) Small lymphocytes do not contain granules in their cytoplasm, and cytotoxic lymphocytes are small lymphocytes that represent a subset of T cells. K cells, although they lack the typical surface markers of lymphocytes, are morphologically identical to small or medium-sized lymphocytes and do not contain granules in their cytoplasm. In contrast to T cells and K cells, NK cells do possess cytoplasmic granules. Although NK cells have been described as "large granular lymphocytes," they are believed to be a cell type that is distinct from mature T cells, B cells, or macrophages. Unlike cytotoxic lymphocytes, both K cells and NK cells possess receptors for the Fc fragment of IgG. However, only K cells require the presence of antibody on the surface of target cells in order to effect cellular killing, a phenomenon known as antibody-dependent cellular cytotoxicity (ADCC) (*p. 160*).

(**220**) Recognition of virally infected cells by means of altered cell-surface HLA antigens is a unique characteristic of cytotoxic lymphocytes. Although natural killer cells can detect and destroy virus-infected cells, they are not dependent on recognition of both viral neoantigens and HLA gene products to achieve their cytotoxic effect (*pp. 162, 278*).

221. (D); 222. (E); 223. (C); 224. (B); 225. (D); 226. (B); 227. (A); 228. (A); 229. (E); 230. (C); 231. (E); 232. (B)

Disease processes and tissue injuries of specific type are usually associated with a characteristic pattern of inflammation that helps the pathologist to identify and diagnose them.

(**221 and 225**) Cat scratch lymphadenitis and brucellosis characteristically produce granulomatous inflammation in involved tissues. Granulomas of cat scratch lymphadenitis are distinctive in the later phases of the disease because of their coalescence to form large stellate structures that contain neutrophils and necrotic debris in their centers. Chronic brucellosis causes well-formed granulomas, with or without central necrosis, that may occur in organs throughout the body. Thus, it can be difficult to differentiate from tuberculosis. Granulomatous inflammation in infectious diseases is the result of cell-mediated hypersensitivity in which activated, sensitized T cells release lymphokines and other effector molecules that attract macrophages and mediate granuloma formation (*pp. 291, 331*).

(**222 and 229**) The immune system is also the major host defense against viral infections. Inflammatory responses usually play only a minor or secondary role. Thus, the cellular infiltrates that are seen in acute viral pneumonia and acute viral hepatitis are composed predominantly of the mononuclear cells that constitute the effector cells of the immune system: lymphocytes, plasma cells, and monocytes. These same cell types also predominate in chronic inflammatory reactions. Therefore, even though they are acute in nature, viral pneumonia and viral hepatitis elicit cellular responses that are identical to those seen in chronic inflammatory conditions (*pp. 737, 906, 907*).

(**223, 230, 231**) Acute appendicitis and acute ascending cholangitis are examples of suppurative (purulent) inflammation. Bacterial invasion, usually following luminal obstruction, is thought to play a major role in both of these processes. Masses of polymorphonuclear leukocytes are attracted to the site of infection, producing purulent exudate (pus). In contrast to the suppurative cholangitis produced by the bile duct obstruction and ascending infection, nonsuppurative inflammation of bile ducts is the hallmark of primary biliary cirrhosis. In this disease, bile duct inflammation and destruction are immunologically mediated (a direct immunologic attack on bile ducts), and mononuclear cell infiltrates in and around the walls of the intrahepatic bile ducts (nonsuppurative cholangitis) are characteristic (*pp. 875, 928–930, 991*).

(**224, 226, 232**) Fibrinous inflammation is characterized by the exudation of large amounts of plasma proteins, including fibrinogen, and the precipitation of large masses of fibrin. Cellular infiltrates may be minimal in this type of inflammation, which occurs primarily as a result of alterations in vascular integrity and increased permeability. Examples of this type of inflammation include rheumatic pericarditis, uremic pericarditis, and adult hyaline membrane disease (adult respiratory distress syndrome with diffuse alveolar damage). In diffuse alveolar damage the amount and type of accompanying cellular inflammation may vary somewhat, but the hyaline membranes that are the characteristic histologic features of this disorder are composed predominantly of fibrin (*pp. 603, 714, 997*).

(**227 and 228**) Serous inflammation is characterized by an outpouring of watery fluid representing either a leakage of serum from blood vessls or the secretion products of serous cells. Skin blisters resulting from mechanical friction or shallow thermal burns are common examples of serous inflammation. This type of inflammation is most often seen in mild injuries and often occurs early in the development of other types of acute inflammatory reactions before cellular infiltrates become prominent (*pp. 65–66*).

233. (E); 234. (D); 235. (E); 236. (E); 237. (A); 238. (C); 239. (D)

A large number of chemical agents are known to induce cancers in experimental animals and to induce neoplastic transformation of cells *in vitro*. Many human cancers are also linked by strong epidemiologic evidence to chemical carcinogens.

(**233**) Aflatoxin B_1, a compound produced by some strains of the fungus *Aspergillus flavus*, is a contaminant of improperly stored grains and peanuts. It has been linked to the induction of hepatocellular carcinoma (*p. 238*).

(**234 and 239**) Beta-naphthylamine is an azo dye that is commonly used in the aniline dye and rubber industries. This chemical has been known to increase by 50-fold the incidence of bladder cancer among exposed industrial workers. Some azo dyes have been used as food coloring agents such as those that color margarine yellow or maraschino cherries red, but these substances are now federally regulated because of the concern over their carcinogenic potential. Benzidine, an aromatic amine, is a common chemical used by biochemists, dye workers, and wood chemists. This chemical has also been shown by epidemiologic studies to be linked to bladder cancer in men (*pp. 238, 460–461*).

(**235**) Busulfan is an alkylating agent commonly used in the chemotherapy of lymphoid neoplasms, leukemia, and other forms of cancer. Like the other chemotherapeutic alkylating agents, however, it represents a double-eged sword. Although the alkylating agents exert their therapeutic effect by damaging DNA in tumor cells, they are also capable of damaging the DNA of normal cells. Thus, alkylating agents may function as direct-acting carcinogens (*p. 237*).

(**236**) Vinyl chloride is a chemical used in the manufacture of rubber, polyvinyl resins, and organic chemicals that is associated with a rare tumor of the liver, hepatic angiosarcoma. This highly aggressive neoplasm has also been linked to arsenic or Thorotrast exposure (*pp. 460–461, 939*).

(**237**) Metals such as chromium and nickel that may be volatilized and inhaled in industrial environments have been linked to an increased incidence of lung cancer among exposed workers (*p. 238*).

(**238**) Nitrosamines have been linked to carcinoma of the stomach and less strongly to carcinoma of the pancreas. These compounds appear to be derived from a dietary source. Nitrites used as food preservatives may combine with amines from digested proteins in the acid environment of the stomach to form nitrosamines. Thus, foods that are high in nitrites, such as processed meat and frankfurters, have been regarded as suspect (*pp. 238, 426*).

240. (E); 241. (E); 242. (A); 243. (B); 244. (D); 245. (E); 246. (C)

The diagnosis, either clinical or pathological, of many types of neoplasms can be greatly aided by the detection of an associated tumor cell product. When dealing with an anaplastic tumor showing little or no evidence of differentiation, the identification of cell elements or products that are known to be restricted to certain cell types can be essential in diagnosing the histogenetic origin of the malignancy. Often, effective treatment hinges on the precise identification of tumor type, and immunohistochemical methods must be used to identify such tumor markers in biopsy tissue.

(**242**) Hepatomas and yolk sac tumors of germ cell origin are examples of tumors that characteristically produce alpha-fetoprotein (AFP). Since metastatic tumor is by far more common than primary malignancy in the liver, the presence of AFP can help to positively identify the less common primary hepatoma. In 85% of cases, hepatomas produce substantial amounts of this substance (*p. 268*).

(**243**) Like many well-differentiated adenocarcinomas, colon cancers commonly produce a glycoprotein normally found in embryonic tissues of the gut known as carcinoembryonic antigen (CEA). Blood levels of CEA are often elevated in patients with colonic carcinoma and fall below detectable levels after complete resection of the primary tumor. Monitoring of the blood levels of CEA following surgical resection has been used clinically to detect possible recurrences of the tumor (*p. 268*).

(**244**) The production of large amounts of human chorionic gonadotropin (HCG) is characteristic of choriocarcinoma, a malignant tumor of placental or germ cell origin. Detection of HCG is commonly used in the initial diagnosis of this malignancy or in diagnosing recurrences. Although multinucleate, syncytiotrophoblastic-type cells can occur in such diverse tumors as seminoma or gastric carcinoma, these cells usually fail to generate the high serum levels of HCG so commonly found with choriocarcinoma (*pp. 1152, 1161*).

(**246**) In addition to hormones and oncofetal antigens, the identification of intermediate filaments can be helpful in determining the tissue of origin of a tumor. Desmin, for example, is a cytoskeletal intermediate filament found only in muscle cells and fibroblasts. Thus, the detection of desmin in the cytoplasm of an anaplastic sarcoma can help to identify it as either a rhabdosarcoma, leiomyosarcoma, or fibrosarcoma, and sarcomas of other mesenchymal cell types can then be eliminated from the differential diagnosis (*p. 28*).

(**240, 241, 245**) Lymphomas, ganglioneuroblastomas, and medullary carcinomas of the thyroid do not produce any of the substances listed as choices. They can be identified by other specific markers, however. Lymphomas are often distinguished by their expression of lymphocyte-specific cell surface antigens recognized by monoclonal antibodies such as OKT and Leu. Ganglioneuroblastoma commonly produces neuron-specific enolase. Medullary carcinoma of the thyroid can be identified by its production of calcitonin and/or amyloid (*pp. 159, 1222–1223, 1406*).

247. (B); 248. (E); 249. (A); 250. (A); 251. (B); 252. (E); 253. (E); 254. (E); 255. (D); 256. (E)

(**249 and 250**) Although oncogenic viruses are known to be capable of inducing malignant tumor formation in a wide variety of animals including primates, the evidence linking viruses to carcinogenesis in humans is severely limited and usually indirect. Perhaps the best known association at present is that between the Epstein-Barr virus and the African type of Burkitt's lymphoma. This virus is also associated with undifferentiated nasopharyngeal carcinoma (*pp. 245, 662, 764*).

(**247**) Uterine cervical carcinoma has been linked to two classes of viruses: human papilloma virus (HPV) and herpes simplex virus Type II (HSV II). The exact role played by these viruses in the causation of this malignancy are as yet unclear, and it is possible that they act synergistically (*pp. 1124–1125*).

(**251**) HPV is also linked to another type of squamous cell carcinoma, that which arises in the cutaneous or mucosal warts produced by this virus. As in the uterine cervix, most of the lesions produced by HPV are benign. However, the mucosal lesions (condylomata acuminata) occasionally give rise to squamous cell carcinoma. In the rare clinical disease known as epidermodysplasia verruciformis, HPV-induced cutaneous warts often progress to squamous cell carcinoma, especially when one particular subtype of papilloma virus is the causative agent (*pp. 244–245*).

(**255**) The evidence suggesting a causal relationship between the hepatitis B virus and hepatocellular carcinoma is substantial. There is also strong evidence linking the naturally occurring chemical carcinogen aflatoxin with hepatoma induction, and it may be that these two carcinogenic agents act in concert in some cases (*pp. 935–938*).

(**254 and 256**) It is of interest that none of the influences related to induction of hepatoma has any bearing on the development of cholangiocarcinoma. Like angiosarcoma of the liver, cholangiocarcinoma has been linked with previous exposure to Thorotrast, formerly used in radiography of the biliary tract. However, neither one of these tumors is known to be causally related to viral infection *(pp. 938–939)*.

(248, 252, 253) Although breast cancer can be virally induced in the mouse by an oncogenic RNA virus known as the mouse mammary tumor virus (MMTV), there is no evidence that human breast cancer is virally induced. Similarly, although a number of viruses are capable of inducing sarcomas in animals of various species (in hamsters sarcomas can be induced by various strains of adenovirus), human sarcomas are not known to be virally caused. At least one form of human T-cell lymphoma/leukemia has been shown to be virally induced, however. The causative agent is the C retrovirus known as HTLV. A subtype of this virus is now known to be the causal agent in another devastating human disease, the acquired immune deficiency syndrome (AIDS) *(pp. 243–246)*.

257. (E); 258. (A); 259. (A); 260. (A); 261. (A); 262. (C); 263. (A); 264. (E); 265. (A); 266. (E)

A paraneoplastic syndrome is a symptom complex occurring in a patient with a malignant tumor that can be ascribed neither to the effects of tumor spread nor to the production of indigenous tumor hormones. Paraneoplastic syndromes occur in about 15% of patients with advanced malignancies. They can be difficult to control clinically and, depending on the type of syndrome, can even cause the death of the patient.

(258, 259, 260, 261, 263, 265) Bronchogenic carcinoma is the most common form of underlying malignancy in many of the major types of paraneoplastic syndromes. Hypercalcemia, caused by the elabora-

tion of parathyroid hormone by the tumor, occurs most commonly with oat cell or squamous cell carcinomas of the lung. Hyponatremia, caused by tumor cell secretion of antidiuretic hormone, is also seen most commonly in patients with bronchogenic carcinoma. Hypertrophic osteoarthropathy with clubbing of the fingers is seen almost exclusively in patients with bronchogenic carcinoma. The less well understood cancer-associated dermatomyositis and myasthenia gravis syndromes both occur most commonly in lung cancer patients. Although the nephrotic syndrome, thought to be induced by immune complexes containing tumor antigens, may occur with gastric or colon carcinomas among other malignancies, it is most often caused by lung cancer.

(262) When polycythemia occurs as a paraneoplastic syndrome, it is most often caused by the elaboration of erythropoietin by renal cell carcinoma. This syndrome also occurs occasionally in association with cerebellar hemangioma and hepatocellular carcinoma, however.

(257, 264, 266) None of the tumor types listed as choices constitutes the major form of underlying cancer associated with the paraneoplastic syndromes of acanthosis nigricans, anemia, or hypoglycemia. Gastric carcinoma is the tumor most often associated with the malignant form of acanthosis nigricans. Although the causal mechanism is unknown, carcinoma of thymic origin is the most common type of tumor associated with the paraneoplastic syndrome of anemia. Hypoglycemia, usually caused by the production of insulin or an insulin-like substance by tumor cells, occurs most commonly and curiously with sarcomas, especially fibrosarcoma *(p. 256)*.

2

PEDIATRIC AND GENETIC DISEASES

DIRECTIONS: For Questions 1 to 11, choose the ONE BEST answer to each question.

1. The leading cause of death in infancy (under 1 year of age) is:

    A. Congenital anomalies
    B. Hyaline membrane disease
    C. Pneumonia
    D. Accident
    E. Malignant neoplasms

2. Five minutes after birth, an infant appears pale and blue, has a heart rate of 90, and has slow irregular respirations. His muscles are limp and he makes no response to a nasal catheter. His Apgar score is:

    A. 0
    B. 1
    C. 2
    D. 3
    E. 4

3. Which one of the following statements about the therapy of Rh incompatibility (Rh hemolytic disease) is correct?

    A. Antigammaglobulin antibody is administered to the affected infant of a sensitized mother after birth
    B. Antigammaglobulin antibody is administered to the affected infant of a sensitized mother in utero
    C. Anti-D immunoglobulin is given to a nonsensitized mother just before delivery
    D. Anti-D immunoglobulin is given to a sensitized mother before birth
    E. Anti-D immunoglobulin is given to a sensitized mother throughout the last trimester of pregnancy

4. The lesion pictured in Figure 2–1 arose on the face of a young child and grew rapidly to a large red-blue mass. This lesion:

    A. Is known as a choristoma
    B. Will most likely regress spontaneously
    C. Is best treated by surgical excision
    D. Is best treated by radiation therapy
    E. Tends to metastasize to local lymph nodes

5. Conditions associated with impaired intrauterine fetal growth and low birth weight include all of the following EXCEPT:

    A. First pregnancy
    B. Chromosomal disorders of the fetus
    C. Small placentas
    D. Toxemia of pregnancy
    E. Maternal alcohol abuse

6. Congenital malformations are associated with all of the following conditions EXCEPT:

    A. Fetal chromosomal abnormalities
    B. Maternal thalidomide use

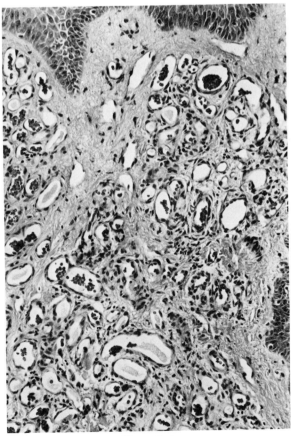

Figure 2–1

C. Rubella infection in the first 8 weeks of pregnancy
D. Cytomegalovirus infection in the second trimester of pregnancy
E. Heavy cigarette smoking throughout pregnancy

7. In severe cases of erythroblastosis fetalis, all of the following findings are characteristic EXCEPT:

A. Anasarca
B. Yellow pigmentation of the brain
C. Extramedullary hematopoiesis
D. Enlarged placenta
E. Dark urine

8. All of the conditions listed below are commonly associated with the disease process illustrated by the micrograph of pancreas in Figure 2–2 EXCEPT:

A. Diabetes mellitus
B. Meconium ileus
C. Male infertility
D. Pseudomonas pneumonia
E. Vitamin K deficiency

9. Malignancies that commonly occur in children under 5 years of age include all of the following EXCEPT:

A. Leukemia
B. Wilms' tumor
C. Retinoblastoma
D. Rhabdomyosarcoma
E. Osteosarcoma

10. Principal characteristics of the group of genetic disorders known as the mucopolysaccharidoses include all of the following EXCEPT:

A. Hepatomegaly
B. Muscular weakness
C. Skeletal deformities
D. Coronary artery disease
E. Cardiac valvular lesions

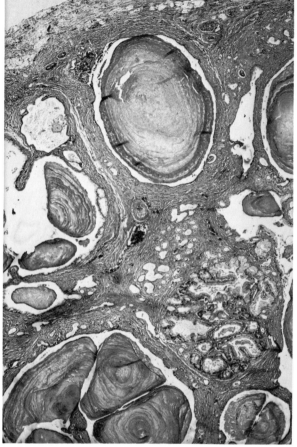

Figure 2–2

11. All of the following statements about congenital heart disease are true EXCEPT:

A. Most of the cases are associated with chromosomal abnormalities
B. Males are more commonly affected
C. The most common clinical presentation is cyanosis
D. Impaired growth and development are common
E. Affected individuals are at increased risk of developing any disease of childhood

DIRECTIONS: For Questions 12 to 17, ONE or MORE of the completions given correctly finishes the incomplete statement. Choose:

A—if only *1,2, and 3* are correct
B—if only *1 and 3* are correct
C—if only *2 and 4* are correct
D—if only *4* is correct
E—if all are correct

12. A 2000-gm infant delivered at 39 weeks gestational age:

1. Is considered preterm
2. Is appropriate weight for gestational age
3. Is at high risk for hyaline membrane disease
4. Has a greater than 95% chance of survival

A. 1,2,3   B. 1,3   C. 2,4   D. 4 Only   E. All

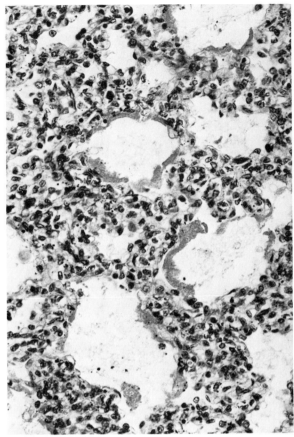

Figure 2–3

Questions 13 and 14 refer to Figure 2–3.

13. The condition shown in Figure 2–3 is associated with:

1. Diabetes in the mother
2. Infants of male sex
3. Delivery by cesarean section
4. Preterm delivery

    A. 1,2,3   B. 1,3   C. 2,4   D. 4 Only   E. All

14. The major complication(s) in infants recovering from this condition is/are:

1. Patent ductus arteriosus
2. Intraventricular cerebral hemorrhage
3. Necrotizing enterocolitis
4. Respiratory infection

    A. 1,2,3   B. 1,3   C. 2,4   D. 4 Only   E. All

15. Enzymatic deficiencies that produce progressive mental deterioration and lead to death in infancy include:

1. Galactosemia
2. Niemann-Pick disease
3. Tay-Sachs disease
4. McArdle's syndrome

    A. 1,2,3   B. 1,3   C. 2,4   D. 4 Only   E. All

16. The sudden infant death syndrome:

1. Usually occurs in infants with congenital malformations
2. Is associated with maternal narcotic abuse
3. Tends to occur in infants who are postmature at birth
4. Usually occurs between the ages of 2 and 4 months

    A. 1,2,3   B. 1,3   C. 2,4   D. 4 Only   E. All

17. Neurofibromatosis (von Recklinghausen's disease) is associated with:

1. Mental retardation
2. Scoliosis
3. Hemangioblastomas of the central nervous system
4. Pigmented macular skin lesions

    A. 1,2,3   B. 1,3   C. 2,4   D. 4 Only   E. All

DIRECTIONS: For Questions 18 to 37, you are to decide whether EACH choice is TRUE or FALSE.

For each of the following statements about erythroblastosis fetalis (hemolytic disease of the newborn), choose whether it is TRUE or FALSE.

18. ABO hemolytic disease requires no prior sensitization of the mother

19. Most antibodies generated in Rh hemolytic disease are of the IgM type

20. ABO hemolytic disease occurs almost exclusively in infants of type O mothers

21. Maternal Rh sensitization occurs more readily when the fetus is also ABO incompatible

22. The magnitude of the antibody response in Rh hemolytic disease is independent of the dose of the immunizing antigen

For each of the following statements about the ductus arteriosus, choose whether it is TRUE or FALSE.

23. Functional closure normally occurs within the first 24 hours of postnatal life

24. Closure is delayed in premature infants

25. Prostaglandins are essential to normal closure
26. Patent ductus arteriosus presents with cyanosis during infancy
27. Patent ductus arteriosus creates an early systolic blowing murmur

For each of the following statements about coarctation of the aorta, describe whether it is TRUE or FALSE.

28. It occurs commonly in Turner's syndrome
29. It occurs as a solitary defect about 75% of the time
30. Preductal coarctation causes right ventricular hypertrophy *in utero*
31. Notching of the inner surfaces of the ribs by X-ray is associated with preductal coarctation

32. The lesion often recurs after surgical resection

For each of the following statements about the tetralogy of Fallot, choose whether it is TRUE or FALSE.

33. The severity of clinical symptoms is most directly related to the degree of right ventricular outflow obstruction
34. A patent ductus arteriosus is requisite to survival in most cases
35. The intensity of the heart murmur is directly proportional to the severity of the right ventricular outflow obstruction
36. Polycythemia is a common complication
37. Early corrective surgery is the treatment of choice

DIRECTIONS: For Questions 38 to 59, the set of lettered headings is followed by a list of numbered words or phrases. For each numbered word or phrase choose:

        A—if the item is associated with (A) only
        B—if the item is associated with (B) only
        C—if the item is associated with *both* (A) and (B)
        D—if the item is associated with *neither* (A) nor (B)

For each of the characteristics listed below, choose whether it describes phenylketonuria, alkaptonuria, both, or neither.

    A. Phenylketonuria
    B. Alkaptonuria
    C. Both
    D. Neither

38. A defect in tyrosine metabolism causes the disease
39. Affected infants appear normal at birth
40. Urine turns black on standing
41. Untreated patients often develop mental retardation
42. Vertebral arthritis characteristically develops

For each of the characteristics listed below, choose whether it describes Marfan's syndrome, the Ehlers-Danlos syndromes, both, or neither.

    A. Marfan's syndrome
    B. Ehlers-Danlos syndromes
    C. Both
    D. Neither

43. Occur(s) as congenital but not hereditary disorder(s)
44. Characterized by a primary defect in collagen structure
45. Associated with a high frequency of aortic aneurysms

46. Characterized by long slender extremities
47. Typically produces joint inflexibility

For each of the following statements, choose whether it describes atrial septal defect, ventricular septal defect, both, or neither.

    A. Atrial septal defect (ASD)
    B. Ventricular septal defect (VSD)
    C. Both
    D. Neither

48. The lesion is the most common congenital cardiac defect
49. The defect is commonly first recognized in adult life
50. A small defect predisposes to bacterial endocarditis
51. Pulmonary hypertension commonly develops
52. The defect develops between the second and eighth weeks of embryogenesis
53. The defect is a feature of tetralogy of Fallot
54. Early surgical closure reduces morbidity

For each of the following characteristics, choose whether it describes tricuspid atresia, pulmonary valve atresia, both, or neither.

    A. Tricuspid valve atresia
    B. Pulmonary valve atresia
    C. Both
    D. Neither

55. Commonly associated with a hypoplastic right ventricle
56. Commonly associated with an atrial septal defect
57. Frequently associated with a ventricular septal defect

58. Accounts for as much as 15% of congenital cyanotic heart disease
59. Depends upon a patent ductus arteriosus to provide blood flow to the lungs

DIRECTIONS: Questions 60 to 68 are matching questions. For each numbered item, choose the most likely associated lettered item from those provided. Each numbered item has ONLY ONE answer. Within each group, each lettered item may be the answer to one, more than one, or none of the numbered items.

For each of the sexual disorders listed below, choose whether the most common associated karyotype is 45,XO, 46,XY, 47,XXY, or none of these.

    A. 45,XO
    B. 46,XY
    C. 47,XXY
    D. None of these

60. Klinefelter's syndrome
61. Turner's syndrome
62. True hermaphroditism
63. Testicular feminization syndrome

For each of the features listed below, choose whether it is characteristic of Fabry's disease, Lesch-Nyhan syndrome, von Hippel–Lindau disease, Wilson's disease, or none of these.

    A. Fabry's disease
    B. Lesch-Nyhan syndrome
    C. Von Hippel–Lindau disease
    D. Wilson's disease
    E. None of these

64. Gout and self-mutilative behavior
65. Progressive renal failure and angiokeratomas
66. Xanthomas and accelerated atherosclerosis
67. Cirrhosis and cavitation of the brain
68. Retinal angiomas and renal cell carcinoma

2

PEDIATRIC AND GENETIC DISEASES

ANSWERS

1. (A) In the United States, more than 20 times the number of deaths occur in infancy (less than 1 year of age) than in any other period of childhood. Among neonates (less than 4 weeks of age), survival correlates with birth weight, and the leading causes of death are asphyxia, immaturity, and hyaline membrane disease. After 4 weeks of age, however, congenital anomalies cause increasing numbers of deaths and ultimately comprise the leading cause of death in infancy. Pneumonia, although an important cause of mortality in infancy, causes less than half as many infant deaths as congenital anomalies. Accidents and malignant neoplasms cause only a small fraction of the total number of deaths in infancy, but in the older pediatric age group they assume major importance. In fact, accidents have become the leading cause of death among children from 1 to 14 years of age (*pp. 474–475*).

2. (C) The Apgar score is a useful clinical method for evaluating the physiologic condition of a newborn infant on a simple rapid basis. Five parameters are evaluated: heart rate, respiratory effort, muscle tone, response to nasal catheter, and color. The infant is evaluated at 1 and 5 minutes of life and each item is given a score of 0, 1, or 2. A score of 2 is normal, a score of 0 indicates absence of that function, and a score of 1 is an intermediate response. Thus, an infant with a heart rate of less than 100 (score 1), slow irregular respirations (score 1), and absence of muscle tone, pink color, or response to a nasal catheter (scores of 0) would have an overall Apgar score of 2. The Apgar score correlates well with the chances of survival during the first 28 days of life. Infants with Apgar scores of 0 or 1 at 5 minutes have a 50% risk of mortality during the first months of life. Prognosis improves with increasing Apgar scores, and mortality is almost 0% when the score is 7 or greater (*pp. 477–478*).

3. (C) The principle of the therapeutic approach to Rh incompatibility is to *prevent* maternal sensitization to the D antigen. Thus, prior to delivery, anti-D immunoglobulin is administered to the nonsensitized, Rh-negative mother. The administered antibody coats the fetal red cells that leak into the maternal circulation. Thus, the antigenic determinants become masked and fail to stimulate the maternal immune system. This treatment must be given for the first and every subsequent pregnancy of the unsensitized mother. There is no theoretical or practical use for this treatment in the sensitized mother (*p. 489*).

4. (B) The lesion pictured in the micrograph is a benign tumor of blood vessels known as a capillary hemangioma. Hemangiomas are the most common tumors of infancy. Since this lesion is benign and tends to regress spontaneously, it does not require surgical excision or radiation therapy and, of course, does not metastasize. A choristoma is the name applied to microscopically normal cells or tissues that are present in an abnormal location (e.g., a pancreatic rest in the duodenal submucosa). Although benign, a hemangioma is a true tumor and would therefore not be classifiable as a choristoma (*pp. 497, 539–540*).

5. (A) Low birth weight in small-for-gestational-age infants is frequently the result of impaired intrauterine growth. Impaired growth in utero may be caused by a variety of fetal, placental, or maternal factors. Fetal conditions that commonly reduce growth potential despite an adequate supply of nutrients from the mother include chromosomal disorders, congenital anomalies, and congenital infections. Small placentas and other placental conditions (infections, tumors, or vascular lesions) may produce placental insufficiency and retard intrauterine growth. Most commonly, however, impaired intrauterine growth is caused by maternal conditions that limit or interfere with fetal nourishment or oxygenation. In this category, maternal vascular diseases such as toxemia of pregnancy or chronic systemic hypertension are common underlying causes. Additional important maternal causes of impaired intrauterine growth include alcohol abuse, cigarette smoking, and narcotic abuse. First pregnancy, however, is not in itself associated with impaired intrauterine fetal growth. On the contrary, it is more likely that the small uterus of a first pregnancy may constrain a normally growing fetus and cause fetal deformation (*pp. 476, 482*).

6. (E) Congenital malformations are structural defects that are present at birth. Major malformations result from a defect in embryogenesis and are present in as many as 2% of newborn infants. The cause of most (65 to 70%) congenital malformations in humans is unclear, but the remainder are known to be related to either genetic or environmental factors. Fetal chromosomal abnormalities are among the most common genetic causes of congenital malformation. Environmental causes include infection, drugs, chemicals, and irradiation. Maternal thalidomide use is an infamous cause of malformation. Rubella and cytomegalovirus are two of the most common infectious agents known to cause congenital malformations. Although heavy cigarette smoking throughout pregnancy is associated with infants that are small for gestational age, there is no definitive evidence that it leads to congenital malformations *(pp. 479–481)*.

7. (E) In cases of severe erythroblastosis fetalis, (see Questions 18–22), hemolysis is extensive, and the oxygen-carrying capacity of the blood is severely impaired. Thus, the heart may suffer hypoxic damage, leading to circulatory failure. Circulatory failure, in turn, exacerbates the anemia-induced hypoxic damage to other organs. The liver, with its high metabolic rate, is especially prone to injury, and hepatic failure with resultant edema (anasarca) often ensues. Unconjugated hyperbilirubinemia, the hallmark of any hemolytic disease with jaundice, has severe consequences in the neonate that would not occur in an older child or an adult. In the neonate, unconjugated bilirubin, which is markedly lipophilic, passes readily through the immature blood-brain barrier, causing toxic damage to the brain and spinal cord. The brain becomes edematous and has a characteristic bright yellow pigmentation (kernicterus). Kernicterus is the most serious complication of erythroblastosis fetalis. The marked increase in erythropoietic activity in this hemolytic state characteristically induces extramedullary hematopoiesis in the spleen and liver and possibly other tissues as well. Enlarged, heavy, edematous placentas are also highly characteristic of severe erythroblastosis fetalis with liver damage, hypoalbuminemia, and fetal edema.

Dark urine is a consequence of spillover into the urine of water-soluble conjugated bilirubin. This occurs in disorders in which bilirubin is conjugated but not excreted (e.g., cholestatic jaundice). In erythroblastosis fetalis, however, jaundice is caused by an excess production of *unconjugated* bilirubin and is not productive of dark urine *(pp. 487–488)*.

8. (A) Although the pathologic changes in the pancreas pictured in the micrograph are characteristic of cystic fibrosis, they make it difficult to identify the tissue. Markedly dilated pancreatic ducts plugged with inspissated secretions dominate the pathologic picture. The obstruction leads to atrophy of the exocrine pancreas and its replacement by fibrous tissue. As is typical of any form of pancreatic ductal obstruction with secondary pancreatic atrophy, the endocrine pancreas is largely spared. Diabetes mellitus, therefore, is not commonly associated with cystic fibrosis or any other form of pancreatic ductal obstruction. The major defect in cystic fibrosis is the production in glandular structures of a highly cystic mucus that is difficult to mobilize and that tends to form plugs. Tissues that are organized around mucin-secreting tubal structures such as the bronchial tree, the gastrointestinal mucosa, and the excretory ducts of the male genital system are primarily involved in this disease process. In newborns with this disease, small bowel obstruction known as meconium ileus may occur as a consequence of abnormal gastrointestinal mucous secretion and the absence of pancreatic amylases. Obstruction of Wolffian duct derivatives (the epididymis and vas deferens) produces azoospermia and infertility in 95% of males with this disease. Pulmonary abnormalities are present in almost every case of cystic fibrosis. The bronchial tree becomes plugged with tenacious mucous secretions. Superimposed infections give rise to severe chronic bronchitis and marked bronchiectasis. *Pseudomonas aeruginosa* and *Staphylococcus aureus* are the two most common pathogens responsible for lung infections in this setting. Deficiency of vitamin K, a fat-soluble vitamin, often occurs as part of the malabsorption syndrome that results from the loss of pancreatic exocrine secretions *(pp. 493–495)*.

9. (E) Although benign tumors are far more common in infancy and childhood than malignant neoplasms, several malignancies exhibit sharp peaks in incidence in children under 5 years of age. Primary among these are leukemia (particularly acute lymphocytic leukemia), Wilms' tumor (nephroblastoma), retinoblastoma, and rhabdomyosarcoma as well as neuroblastoma, hepatoblastoma, teratoma, and ependymoma. Osteosarcoma is virtually nonexistent in this age group and characteristically occurs in children 10 to 15 years of age. Knowledge of the characteristic age distribution in childhood neoplasms can be helpful in diagnosing malignant processes in early childhood *(pp. 498–499)*.

10. (B) The mucopolysaccharidoses are a group of genetic disorders resulting from deficiencies of specific lysosomal enzymes involved in the degradation of mucopolysaccharides. Mucopolysaccharides typically accumulate in the mononuclear phagocyte system, causing hepatosplenomegaly. Accumulation in endothelial cells, intimal smooth muscle cells, and fibroblasts throughout the body is also common. The cardiovascular system is usually involved, and coronary artery and cardiac valvular lesions are produced. Skeletal and facial deformities also occur; the head is typically large and long, and the nose is broad and flat. Muscular weakness, however, is a symptom not characteristic of the mucopolysaccharidoses. It is, instead, one of the cardinal symptoms of glycogen storage diseases *(pp. 148–151)*.

11. (A) Only about 5% of cases of congenital heart disease are associated with chromosomal abnormality. Yet some genetic factors appear to play a role in the etiology of congenital heart disease, since about one-third of affected individuals have one or more relatives with congenital heart disease. In addition, congenital heart disease appears more frequently in males, suggesting a sex-linked genetic influence. Although congenital heart disease covers a spectrum of disorders, most of the anomalies produce some degree of cyanosis and commonly lead to impaired growth and development of the affected child. In addition to the direct consequences of the cardiac defect, affected children are at higher risk of developing any of the acquired diseases of childhood (*p. 586*).

12. (D) Only infants delivered before the 37th or 38th week of gestation are considered preterm. Infants born between the 38th and 42nd weeks of gestation are considered term infants. Their birth weight is considered appropriate for gestational age if it falls between the 10th and the 90th percentiles of weights within that gestational age group. For a term infant at 39 weeks, an appropriate birth weight would range from approximately 2300 to 3600 grams, and a 2000-gram infant would be considered small for its gestational age.

Classifying infants on the basis of both their birth weight and their gestational age in this way is more accurately predictive of infant morbidity and mortality than classification by either parameter alone. For example, a 2000-gram infant born at 34 weeks of gestation has an 8% mortality rate, and yet an infant of the same birth weight born at 39 weeks of gestation has only a 2% risk of mortality. Certain causes of infant morbidity are associated only with preterm delivery (irrespective of birth weight) and result from functional and structural immaturity of various organ systems. Hyaline membrane disease of the newborn, caused by functional immaturity of type II pneumocytes, is a prime example. A full-term infant would not be at increased risk for hyaline membrane disease (*pp. 474–476*).

13. (E) The micrograph of lung illustrates the classic microscopic features of respiratory distress syndrome of the newborn. This disorder is the result of structural and functional immaturity of the lungs, almost always occurring in infants delivered before term. The fundamental defect is deficient surfactant production by immature type II pneumocytes. As a consequence, the work of expanding the air spaces increases dramatically, and widespread atelectasis ensues. The resultant hypoxemia and acidosis not only further impair surfactant production but lead to pulmonary vasoconstriction and hypoperfusion. Capillary endothelial cells then suffer anoxic damage, and plasma proteins (particularly fibrinogen) leak into the alveolar spaces to form thick hyaline membranes, the characteristic pathologic feature of this disorder. Respiratory distress syndrome of the newborn occurs six times more frequently in infants of diabetic mothers compared with those of normal mothers and twice as often in male infants as female. Delivery by cesarean section when performed before the 38th week of gestation is also associated with a higher risk of respiratory distress syndrome in the infant. By far the most common association with respiratory distress syndrome of newborns, however, is preterm delivery (*pp. 483–484*).

14. (A) In general, infants with respiratory distress syndrome have an excellent chance of recovery if ventilatory therapy is successful in maintaining their life for the first 3 to 4 days. Unfortunately, however, recovery from respiratory distress syndrome is associated with a variety of complications. Most significantly, the infant is at increased risk of patent ductus arteriosus, intraventricular cerebral hemorrhage, and necrotizing enterocolitis. The first results from delayed closure of the ductus because of immaturity, hypoxia, and acidosis. Intraventricular hemorrhage is a consequence of anoxia and immaturity of the brain as well as the disproportionately large amount of cerebral blood flow through the periventricular circulation where the vessel walls are fragile. The pathogenesis of necrotizing enterocolitis is less well understood but is thought to be related to intestinal ischemia resulting from hypoxia and secondary bacterial invasion. Interestingly, it is the *extra*pulmonary consequences of hypoxia that pose the greatest risk to life in the recovery phase of neonatal respiratory distress syndrome. Although respiratory infection may occur in this setting, it is not a major complicating factor. Pneumonia in the newborn is usually a consequence of complications of pregnancy or labor with resultant aspiration of infected amniotic fluid by the fetus (*pp. 484–485*).

15. (A) Galactosemia, Niemann-Pick disease, and Tay-Sachs disease all produce progressive mental deterioration in the affected infant. Although benign variants of galactosemia exist, the most common form involves a lack of galactose-1-phosphate uridyl transferase with resultant galactosemia and progressive mental retardation. The pathophysiologic basis of the mental retardation in galactosemia is as yet poorly understood. In Niemann-Pick disease and Tay-Sachs disease, however, it is the accumulation of sphingomyelin and G_{M2} gangliosides respectively in the central nervous system of affected infants that leads to the progressive mental retardation characteristic of these diseases. McArdle's syndrome does not involve the central nervous system at all. It is a condition produced by a deficiency of phosphorylase in striated muscle, and in general its only symptoms are muscular weakness following periods of physical activity (*pp. 142–146, 153, 491–492*).

16. (C) The sudden infant death syndrome (SIDS) is an enigmatic disorder. Its very definition reflects the almost complete lack of understanding of this process: "the sudden and unexpected death of an infant who was either well or almost well prior to death, and whose death remains *unexplained* after the performance of an adequate autopsy." There is no evidence that these deaths occur more frequently in infants with congenital malformations than in normal infants. Epidemiologic studies have shown that the risk of SIDS is increased if the mother has abused narcotics or smoked cigarettes. SIDS also occurs more frequently in infants who are *pre*mature and are the offspring of young mothers. Most infants stricken by SIDS are between the ages of 2 and 4 months and usually die at home during the night after a period of sleep. It is currently thought that SIDS results from an instantaneous interruption of some basic physiologic function, either cardiac or respiratory, but the cause of the dysfunction is still far from clear (*pp. 495–496*).

17. (C) Neurofibromatosis (von Recklinghausen's disease) is a syndrome with two major features: multiple neural tumors (neurofibromas) throughout the body and pigmented skin lesions. Skeletal abnormalities such as scoliosis also commonly occur in this syndrome. Notably, patients with this syndrome are usually of normal mentality. Hemangioblastomas of the central nervous system do not occur in von Recklinghausen's disease but are characteristic of another rare autosomal disorder known as von Hippel–Lindau's disease (*pp. 138–139*).

18. (True); 19. (False); 20. (True); 21. (False); 22. (False)
When the red blood cells of a fetus display antigenic determinants inherited from the father that differ from those of the mother, a maternal immune reaction against the fetal erythrocyte antigens may occur. The maternal antibodies cross the placenta and cause hemolysis in the infant (erythroblastosis fetalis). Although in theory many erythrocyte antigens could produce this phenomenon, in practice only ABO and Rh antigens cause significant amounts of hemolytic disease of the newborn.

(18 and 19) One of the major differences between the immunologic disease produced by ABO antigens and Rh antigens is the role of prior maternal sensitization. In Rh hemolytic disease, an Rh-negative mother is exposed to the red cells of the Rh-positive infant during delivery when the infant erythrocytes leak into the maternal circulation. The IgG antibodies formed in response to this exposure cross the placenta and cause disease in Rh-positive fetuses of *subsequent* pregnancies. Antibodies to A and B antigens, in contrast, occur naturally in all individuals lacking one or both (type O individuals) of these antigens. No previous sensitization is required.

(20) Naturally occurring antibodies to A and B antigens are mostly of the IgM type and do not cross the placenta. Type O individuals, however, often make IgG antibodies to these antigens as well. Thus, hemolytic disease occurs almost exclusively in infants

of type O mothers. Luckily, disease produced by ABO incompatibility is rarely severe.

(21) The incidence of maternal immunization against Rh antigens is greatly *reduced* if concurrent ABO incompatibility exists. This is thought to occur because leaked fetal red cells are promptly coated with agglutinating IgM antibodies against A and/or B antigens and rapidly removed from the maternal circulation by the mononuclear phagocyte system before sensitization to Rh antigen can occur. **(22)** Besides ABO incompatibility, another important factor modulating the maternal immune response is the dose of the immunizing antigen. The magnitude of the subsequent response is directly proportional to the magnitude of exposure to the immunogen. Thus, obstetric complications that increase the risk of placental hemorrhage (e.g., placenta previa, cesarean section, or toxemia of pregnancy) increase the risk of immunization (*pp. 486–487*).

23. (True); 24. (True); 25. (False); 26. (False); 27. (False)
(23) The ductus arteriosus is a vascular channel that connects the pulmonary artery with the aorta and serves to divert blood flow from the pulmonary vascular system during intrauterine life. Normally, during the first day of postnatal life, muscular contraction of the ductus arteriosus occurs and produces functional closure of the conduit.

(24) In premature infants, this muscular contraction and functional closure are delayed. **(25)** Physiologic stimuli that cause the ductus to remain open include low arterial oxygen tensions and vasodilators, including prostaglandins. Vasodilatory prostaglandins, then, would delay normal closure.

(26) Most commonly, patent ductus arteriosus produces no functional defect at birth. During infancy, when the shunt is left-to-right, there is no cyanosis. It is only with the ultimate production of pulmonary hypertension and reversal of the shunt from right-to-left that cyanosis develops.

(27) The murmur of patent ductus arteriosus is a harsh, continuous sound that is described as "machinery-like" (*pp. 588–589*).

28. (True); 29. (False); 30. (True); 31. (False); 32. (False)
(28) Coarctation (constriction) of the aorta is the third most common congenital cardiovascular anomaly and comprises about 10% to 15% of all congenital cardiovascular defects. Females with Turner's syndrome often have coarctation of the aorta. However, the defect, overall, is two to three times more common in males.

(29) Although coarctation of the aorta may sometimes occur as a solitary defect, in 75% of the cases it occurs in association with other congenital cardiovascular defects.

(30) The position of the defect has a profound effect on the prognosis. Coarctations located proximal to the ductus arteriosus carry an ominous prognosis. In such cases, the right side of the heart must supply the entire systemic circulation through the ductus arteriosus. Consequently, right ventricular hypertrophy occurs early, often *in utero*. Postpartum survival depends upon the patency of the ductus arteriosus, but heart failure commonly supervenes, and many infants die in the neonatal period.

(31) When the coarctation is located distal to the ductus arteriosus (postductal coarctation), blood flow to the head and upper extremities is unimpaired, but blood flow to the lower half of the body depends upon the development of collateral flow that bypasses the aortic obstruction. Blood is frequently diverted through the intercostal arteries, a common collateral bypass route. As they undergo enlargement, the intercostal arteries tend to produce erosion of the inner surface of the ribs that commonly appears radiographically as "notching." (32) Surgical correction is the definitive treatment and is curative in most cases. The defect does not tend to recur once it has been surgically resected *(pp. 589–590)*.

33. (True); 34. (False); 35. (False); 36. (True); 37. (True)

(33) Of the four features that comprise the tetralogy of Fallot—(1) ventricular septal defect, (2) an overriding aorta, (3) right ventricular outflow obstruction, and (4) right ventricular hypertrophy—it is the degree of obstruction to the outflow from the right ventricle that determines the severity of the clinical symptoms. (34) The right ventricular outflow obstruction, which usually consists of a narrowing of the infundibulum of the right ventricle (with or without pulmonary valvular stenosis), limits flow through the pulmonary arterial system. Patency of the ductus arteriosus does not alleviate this physiologic deficit and therefore does not affect survival.

(35) The heart murmur of tetralogy of Fallot is one produced by the right ventricular outflow obstruction and is *inversely* proportional to its severity. (36) Reduction of flow through the pulmonary system and shunting of blood through the ventricular septal defect leads to profound cyanosis. The low oxygen tension is a stimulus to erythropoietin production, and thus polycythemia is a common part of the clinical picture. (37) Corrective surgery should be performed as soon as possible in patients with tetralogy of Fallot, since the right ventricular outflow obstruction (infundibular narrowing) tends to increase with time. Untreated, most patients die before age 10 from cyanosis and congestive heart failure *(p. 590)*.

38. (C); 39. (C); 40. (B); 41. (A); 42. (B)

(38) Phenylketonuria and alkaptonuria are diseases that are both caused by inborn errors of tyrosine metabolism. (39) The defect in phenylketonuria (PKU) is a total lack of hepatic phenylalanine hydroxylase, preventing the conversion of phenylalanine to tyrosine. The defect in alkaptonuria is the lack of

homogentisic oxidase, blocking the metabolism of phenylalanine-tyrosine at the level of homogentisic acid. In both diseases, the affected infant appears normal at birth.

(40) In alkaptonuria, homogentisic acid accumulates in the body and spills over into the urine. If the urine is allowed to stand, the homogentisic acid oxidizes, and the urine turns black. (42) The retained homogentisic acid in the body characteristically binds to connective tissues, tendons, and cartilage, producing a characteristic blue-black pigmentation (ochronosis) and arthritis.

(41) The build-up of dietary phenylalanine in infants with phenylketonuria has more profound consequences. Unless treated with dietary restriction, hyperphenylalaninemia leads to mental deterioration and retardation in most patients *(pp. 142, 490–491)*.

43. (D); 44. (C); 45. (C); 46. (A); 47. (D)

(43) Marfan's syndrome and Ehlers-Danlos syndromes are hereditary disorders of connective tissue. Marfan's syndrome is an uncommon autosomal dominant syndrome. The Ehlers-Danlos syndromes encompass seven variants with distinctive modes of inheritance. Of these seven variants, only one type is X-linked; three are autosomal dominant and three are autosomal recessive.

(44) Both Marfan's syndrome and the Ehlers-Danlos syndromes are characterized by a primary defect in collagen structure. Reduced tensile strength of connective tissue is the result. The precise biochemical defects in these disease processes have not been elucidated.

(45) In both syndromes, aortic aneurysms occur with a high frequency and constitute the major life-threatening complication. (46) The skeletal abnormalities of Marfan's syndrome are, however, distinctive. Individuals with Marfan's syndrome characteristically have long slender extremities with particular elongation of the fingers and tall stature. (47) Although joint disorders are characteristic of both Marfan's and Ehlers-Danlos syndromes, they are typified by joint ligament laxity and hypermobility of the joints rather than the inflexibility that occurs in most other joint diseases *(pp. 137–138, 155)*.

48. (B); 49. (A); 50. (B); 51. (C); 52. (C); 53. (B); 54. (B)

(48 and 49) Atrial septal defect (ASD) constitutes the most frequent congenital cardiac anomaly to remain asymptomatic through childhood. ASD is usually first recognized in the adult. Overall, however, ventricular septal defect (VSD) is the most common congenital cardiac anomaly. VSD is commonly symptomatic in childhood, even from birth, depending on the size of the defect.

(50) Infective endocarditis is rare with ASD of any size. Small or moderate-sized VSD, however, poses a well-defined risk of superimposed bacterial endocarditis. (51) The end result of septal defects in the

heart, whether atrial or ventricular, is a left-to-right shunt that increases flow through the pulmonary system and ultimately induces pulmonary hypertension and respiratory difficulty.

(**52**) Normally by the eighth week of gestational life, both the atrial and septal walls of the heart have completed their development. Defects in the development of either the atrial septum or the ventricular septum are thus produced between the second and eighth weeks of embryogenesis. (**53**) VSD is frequently associated with other structural cardiac anomalies. VSD constitutes one of the four cardiac defects in the syndrome known as tetralogy of Fallot, in which it is accompanied by an overriding aorta, right ventricular outflow obstruction, and right ventricular hypertrophy (see Question 33).

(**54**) Surgical closure of an ASD is not generally indicated during infancy. Most are well tolerated during the first decade of life before pulmonary hypertension develops. Thus, the threat to life during infancy is less than that of the operative mortality associated with surgical closure. Ventricular septal defects that are functionally significant, however, may lead to right ventricular enlargement and pulmonary hypertension with cyanosis. They may, furthermore, predispose to infective endocarditis. Surgical closure in this case would offset the risk of operative mortality (*pp. 587–588*).

55. (C); 56. (C); 57. (A); 58. (A); 59. (C)

(**55 and 56**) Tricuspid valve atresia and pulmonary valve atresia are both commonly associated with a hypoplastic right ventricle and an atrial septal defect. (**57**) In addition, tricuspid valve atresia is frequently associated with a ventricular septal defect. (**58**) Although neither is a common congenital cardiac defect, pulmonary valve stenosis or atresia accounts for 5 to 15% of congenital cardiac defects, whereas tricuspid atresia accounts for only about 2%. (**59**) Since both tricuspid atresia and pulmonary atresia severely reduce flow through the pulmonary arterial system, a septal defect and patent ductus arteriosus are necessary to provide blood flow to the lungs (*pp. 590–591*).

60. (C); 61. (A); 62. (D); 63. (B)

(**60**) Cytogenetic disorders involving sex chromosomes occur more frequently than those involving autosomal aberrations. One of the most common is Klinefelter's syndrome, with an approximate incidence of 1 in every 600 male births. The characteristic karyotype of Klinefelter's syndrome is 47,XXY, although numerous multiple X chromosome variants and mosaics may also occur. Since the major manifestation of Klinefelter's syndrome is hypogonadism, the disorder is rarely diagnosed before puberty.

(**61**) Turner's syndrome, occurring approximately once in every 3000 female births, is generally associated with a 45,XO karyotype. The major manifestation of Turner's syndrome is gonadal (ovarian) dysgenesis, but the disorder is commonly recognized from birth by the accompanying characteristic manifestations, webbing of the neck and peripheral lymphedema.

(**62**) True hermaphroditism is a rare disorder that is most often associated with a 46,XX karyotype, although some mosaics have been described. The disorder is characterized by the presence of both ovarian and testicular tissue; external genitalia are usually ambiguous.

(**63**) The syndrome of testicular feminization is characteristically associated with a 46,XY karyotype. This disorder is a form of male pseudohermaphroditism and is characterized by a female phenotype with good breast development but absence of uterus and tubes. Bilateral inguinal testes are usually present (*pp. 129–134*).

64. (B); 65. (A); 66. (E); 67. (D); 68. (C)

(**64**) The Lesch-Nyhan syndrome is an X-linked disorder that is characterized by a deficiency of hypoxanthine-guanine phosphoribosyl transferase, an enzyme involved in purine metabolism. Without this enzyme, there is deficient production of the nucleotides that *inhibit* the enzyme governing the rate-limiting step of *de novo* uric acid synthesis. Thus, uric acid is synthesized in excess, and gout is produced. A variety of neurologic problems whose pathogenesis is less well understood also occur. Principal among them are self-mutilation, aggressive behavior, mental retardation, spastic cerebral palsy, and choreoathetosis.

(**65**) Fabry's disease is an X-linked disorder of ceramide trihexoside (a glyco-sphingolipid) metabolism, resulting in the systemic accumulation of this compound. Although the cardiovascular system, the central nervous system, and the reticuloendothelial systems are all affected, the kidney is the most severely involved organ, and most patients die of progressive renal failure in middle life. However, another aspect of Fabry's disease may dominate the clinical picture; namely, red-blue elevated skin nodules known as angiokeratomas. Histologically, an angiokeratoma consists of a dermal cavernous hemangioma with hyperkeratotic thickening of the overlying epidermis. Although they are a characteristic finding in Fabry's disease, their relationship to the underlying storage disorder is obscure.

(**66**) Xanthomas and accelerated atherosclerosis are the features of familial hypercholesterolemia, an autosomal dominant disorder that is possibly the most common disease with Mendelian inheritance. Familial hypercholesterolemia results from loss of feedback control mechanisms that regulate cholesterol synthesis. Deposition of cholesterol in skin (xanthomas), coronary arteries, peripheral vessels, and other organs typically results. Death from coronary artery disease and myocardial infarction at an early age is a common consequence.

(67) Wilson's disease is a rare inborn error of copper metabolism. Excess deposits of copper accumulate in the brain, liver, and cornea to produce the three characteristic pathologic consequences of this disorder: degenerative changes in the brain with focal cavitation, liver damage with cirrhosis, and the pathognomonic green-brown ring at the limbus of the cornea (Kayser-Fleischer ring). Characteristically, hepatic disease occurs long before the ocular or neurologic disease becomes clinically evident. The disease is important to recognize because it can be treated effectively with a low-copper diet and chelating agents.

(68) Von Hippel–Lindau disease is a rare autosomal dominant disorder characterized by the occurrence of multiple benign and malignant neoplasms throughout the body. The most commonly occurring tumors in this disorder are retinal and cerebellar hemangioblastomas. Renal cell carcinomas, adrenal pheochromocytomas, angiomas of the liver and kidney, and adenomas of the kidney and epididymis are also common. Renal cell carcinomas occur in about 25% of cases and in this subgroup are the major cause of death (*pp. 139–140, 152, 932–933, 1358*).

3

NUTRITIONAL DISEASES

DIRECTIONS: For Questions 1 to 14, choose the ONE BEST answer to each question.

1. All of the following conditions are frequently associated with secondary malnutrition EXCEPT:

A. Diabetes mellitus
B. Membranous nephritis
C. Crohn's disease
D. Anticonvulsant medication
E. Hypothyroidism

2. All of the following statements about hypovitaminosis A are true EXCEPT:

A. It is the primary cause of blindness in Central America
B. It is characterized by failure of epidermal squamous cells to keratinize adequately
C. It is associated with epithelial metaplasia in the gastrointestinal tract
D. It predisposes to respiratory tract infections
E. It causes impaired vision in dim light

3. Hypovitaminosis A occurs in association with all of the following conditions EXCEPT:

A. Pseudomembranous colitis
B. Chronic pancreatitis
C. Whipple's disease
D. Abetalipoproteinemia
E. Cirrhosis

4. Deficiency of vitamin D is associated with all of the following conditions EXCEPT:

A. Strict vegetarianism
B. Celiac disease (nontropical sprue)
C. Cirrhosis
D. Hypoparathyroidism
E. Chronic renal failure

5. All of the following statements about vitamin E are true EXCEPT:

A. There is no known deficiency state in the human adult
B. There is no known toxicity state in the human adult
C. It is effective in the treatment of retrolental fibroplasia in premature infants

D. It is effective in the treatment of male infertility
E. It is believed to function biologically as an antioxidant

6. All of the following statements about thiamine deficiency (beriberi) are true EXCEPT:

A. It is associated with diets of polished rice
B. It is associated with diuretic therapy
C. It is associated with diets of raw fish
D. It is common among alcoholics
E. It is common among patients with pancreatic insufficiency

7. Absorption of vitamin B_{12} is dependent on all of the following factors EXCEPT:

A. Intrinsic factor
B. R-binder proteins
C. Pancreatic proteases
D. Bile salts
E. Calcium

8. At the cellular level, deficiency of vitamin B_{12} will cause all of the following EXCEPT:

A. Increased intrinsic factor production
B. Folate deficiency
C. Synthesis of abnormal fatty acids
D. Reduced adenine synthesis
E. Reduced thymidine synthesis

9. Patients with scurvy frequently develop defects of all of the following functions EXCEPT:

A. Phagocytotic activity of macrophages
B. Iron absorption
C. Collagen cross-linking
D. Formation of hydroxyproline
E. Platelet adhesion

10. Neurologic dysfunctions are known to result from deficiencies of all of the following nutrients EXCEPT:

A. Pyridoxine (vitamin B_6)
B. Niacin
C. Copper
D. Vitamin B_{12}
E. Folate

11. All of the following statements about iron as a nutrient are true EXCEPT:

   A. Daily adult requirements are twice as great for young women as young men
   B. Dietary iron is efficiently (80% to 90%) absorbed
   C. Deficiency in adult males is often due to gastrointestinal blood loss
   D. Only the divalent form of inorganic iron can be absorbed
   E. Atrophic gastritis is frequently associated with iron deficiency anemia

12. All of the following conditions are associated with obesity ("overnutrition") EXCEPT:

   A. Hypertension
   B. Diabetes mellitus
   C. Hyperlipidemia
   D. Gallstones
   E. Rheumatoid arthritis

13. Epidemiologic or experimental evidence exists for each of the dietary element–organ cancer associations listed below EXCEPT:

   A. Animal fats–breast carcinoma
   B. Animal fats–colonic carcinoma
   C. Animal fats–gastric carcinoma
   D. Sodium nitrite food preservatives–gastric carcinoma
   E. Hydrocarbons of smoked foods–gastric carcinoma

14. Which of the following statements about vitamin K deficiency is TRUE?

   A. It causes defects in both the intrinsic and extrinsic coagulation pathways
   B. It produces defects in platelet functioning
   C. It is associated with strict vegetarian diets
   D. Intestinal bacteria produce enough vitamin K to prevent deficiency under normal conditions
   E. It develops less frequently in breast-fed infants than in bottle-fed infants

DIRECTIONS: For Questions 15 to 17, ONE or MORE of the completions given correctly finishes the incomplete statement. Choose:

     A—if only *1,2, and 3* are correct
     B—if only *1 and 3* are correct
     C—if only *2 and 4* are correct
     D—if only *4* is correct
     E—if all are correct

15. Vitamins that are ingested in an inactive form and require metabolic conversion to an active form include:

   1. Vitamin K
   2. Vitamin E
   3. Vitamin C
   4. Vitamin D

     A. 1,2,3 B. 1,3 C. 2,4 D. 4 Only E. All

16. Pellagra is associated with which of the following conditions?

   1. Diets consisting primarily of maize
   2. Cirrhosis
   3. Functioning carcinoid tumors
   4. Hartnup disease

     A. 1,2,3 B. 1,3 C. 2,4 D. 4 Only E. All

17. Which of the following conditions is/are often associated with a vitamin B_{12} deficiency?

   1. Strict vegetarianism
   2. Achlorhydria
   3. Celiac disease (nontropical sprue)
   4. Jejunal resection

     A. 1,2,3 B. 1,3 C. 2,4 D. 4 Only E. All

DIRECTIONS: For Questions 18 to 55, the set of lettered headings is followed by a list of numbered words or phrases. For each numbered word or phrase choose:

A—if the item is associated with (A) only
B—if the item is associated with (B) only
C—if the item is associated with *both* (A) and (B)
D—if the item is associated with *neither* (A) nor (B)

For each of the characteristics listed below, choose whether it describes kwashiorkor, marasmus, both, or neither.

A. Kwashiorkor
B. Marasmus
C. Both
D. Neither

18. Total caloric intake is inadequate
19. Affected infants appear cachectic and ravenously hungry
20. Anemia is frequently present
21. Desquamative skin lesions are pathognomonic
22. Fatty change is usually seen in the liver
23. Intercurrent infection exacerbates the condition
24. Both B- and T-lymphocyte functions are depressed

For each of the characteristics listed below, choose whether it describes rickets, osteomalacia, both, or neither.

A. Rickets
B. Osteomalacia
C. Both
D. Neither

25. Osteoid mineralization is retarded
26. Endochondral ossification is retarded
27. Osteitis fibrosa frequently occurs concomitantly
28. The disease has a hereditary autosomal recessive form
29. The disease has a hereditary X-linked form
30. Tetracycline administration is useful for treatment

For each of the characteristics listed below, choose whether it relates to calcium, phosphate, both, or neither.

A. Calcium
B. Phosphate
C. Both
D. Neither

31. Decreased serum levels induce synthesis of $1,25-(OH)_2D_3$
32. Intestinal absorption is increased by vitamin D

33. Renal reabsorption is increased by vitamin D
34. Increased renal excretion occurs in the Fanconi syndrome
35. Lamellar osteoid seams appear in bone in deficiency states
36. Anticonvulsant drugs cause decreased intestinal absorption
37. Serum levels affect calcitonin secretion

For each of the following features of cardiac disease in the alcoholic patient, choose whether it is characteristic of alcoholic cardiomyopathy, beriberi heart disease, both, or neither.

A. Alcoholic cardiomyopathy
B. Beriberi heart disease
C. Both
D. Neither

38. Produces a dilated and flabby heart
39. Characterized microscopically by small foci of ischemic myocardial necrosis
40. Characterized clinically by low output heart failure
41. Associated with peripheral edema
42. Associated with skeletal muscle weakness
43. Associated with the Wernicke-Korsakoff syndrome

For each of the following conditions, choose whether it is associated with vitamin B_{12} deficiency, folate deficiency, both, or neither.

A. Vitamin B_{12} deficiency
B. Folate deficiency
C. Both
D. Neither

44. Occurs in pernicious anemia
45. Commonly caused by alcoholism
46. Typically produces glossitis
47. Typically produces sideroblasts in the bone marrow
48. Results in hypersegmentation of neutrophils

For each of the physiologic processes listed below, choose whether it requires vitamin C, vitamin D, both, or neither.

A. Vitamin C
B. Vitamin D
C. Both
D. Neither

49. Osteoid production
50. Osteoid mineralization
51. Bone resorption
52. Bone remodeling
53. Cartilage resorption in endochondral bone growth
54. Tooth formation
55. Wound healing

DIRECTIONS: Questions 56 to 82 are matching questions. For each numbered item, choose the most likely associated lettered item from those provided. Each numbered item has ONLY ONE answer. Within each group, each lettered item may be the answer to one, more than one, or none of the numbered items.

For each of the vitamins listed below, choose whether its principal storage site is within striated muscle, adrenal cortex, liver, all body tissues in even distribution, or none of these.

A. Striated muscle
B. Adrenal cortex
C. Liver
D. Evenly distributed in all tissues
E. None of the above

56. Vitamin A
57. Vitamin B_1 (thiamine)
58. Vitamin D
59. Folate
60. Vitamin B_6 (pyridoxine)
61. Vitamin C
62. Riboflavin

For each of the following characteristics, choose whether it is associated with riboflavin, niacin, pyridoxine, all of these, or none of these.

A. Riboflavin
B. Niacin
C. Pyridoxine (vitamin B_6)
D. All of the above
E. None of the above

63. The molecule is a coenzyme in cellular oxidative metabolism
64. The human body is capable of endogenous synthesis of the vitamin
65. Dietary intake of tryptophan determines the dietary requirement for the vitamin
66. It is particularly important in tryptophan metabolism
67. A deficiency state causes a macrocytic anemia
68. A deficiency state causes a dermatitis
69. A deficiency state is associated with dementia

70. Parenteral administration commonly produces toxic effects

For each of the hematologic abnormalities listed below, choose whether it is associated with iron deficiency, vitamin B_{12} deficiency, starvation, none of these, or all of these.

A. Iron deficiency
B. Vitamin B_{12} deficiency
C. Starvation
D. None of the above
E. All of the above

71. Increased hemolysis
72. Increased osmotic fragility of erythrocytes
73. Hypochromic, microcytic anemia
74. Normochromic, macrocytic anemia
75. Hypochromic, normocytic anemia

For each of the characteristics listed below, choose whether it is associated with zinc, copper, selenium, all of these, or none of these.

A. Zinc
B. Copper
C. Selenium
D. All of the above
E. None of the above

76. It functions as a component of a metalloenzyme
77. Deficiencies are common in patients receiving total parenteral nutrition
78. In children, deficiency causes growth retardation
79. Deficiency causes anemia
80. Deficiency causes cardiomyopathy
81. It is required for the formation of cross-linkages in collagen
82. It is required for the formation of cross-linkages in elastin

3

NUTRITIONAL DISEASES

ANSWERS

1. (E) Diabetes mellitus causes derangements in the metabolism of all foodstuffs including fats, carbohydrates, and proteins that may produce secondary deficiencies of these basic nutrients. In addition, loss of minerals and electrolytes may occur in the urine as glycosuria induces an osmotic diuresis. Membranous nephropathy, as a cause of the nephrotic syndrome, is associated with excessive protein losses and secondary protein malnutrition. Crohn's disease causes small intestinal mucosal abnormalities resulting in an inadequate absorptive surface and a malabsorption syndrome. The accompanying diarrhea may affect the absorption of many nutrients, but vitamin B_{12} deficiency is often a specific manifestation, since the ileum, the primary site of vitamin B_{12} absorption, is the region of the small bowel most frequently affected by Crohn's disease. Anticonvulsant medications (e.g., phenytoin and phenobarbital) are associated with a variety of secondary vitamin deficiency states, although the mechanisms by which these are produced remain largely unknown. Folate, vitamin D, and vitamin K are the nutrients most often depleted by long-term anticonvulsant therapy. Although hypothyroidism may rarely produce a malabsorptive syndrome, it is not usually associated with secondary malnutrition. Hyperfunction of the thyroid, however, frequently produces a clinical picture of malnutrition. This is the result of numerous factors, including anorexia, increased metabolic demands, and diarrhea with nutrient losses (*pp. 400, 841, 947, 1011–1012, 1203–1204*).

2. (B) Vitamin A is known to be requisite to: (1) the processes of maturation and differentiation of epithelial cells, both glandular and squamous, and (2) the production of photosensitive pigments in the retina. Deficiencies of the vitamin lead to decreased production of rhodopsin in rods (impairing vision in dim light) and iodopsin in cones and can, therefore, produce blindness. Indeed, it is the leading cause of blindness in Central America, the Middle East, and India. Keratinization and softening of the cornea (keratomalacia) can also result from hypovitaminosis A and contribute to the visual defects. Other squamous epithelial surfaces also undergo *excessive* (rather than reduced) keratinization, and glandular or ciliated surfaces (e.g., gastrointestinal and bronchial mucosae) undergo squamous metaplasia. Squamous metaplasia in the bronchial tree destroys the natural host defense provided by ciliated epithelial surfaces

and increases susceptibility to respiratory tract infection (*pp. 404–405*).

3. (A) Vitamin A is a fat-soluble vitamin. Therefore, a primary deficiency of the vitamin may occur in any disease causing impaired absorption of fat. In chronic pancreatitis, the resultant pancreatic insufficiency leads to defective intraluminal hydrolysis, solubility, and subsequent absorption of fat. Whipple's disease, an acquired small bowel disease of as yet unknown etiology, causes fat malabsorption. In this disease, the small bowel mucosa is grossly thickened by large aggregates of distended macrophages that cause lymphatic obstruction and compromise transport of absorbed fat. The mucosal absorptive cell is the site of the primary defect in abetalipoproteinemia. This form of malabsorption is hereditary rather than acquired and is characterized by an inability to synthesize beta lipoproteins. Since beta lipoproteins are required for the export of triglycerides from intestinal absorptive cells, fats accumulate within the mucosal cells. A severe hypolipidemia and consequent hypovitaminosis A result. The diffuse hepatic parenchymal damage of cirrhosis may cause hypovitaminosis A by two separate mechanisms: (1) reduction of synthesis of plasma transport proteins required for distribution of vitamin A to the tissues and (2) compromise of hepatic retinyl ester stores (the principal reservoir of vitamin A in the body). Pseudomembranous colitis is not usually associated with defects in nutrient absorption. The disease process (the result of clostridial overgrowth) is not chronic and is entirely limited to the mucosa of the colon. Nutrient absorption in the small bowel takes place normally. Therefore, absorption, transport, or storage of vitamin A is unaffected. (*pp. 403, 846–851*).

4. (D) Vitamin D is a biochemical relative of cholesterol, and its principal dietary sources are animal products. Strict vegetarian diets therefore can lead to vitamin D deficiency. This is especially true if endogenous sources of vitamin D are inadequate, as they are for most people living in the northern hemisphere where exposure to sunlight is limited. Since dietary vitamin D is absorbed in the small intestine like other fats, diseases such as celiac sprue (nontropical sprue) that severely reduce the bowel's absorptive surface compromise uptake of vitamin D. The liver plays three key roles in vitamin D metabolism: (1) synthesis of serum transport proteins for vitamin D, (2) storage of the vitamin, and (3) 25-hydroxylation of vitamin D_3, the first step in the metabolic conversion of vitamin D_3 (endogenous or exogenous) to its metabolically active form. Thus hepatic parenchymal disease, such as cirrhosis, is often associated with a vitamin D deficiency state. The second step in conversion of D_3 to its active form, 1-hydroxyl, takes place in the kidney. Severe renal parenchymal disease with chronic renal failure therefore can lead to a functional vitamin D deficiency.

The parathyroid glands have no direct effect on vitamin D metabolism. Indirectly, however, hypoparathyroidism would be expected only to *stimulate* vitamin D metabolism in response to the consequent fall in serum calcium concentration *(pp. 406–408, 996–997).*

5. (D) Although vitamin E is recognized as an essential nutrient for man, little else about this element has been definitively characterized to date. No vitamin E deficiency or toxicity states are known to occur clinically, although well-defined deficiency syndromes have been created experimentally in animals. In man, the primary biologic role of vitamin E is that of an antioxidant. It is especially important in the neutralization of free radicals that are continuously generated (and highly destructive) at the cellular level. The therapeutic value of vitamin E has been demonstrated for several diseases known to be caused or complicated by oxidative injury. In particular, vitamin E has proven effective in the treatment of retrolental fibroplasia in premature infants exposed to high oxygen tensions in incubators. Although male sterility results from vitamin E deprivation in experimental animals, the vitamin has not been demonstrated to be essential to fertility in man nor has human male infertility been successfully treated with vitamin E *(pp. 411–412).*

6. (E) Thiamine (vitamin B_1) deficiency is the cause of a disease known as beriberi. Primary dietary deficiency of thiamine occurs in populations whose diet consists largely of polished rice or milled grains, since the discarded husks contain most of the grains' thiamine. Increased losses of this water-soluble vitamin with diuretic therapy also cause deficiencies. Thiamine losses also occur as a consequence of direct enzymatic degradation of the vitamin by thiaminases contained in raw foods such as fish, shellfish, or meat. A diet consisting mainly of these foods therefore may cause beriberi. Alcoholism is the most universal cause of beriberi. Poor general nutrition with decreased thiamine intake, coupled with increased losses from vomiting and ethanol-induced diuresis, forms the basis for thiamine deficiency in alcoholic patients. Because thiamine is readily absorbed in the upper intestinal tract without the aid of pancreatic enzymes, pancreatic insufficiency is not associated with thiamine deficiency *(p. 413).*

7. (D) Absorption of vitamin B_{12} is a complex process requiring the interaction of a number of factors. When ingested, the vitamin is attached to animal protein from which it is released in the acid-peptic milieu of the stomach. It then complexes with a secreted gastric protein known as R-binder protein, which has a high affinity for cobalamin at a low pH. Pancreatic proteases in the duodenum, in turn, release cobalamin from the R-binder protein. The vitamin then combines with the glycoprotein synthesized by gastric parietal cells known as intrinsic factor. Specific mucosal cell receptors in the ileum bind the intrinsic factor–vitamin B_{12} complex, but the process requires calcium and a pH greater than 5.6. Once bound, the complex is then taken up and transported across the ileal mucosal cell to the blood, completing vitamin B_{12} absorption. None of the steps in this absorptive process, however, is known to require the presence of bile salts *(pp. 418, 632).*

8. (A) Metabolic derivatives of vitamin B_{12} are required for two important biochemical reactions: (1) the conversion of methylmalonyl coenzyme A to succinyl coenzyme A and (2) conversion of homocysteine to methionine. The first is essential to fatty acid synthesis and the second to both adenine and pyrimidine synthesis. Thus, in vitamin B_{12} deficiency, abnormal fatty acids are synthesized, and purine and thymidine synthesis is reduced. In the reaction generating methionine, tetrahydrofolate is also produced from its methylated form. With the decrease in this vitamin B_{12}–dependent reaction, folate is also "trapped" in the form of methyltetrahydrofolate, and a functional folate deficiency is created. Although the availability of vitamin B_{12} is dependent on the production of intrinsic factor, vitamin B_{12} is not known to exert any feedback control on the elaboration of intrinsic factor by gastric parietal cells. Deficiency therefore would not be expected to increase intrinsic factor production *(pp. 418, 632).*

9. (E) Scurvy, the disease produced by vitamin C deficiency, is an uncommon disorder, since vitamin C is abundant in most foods, easily absorbed throughout the small bowel, and stored in substantial quantity in most tissues. The deficiency state reflects the loss of the primary functions of vitamin C in the body: namely, its participation in several steps of collagen metabolism. Vitamin C is required for collagen cross-linking and the hydroxylation of proline as well as other biochemical events in collagen synthesis. Deficiency of vitamin C has also been found to depress both motility and phagocytotic activity in macrophages and neutrophils, creating an immunologic defect. Iron absorption is also adversely affected by deficiency of vitamin C, since the vitamin is known to facilitate uptake of inorganic (nonheme) iron. Although scurvy is associated with hemorrhagic diatheses, these are the result of vascular fragility caused by defective collagen in blood vessel walls.

Platelet functions, however, are not known to be affected by vitamin C deficiency (*pp. 419–420*).

10. (E) Many nutritional deficiencies have profound effects on the nervous system, which may occasionally dominate the clinical presentation. Pyridoxine is known to participate (as a coenzyme) in numerous metabolic functions in the brain, including the synthesis of neurotransmitters. Consequently, pyridoxine deficiency states produce peripheral neuropathies and occasionally convulsions. Furthermore, pyridoxine-deficient mothers may produce mentally retarded infants. Niacin deficiency is typically associated with degeneration of the ganglion cells of the brain and spinal cord tracts. Ganglion cell degeneration produces dementia that, along with diarrhea and dermatitis, forms the classic symptom triad (the three D's) of pellagra. Copper is an essential component of metalloenzymes involved in the synthesis and maintenance of myelin and the metabolism of neurotransmitters. Copper deficiencies therefore produce various central nervous system abnormalities. Vitamin B_{12} deficiency produces peripheral neuropathy and degeneration of the posterior and lateral spinal columns. The pathogenesis of these lesions is not completely understood but may be related to the derangement of cobalamin-dependent fatty acid biosynthesis and incorporation of abnormal fatty acids into the lipids of myelin. The neurologic manifestations of vitamin B_{12} deficiency help to distinguish it from folate deficiency, which it resembles hematologically. Both vitamin B_{12} and folate deficiencies produce megaloblastic anemia, but only vitamin B_{12} deficiency is associated with neurologic abnormalities (*pp. 416–418, 424*).

11. (B) The total iron content of the body is normally a closely regulated constant. Daily losses of iron from sloughing of various epithelial cells (skin, gastrointestinal, and genitourinary) are quite small. Additional losses in the young adult female are most often related to menses and pregnancy. Women of reproductive age therefore require approximately twice as much iron daily as their male counterparts. Significant iron loss in adult males often reflects occult bleeding from an infectious, inflammatory, or neoplastic process in the gastrointestinal tract.

In general, however, iron is efficiently recycled by the body, and losses are minimal. Uptake of exogenous iron must therefore be maintained within narrow limits in order to preserve iron balance. Only about 5 to 10% of dietary iron is normally absorbed. Although organic iron in the form of heme is readily absorbed, inorganic iron (usually present in dietary sources in trivalent form) must be reduced to a divalent state to be absorbed. Gastric acid is thought to aid the process of inorganic iron reduction, since (1) gastric acid secretion is known to be necessary to adequate iron absorption and (2) atrophic gastritis

with achlorhydria is often associated with iron deficiency anemia (*pp. 422–423*).

12. (E) In the United States, obesity is the single most common nutritional disorder. Obesity is known to predispose to a number of diseases that carry significant risks of morbidity and even mortality. Among the conditions strongly associated with obesity are hypertension, adult onset diabetes mellitus, hyperlipidemia, and cholelithiasis (gallstones). Obesity also predisposes to degenerative osteoarthritis from increased stress on weight-bearing joints but is not etiologically related to rheumatoid arthritis, a disease created by immunologic injury (*pp. 424–425*).

13. (C) Numerous epidemiologic and animal studies investigating the etiologic relationship between various dietary elements and cancer have revealed several associations. Of particular interest to Americans, whose diets are generally high in animal products, is the fact that animal fat has been implicated in the pathogenesis of several cancers, including breast cancer and colon cancer. Although the precise role of dietary animal fats in the causation of these two diseases is not completely understood, the mechanisms are thought to be different. Animal fat with a high cholesterol content is believed to provide increased substrate for the synthesis of estrogens known to be related to the genesis of mammary carcinoma. As a factor in the pathogenesis of colon cancer, however, animal fats are thought to induce increased secretion of bile salts that are metabolized by anaerobic bacteria in the intestinal flora to carcinogenic compounds. The supply of bile salts is also abetted by dietary cholesterol, since cholesterol is the precursor molecule from which several bile salts are synthesized. Gastric carcinoma, however, is thought to be related to the direct carcinogenic effects of chemical substances contained within foodstuffs that have been preserved by smoking (introduction of hydrocarbons) or by the addition of nitrite compounds. Nitrites in foods are thought to combine with amines from digested proteins to produce nitrosamines—compounds known to be carcinogenic. No association has been established between gastric carcinoma and animal fats in the diet, however (*pp. 426–427, 821*).

14. (A) Vitamin K is a cofactor for a hepatic carboxylase that converts the inactive proenzyme forms of clotting factors II (prothrombin), VII, XI, and X to their functionally active state. Vitamin K–dependent carboxylation of these factors is required for calcium binding activity. Factor VII is activated in the extrinsic pathway, factor XI in the intrinsic pathway, and factors X and II in both (in the final common pathway). Thus, inactivity of these vitamin K–dependent clotting factors would cause defects in both pathways. However, vitamin K deficiency would not be ex-

no Vit K effect on platelets

pected to affect platelet function, since the vitamin plays no known role in platelet biology.

The dietary form of vitamin K is phylloquinone, or vitamin K₁, which is especially plentiful in leafy green vegetables. Therefore, strict vegetarianism, although associated with deficiencies of most other fat-soluble vitamins, would not be expected to cause a vitamin K deficiency. Intestinal bacteria also contribute to the daily supply by synthesizing menaquinone (vitamin K₂) but do not provide enough of this compound to meet the full vitamin K requirements without dietary supplementation. In infancy, when intestinal bacterial colonization is incomplete and hepatic reserves of vitamin K are small, the risk of developing vitamin K deficiency is increased by breast feeding, since human breast milk contains less vitamin K than cow's milk (*p. 412*).

15. (D) Vitamin K and vitamin E (fat-soluble vitamins) and vitamin C (a water-soluble vitamin) are all obtained from dietary sources in their active form and require no metabolic conversion for biologic activity in man. Vitamin K₁ (phylloquinone) is obtained primarily from leafy green vegetables in the diet, whereas vitamin K₂ (menaquinone) is synthesized by microorganisms in the gastrointestinal tract. Vitamin E is also obtained from leafy green vegetables as well as cooking oils and whole grains. Although alpha-tocopherol is the major dietary form of vitamin E, there are actually 8 compounds (4 tocopherols and 4 tocotrienols) that have vitamin E activity. All of these are absorbed directly from the diet and are utilizable in their absorbed form. Vitamin C (ascorbate) is an acid available in many foodstuffs including fruits, vegetables, liver, fish, and milk. It too is absorbed directly in its biologically active form. Vitamin D, however, is absorbed from dietary sources (a variety of animal products) in the form of cholecalciferol, also called vitamin D₃. Vitamin D₃ requires 2 metabolic conversions in order to acquire full biologic activity. Cholecalciferol is first hydroxylated at the 25-carbon position in the liver and again at the 1-carbon position in the kidney, producing $1,25\text{-}(OH)_2D_3$, the active vitamin D hormone (*see Question 4 and pp. 406, 411–412, 419*).

16. (E) Pellagra is the disease state resulting from a deficiency of niacin, a vitamin that is widely distributed in most foods. Deficiencies are primarily encountered among populations whose diets consist primarily of maize. Although maize contains adequate amounts of niacin, it also has a high leucine content. It is now known that leucine acts as an antagonist in the synthesis of NAD (nicotinamide adenine dinucleotide) and its phosphorylated analog NADP, the two major metabolic coenzymes of which niacin is a component. Thus a disorder identical to niacin deficiency develops as a consequence of increased leucine content in the diet. Pellagra is also encountered in patients with chronic debilitating diseases such as

cirrhosis. Since niacin is also synthesized endogenously from tryptophan, diseases that produce tryptophan depletion may cause pellagra. Active carcinoid tumors, for example, greatly increase the utilization to tryptophan from which they synthesize serotonin; thus, patients with the carcinoid syndrome may also develop pellagra. Hartnup disease may also be complicated by pellagra, since this disease causes decreased intestinal absorption of tryptophan (*pp. 415–416*).

17. (A) Vitamin B₁₂ (cobalamin) is a metallo-organic compound for which the only dietary sources are meats and dairy products. Since fruits and vegetables are devoid of vitamin B₁₂, strict vegetarian diets often produce deficiency states. Achlorhydria will result from any process that is destructive to gastric parietal cells such as chronic gastritis or pernicious anemia. Since parietal cells produce intrinsic factor as well as hydrochloric acid, decreased vitamin B₁₂ absorption as well as achlorhydria will result from their destruction. Celiac disease (nontropical sprue) is also a well-known cause of vitamin B₁₂ deficiency. This condition is characterized by a striking loss of small intestinal villi. Drastic reductions in the absorptive surface of the ileum therefore markedly decrease uptake of the vitamin. Because the ileum is the specific site of absorption of the vitamin B₁₂ intrinsic factor complex, jejunal resection would not be expected to produce a vitamin B₁₂ deficiency (*pp. 418–419*).

18. (B); 19. (B); 20. (A); 21. (A); 22. (C); 23. (C); 24. (A)

(18) Marasmus is a condition caused by a marked deficiency in total caloric intake. Kwashiorkor, in contrast, is the consequence of a deficient protein intake irrespective of the total caloric intake.

(19) Both diseases are most frequently seen in children and in their classic forms are readily distinguishable. On one hand, the marasmic child appears obviously wasted and has a voracious appetite. On the other hand, the child with kwashiorkor appears bloated (edematous) and is often anorectic.

(20) Kwashiorkor can be further distinguished by the presence of a normochromic, normocytic anemia and **(21)** skin lesions. When present, cutaneous lesions characterized by pigment changes and desquamation are pathognomonic of kwashiorkor.

(22) Fatty change in the liver, however, is a common finding in both kwashiorkor and marasmus. **(23)** Also common to both conditions is an increase in the severity of the disease state with intercurrent infection. Infectious processes further increase metabolic demand for calories and proteins already in inadequate supply. **(24)** Patients with either marasmus or kwashiorkor are more susceptible to infection in the first place. In severe cases of either disease, thymic atrophy occurs, and the number of circulating T-cells is reduced. Only in kwashiorkor, however, are both

T-cell function (mitogen-stimulated blast transformation) and B-cell function (immunoglobulin production) measurably reduced *(pp, 400–402).*

25. (C); 26. (A); 27. (C); 28. (C); 29. (C); 30. (D)

(**25**) Deficiency of vitamin D can cause skeletal disease in children (rickets) or in adults (osteomalacia). Both disorders are characterized by retarded or inadequate mineralization of newly formed osteoid in bone.

(**26**) The major distinguishing feature between the two conditions is the defective endochondral ossification of epiphyseal cartilage that occurs in rickets. This distinction is somewhat artificial, however, since it is merely a reflection of ongoing bone growth in children whose epiphyses have not yet closed.

(**27**) In both disorders, the lack of vitamin D has profound effects on the regulation of serum calcium concentration. Resultant hypocalcemia stimulates the parathyroid glands to increase production of parathormone, and parathormone, in turn, induces osteoclastic resorption of mineralized bones. Scalloping and thinning of cancellous and cortical bone are produced along with fibrosis of the marrow (osteitis fibrosa).

(**28 and 29**) Two hereditary diseases characterized by defects in vitamin D metabolism reduce rickets and osteomalacia: an autosomal recessive form (vitamin D–dependent rickets) and an X-linked dominant hereditary form (vitamin D–resistant rickets). With the decreasing incidence of dietary vitamin D deficiency in developed nations, these diseases, especially the latter, have emerged as relatively important causes of rickets and osteomalacia.

(**30**) Because of its chelating property, tetracycline can be used to distinguish mineralized from unmineralized osteoid and to quantitate the rate of bone mineralization. In mineralized osteoid, the incorporated antibiotic can be visualized by its fluorescence under ultraviolet light and the amount of mineralized osteoid measured at a known time after administration of the drug. Thus tetracycline is an aid to the diagnosis and evaluation of rickets and osteomalacia but has no known therapeutic effect on these disease processes *(pp. 408–410).*

31. (C); 32. (C); 33. (A); 34. (B); 35. (A); 36. (C); 37. (A)

(**31**) Although the role of phosphate in vitamin D metabolism is poorly understood, it is known to parallel calcium in some of its effects. Hypophosphatemia as well as hypocalcemia will stimulate synthesis of $1,25\text{-}(OH)_2D_3$. Conversely, elevated serum levels of either phosphate or calcium will increase production of the less metabolically active form of the vitamin, $24,25\text{-}(OH)_2D_3$. (**32**) Vitamin D, in turn, plays at least one parallel role in calcium and phosphate homeostasis: control of uptake from dietary sources. Vitamin D increases intestinal absorption of both elements, although it apparently does so through independent mechanisms for each. (**33**) In the role of conservation of renal losses, however, vitamin D affects only calcium handling. The active form, $1,25\text{-}(OH)_2D_3$, increases the reabsorption of calcium in the distal renal tubules but has no known effect on the renal handling of phosphate.

(**34**) Increased phosphate loss occurs in several forms of renal tubular disorders including the Fanconi syndrome and renal tubular acidosis. The resultant hypophosphatemia stimulates synthesis of $1,25\text{-}(OH)_2D_3$, and intestinal absorption of phosphate increases (see **31** and **32**). If losses exceed uptake, however, defects in bony mineralization characterized by widened osteoid seams ensue.

(**35**) In hypophosphatemic states, osteoid seams composed only of woven osteoid are seen in the bone, but in hypocalcemic states lamellar as well as woven osteoid are characteristically present. Excessive woven osteoid results from defective mineralization of newly laid down osteoid matrix. Lamellar osteoid, however, is produced by mobilization of the mineral phase of lamellar bone in response to the parathormone generated in a hypocalcemic state.

(**36**) The intricate mechanisms that control calcium and phosphate homeostasis can be compromised in a variety of ways by drugs. Virtually all anticonvulsant medications, for example, increase hepatic degradation of vitamin D. Thus, intestinal absorption of both calcium and phosphate are affected. In addition, anticonvulsants act directly on intestinal absorptive cells to inhibit calcium transport.

(**37**) Parathormone and calcitonin affect calcium homeostasis only. These hormones raise or lower serum calcium levels in response to hypo- or hypercalcemia respectively but, unlike vitamin D, are not directly involved in regulation of phosphorus *(pp. 406–410).*

38. (C); 39. (D); 40. (A); 41. (C); 42. (C); 43. (B)

(**38**) Alcoholic cardiomyopathy is caused by the direct toxic effect of alcohol and its metabolites on cardiac muscle. Beriberi heart disease is the result of metabolic derangements in the myofibers induced by thiamine deficiency. The two disorders have many similar manifestations and can be difficult to differentiate from one another. Pathologically, both disorders ultimately produce dilated, flabby hearts, but (**39**) ischemic damage or myocardial necrosis is not characteristically present.

(**40**) Alcoholic cardiomyopathy typically causes low output heart failure, whereas beriberi heart disease is associated with high output failure. Beriberi heart disease is accompanied by peripheral vasodilatation and arteriovenous shunting that produce a high output state.

(**41**) With myocardial failure from either disorder, increased venous pressure and fluid retention produce edema. (**42**) Both disorders may also be associated with skeletal muscle weakness, although the pathogenesis may differ in the two conditions. In alcoholism, muscle weakness may result either from the direct toxic effect of ethanol on skeletal muscle fibers (rhabdomyolysis) or from an alcohol-induced polyneuropathy. In beriberi, however, weakness is primarily the result of the peripheral neuropathy caused by myelin degeneration, a characteristic feature of many thiamine deficiency states. (43) The central nervous system is also affected in both beriberi and alcoholism, but the syndrome known as Wernicke-Korsakoff's encephalopathy is caused only by thiamine deficiency. Clinically, it is characterized by mental confusion, nystagmus, extraocular palsies, and prostration. Pathologically, degeneration of the mammillary bodies is the most common finding (*pp. 413, 596–597, 601*).

44. (A); 45. (C); 46. (C); 47. (D); 48. (C)

(44) Pernicious anemia refers specifically to the megaloblastic anemia resulting from gastric atrophy, decreased intrinsic factor production, and impaired vitamin B_{12} absorption (see Chapter 8, Question 69).

(45) Alcoholism may cause deficiencies of both vitamin B_{12} and folate for several reasons. The general nutritional intake, including that of vitamin B_{12} and folate, is inadequate in many alcoholic patients. Alcohol-associated gastritis and pancreatitis may also lead to defective vitamin B_{12} absorption, which requires gastric intrinsic factors and pancreatic proteases.

(46) Glossitis is a feature of both vitamin B_{12} and folate deficiencies. Because both these elements are necessary to the metabolic events of cell division, rapidly dividing cells in the bone marrow and gastrointestinal tract (including oral mucosal cells) are characteristically affected.

(47) The primary manifestation of both vitamin B_{12} and folate deficiencies is megaloblastic anemia with prominent megaloblasts (not sideroblasts) in the bone marrow. Sideroblastic anemias constitute a separate group of disorders characterized by hypochromic, microcytic erythrocytes and red cell precursors (sideroblasts) containing granules of nonheme iron in their cytoplasm. Sideroblastic anemias have a number of causes, but the common defect is impaired iron utilization. The defect in megaloblastic anemias is defective DNA synthesis (see Question 74).

(48) In megaloblastic anemia due to either folate or vitamin B_{12} deficiency, the defect in DNA metabolism is reflected in the myeloid and megakaryocytic as well as the erythroid series. Thus, neutrophils are also larger than normal and have hypersegmented nuclei (see Chapter 7, Question 2) (*pp. 418–419, 633*).

49. (A); 50. (B); 51. (B); 52. (C); 53. (C); 54. (C); 55. (A)

(49) Vitamin C is essential to the synthesis of all collagen (see Question 9), and is, therefore, requisite to the production of osteoid, a specialized type of collagen. (50) The process of mineralization of osteoid, however, is regulated by vitamin D through its effects on calcium and phosphorus metabolism. (51) Bone resorption is also dependent on vitamin D, since only previously mineralized bone can be resorbed by osteoclasts. (52) Bone remodeling is the combined result of both bone formation and resorption; thus, both vitamin C and vitamin D are required.

(53) In endochondral bone formation, cartilage at the expanding edge of the epiphysis is replaced by osteoid, which is then mineralized. In this process, the cartilage must first undergo provisional mineralization before it can be resorbed and replaced by osteoid. Like mineralization of osteoid, mineralization of cartilage is a vitamin D–dependent process. (54) Tooth enamel formation is also a complex process requiring both collagen matrix synthesis and subsequent mineralization. Therefore, tooth enamel formation, like normal bone formation, is dependent on both vitamins.

(55) Only vitamin C is essential for wound healing, since this is a process based almost completely on collagen and new vessel (hence vascular wall and basement membrane collagen) formation (*pp. 408–409, 419–420, 887–889*).

56. (C); 57. (A); 58. (C); 59. (C); 60. (A); 61. (B); 62. (D)

Recognition of the primary tissue storage sites for vitamins is important, since disease involving those tissues can lead to depletion of vitamin stores and subsequent deficiency states. (56, 58, 59) The liver is the primary storage site for folate and for the fat-soluble vitamins including vitamins A and D. (57 and 60) Two of the water-soluble B vitamins, B_1 (thiamine) and B_6 (pyridoxine), are stored primarily in striated muscle. (62) Riboflavin, another of the B group vitamins, appears to have no primary tissue storage site and is distributed evenly among the body tissues. (61) Vitamin C is unique among the vitamins in having the adrenal cortex as its primary site of storage (*pp. 403, 414, 417, 419*).

63. (D); 64. (B); 65. (B); 66. (C); 67. (E); 68. (D); 69. (B); 70. (B)

(63) Riboflavin, niacin, and pyridoxine are all B vitamins that function as coenzymes in a variety of important reactions in cellular oxidative metabolism. (64) Niacin is unique among the B vitamins, because it can be synthesized endogenously from tryptophan. (65) Thus, the dietary requirements for niacin vary inversely with the tryptophan content of the diet, and a niacin deficiency state (pellagra) usually reflects a deficiency of both niacin and tryptophan. (66) Many of the biochemical reactions in tryptophan metabolism, in turn, require pyridoxine as a cofactor. (67) Experimental deficiency states of any one of these three vitamins—riboflavin, niacin, or pyridox-

ine—may produce an anemia. Clinically, however, anemia rarely occurs in association with deficiencies of these nutrients. Moreover, when anemias do occur, they are usually normocytic. (Macrocytic anemias are associated with deficiencies of two other B group vitamins: cyanocobalamin [vitamin B_{12}] and folate.) (**68**) Dermatitis is a characteristic clinical feature of the deficiency states of all three vitamins. (**69**) Dementia, however, is associated only with niacin deficiency and is usually accompanied by a desquamative dermatitis and diarrhea (the "three D's" of pellagra). (**70**) Because they are water soluble and can be rapidly eliminated in the urine, B group vitamins do not produce persistent toxic disorders. However, parenteral administration of niacin commonly produces transient toxic effects such as abdominal pain and peripheral vasodilatation. Toxic reactions are not associated with either riboflavin or pyridoxine (*pp. 414–417*).

71. (D); 72. (D); 73. (A); 74. (B); 75. (C)

(**71**) Iron deficiency, vitamin B_{12} deficiency, and starvation all produce anemia. The anemia in all three cases is based primarily on red cell production and maturation defects rather than increased erythrocyte destruction. Increased hemolysis is not a feature of any of these conditions. (**72**) Nor is osmotic fragility associated with these anemias. Osmotic fragility reflects a defect (usually hereditary) in the red cell membrane. No membrane defects are known to be produced in the anemias of nutritional deficiency.

(**73**) Iron deficiency is manifested by insufficient production of hemoglobin. Red cells are pale and decreased in size, constituting a hypochromic, microcytic anemia.

(**74**) Vitamin B_{12} deficiency produces a defect in DNA synthesis. Red cell precursors grow in size as their cytoplasm develops, but they cannot divide. Hemoglobin production is not affected, however. Megaloblasts produce abnormally large erythrocytes, and the resultant anemia is characterized as normochromic, macrocytic.

(**75**) For reasons less well understood, the characteristic anemia of starvation is hypochromic and normocytic. Normal red cell morphology is not typical of any of these deficiency states, although a normochromic, normocytic anemia may appear in starvation (*pp. 402, 630, 638*).

76. (D); 77. (D); 78. (A); 79. (B); 80. (C); 81. (B); 82. (B)

(**76**) Deficiencies of zinc, copper, or selenium can have profound effects on cellular metabolism, since these elements are critical components of numerous essential metalloenzymes. (**77**) Because deficiencies of these elements are common among patients receiving total parenteral nutrition, they are of ever-increasing clinical importance. (**78**) Zinc deficiency causes retardation of growth and defective sexual maturation in children and adults. (**79**) Of these elements only copper deficiency is known to cause anemia, however. The copper-requiring protein, ceruloplasmin, is critical to the oxidation of iron required for heme synthesis. (**80**) Deficiency of selenium has been associated with a congestive myopathy known as Keshan disease, which is endemic in selenium-deficient areas of China. The disorder has also been described in patients receiving parenteral nutritional support. (**81 and 82**) Copper is the metallic element in the metalloenzyme lysyl oxidase that is essential to formation of cross-linkages in both elastin and collagen (*pp. 423–424*).

4

INFECTIOUS DISEASES

DIRECTIONS: For Questions 1 to 5, choose the ONE BEST answer to each question.

1. Which of the following is the *least* common cause of "traveler's diarrhea"?

  A. Parvovirus
  B. *Campylobacter jejuni*
  C. *Giardia lamblia*
  D. *Escherichia coli*
  E. Shigella

2. Sexually transmitted chlamydia produce all of the following problems EXCEPT:

  A. Pelvic inflammatory disease
  B. Acute epididymitis
  C. Genital elephantiasis
  D. Condylomata lata
  E. Rectal strictures

3. Ulcerated lesions on the penis occur in the acute form of all the following sexually transmitted infectious diseases EXCEPT:

  A. Herpes genitalis infection
  B. Syphilis

  C. Chancroid
  D. Granuloma inguinale
  E. Gonorrhea

4. Which of the following diseases is a veterinarian at LEAST risk of contracting?

  A. Listeriosis
  B. Brucellosis
  C. Leptospirosis
  D. Toxoplasmosis
  E. Glanders

5. Trichomoniasis is associated with:

  A. Raspberry tongue
  B. Strawberry mucosa
  C. Strawberry gallbladder
  D. Anchovy paste abscesses
  E. None of these

DIRECTIONS: For Questions 6 to 15, ONE or MORE of the completions given correctly finishes the incomplete statement. Choose:

      A—if only *1,2, and 3* are correct
      B—if only *1 and 3* are correct
      C—if only *2 and 4* are correct
      D—if only *4* is correct
      E—if all are correct

6. Mumps in adults:

  1. Is caused by a reovirus
  2. Produces pancreatitis
  3. Produces diagnostic cell inclusions
  4. Usually produces unilateral orchitis

    A. 1,2,3 B. 1,3 C. 2,4 D. 4 Only E. All

7. Which of the following statements about the acquired immune deficiency syndrome (AIDS) is/are true?

  1. Hemophiliacs are at risk
  2. T-suppressor cells are depleted

  3. An aggressive form of Kaposi's sarcoma develops
  4. Leukemia occurs with increased frequency

    A. 1,2,3 B. 1,3 C. 2,4 D. 4 Only E. All

8. Body lice are the principal vectors of transmission of the organisms causing:

  1. Bubonic plague
  2. Relapsing fever
  3. Q fever
  4. Epidemic typhus

    A. 1,2,3 B. 1,3 C. 2,4 D. 4 Only E. All

9. Ticks are the principal vectors of transmission of the organisms causing:

1. Lyme disease
2. Rocky Mountain spotted fever
3. Babesiosis
4. Chagas' disease

    A. 1,2,3   B. 1,3   C. 2,4   D. 4 Only   E. All

10. Organisms that typically invade blood vessel walls include:

1. Pseudomonas
2. Aspergillus
3. Rickettsiae
4. Plasmodia

    A. 1,2,3   B. 1,3   C. 2,4   D. 4 Only   E. All

11. Gonococcal infection:

1. Has an asymptomatic carrier state
2. Is a cause of Fitz-Hugh–Curtis syndrome
3. Causes septic arthritis
4. Is the most common cause of pelvic inflammatory disease

    A. 1,2,3   B. 1,3   C. 2,4   D. 4 Only   E. All

12. Wound infections are one of the most important sources of:

1. Tetanus
2. Diphtheria
3. Gas gangrene
4. Botulism

    A. 1,2,3   B. 1,3   C. 2,4   D. 4 Only   E. All

13. *Bacteria* that *typically* induce granuloma formation include:

1. *Brucella suis* (brucellosis)
2. *Pseudomonas mallei* (glanders)
3. *Francisella tularensis* (tularemia)
4. *Yersinia pestis* (plague)

    A. 1,2,3   B. 1,3   C. 2,4   D. 4 Only   E. All

14. Amebiasis:

1. Is most often asymptomatic
2. Most often affects the left colon
3. Produces flask-shaped ulcers
4. Produces mucosal pseudopolyp formation

    A. 1,2,3   B. 1,3   C. 2,4   D. 4 Only   E. All

15. Which of the following diseases is/are acquired by ingestion of raw or undercooked meat?

1. Schistosomiasis
2. Liver fluke infection
3. Filariasis
4. Tapeworm infection

    A. 1,2,3   B. 1,3   C. 2,4   D. 4 Only   E. All

DIRECTIONS: For Questions 16 to 20, you are to decide whether EACH choice is TRUE or FALSE.

For each of the following statements about infectious mononucleosis, choose whether it is TRUE or FALSE.

16. It is caused by the same virus that causes African Burkitt's lymphoma

17. The abnormal circulating mononuclear cells are infected T lymphocytes

18. Microscopic changes produced in the liver resemble viral hepatitis

19. Microscopic changes produced in the lymph nodes resemble Hodgkin's disease

20. The associated exudative pharyngitis is often culture-positive for beta-hemolytic streptococci

DIRECTIONS: For Questions 21 to 37, the set of lettered headings is followed by a list of numbered words or phrases. For each numbered word or phrase choose:

A—if the item is associated with (A) only
B—if the item is associated with (B) only
C—if the item is associated with *both* (A) and (B)
D—if the item is associated with *neither* (A) nor (B)

For each of the diseases listed below, choose whether it is caused by streptococci, staphylococci, both, or neither.

    A. Streptococci
    B. Staphylococci
    C. Both
    D. Neither

21. Impetigo
22. Erysipelas
23. Erythema nodosum
24. Carbuncles
25. Toxin-induced food poisoning
26. Toxic shock syndrome
27. Glomerulonephritis

For each of the statements listed below, choose whether it describes lepromatous leprosy, tuberculoid leprosy, both, or neither.

    A. Lepromatous leprosy
    B. Tuberculoid leprosy
    C. Both
    D. Neither

28. The causative organism has never been cultured in vitro from individuals with this form of disease
29. Large numbers of organisms are typically found in the lesion
30. Monoclonal hypergammaglobulinemia often occurs
31. The disease is associated with erythema nodosum
32. Nerve involvement is typical

For each of the features listed below, choose whether it is characteristic of nocardiosis, actinomycosis, both, or neither.

    A. Nocardiosis
    B. Actinomycosis
    C. Both
    D. Neither

33. Infection usually occurs in the immunosuppressed
34. Person-to-person spread is the major mode of transmission
35. Abscesses are characteristically produced
36. "Sulfur granules" are typically seen in lesions
37. The causative agent is strictly anaerobic

DIRECTIONS: Questions 38 to 103 are matching questions. For each numbered item, choose the most likely associated lettered item from those provided. Each numbered item has ONLY ONE answer. Within each group, each lettered item may be the answer to one, more than one, or none of the numbered items.

For each of the following features of respiratory viruses, choose whether it describes adenovirus, influenza virus, Coxsackie virus, rhinovirus, or none of these.

    A. Adenovirus
    B. Influenza virus
    C. Coxsackie virus
    D. Rhinovirus
    E. None of these

38. Major cause of the common cold
39. Associated with the Guillain-Barré syndrome
40. Associated with Reye's syndrome in aspirin-treated children
41. Causes herpangina
42. Most common cause of croup (lethal bronchiolitis) in infants
43. Causes epidemic hemorrhagic keratoconjunctivitis
44. Produces characteristic inclusion bodies in infected cells

For each of the features of childhood infectious disease, choose whether it is characteristic of measles (rubeola), German measles (rubella), chickenpox (varicella zoster), all of these, or none of these.

    A. Measles (rubeola)
    B. German measles (rubella)
    C. Chickenpox (varicella zoster)
    D. All of these
    E. None of these

45. The causative organism is a paramyxovirus
46. The disease is highly contagious by droplet aspiration
47. Koplik's spots are clinically diagnostic
48. "Warthin-Finkeldey" cells are a typical histologic feature
49. Maternal disease is associated with congenital malformations
50. Skin lesions are characteristically pustular
51. "Giant cell" pneumonia is sometimes produced
52. A latent phase of infection is a common consequence
53. Recovery confers life-long immunity

For each of the diseases listed below, choose whether it is caused by viral, chlamydial, bacterial, or protozoal infection or whether the causative agent is unknown.

    A. Viral infection
    B. Chlamydial infection
    C. Bacterial infection
    D. Protozoal infection
    E. Causative agent unknown

54. Yellow fever
55. Kawasaki's disease (mucocutaneous lymph node syndrome)
56. Psittacosis
57. Legionnaire's disease
58. Bubonic plague

For each of the bacterial organisms listed below, decide whether it causes pathogenicity in man by one of the mechanisms listed below or whether it acts by none of these mechanisms.

    A. Formation of a phagocyte-resistant capsule
    B. Production of leukocyte-killing substances
    C. Avoidance of immune mechanisms by programmed antigenic variation
    D. Interference with normal phagosome function
    E. None of these

59. Pneumococcus (*Streptococcus pneumoniae*)
60. *Borrelia recurrentis*
61. *Mycobacterium tuberculosis*
62. *Clostridium perfringens*
63. *Vibrio cholerae*
64. *Brucella suis*
65. *Clostridium botulinum*

For each of the following statements about gram-negative bacteria, choose whether it describes *Escherichia coli (E. coli) Proteus mirabilis, Pseudomonas aeruginosa, Klebsiella pneumoniae*, or none of these.

    A. *Escherichia coli (E. coli)*
    B. *Proteus mirabilis*
    C. *Pseudomonas aeruginosa*
    D. *Klebsiella pneumoniae*
    E. None of these

66. Not a source of endotoxin
67. Grows best in anaerobic conditions
68. Characteristically forms numerous small abscesses with lung infection
69. Most common cause of urinary tract infection
70. Typically causes copious slimy mucoid exudates with lung infection
71. Most common cause of sepsis in burn patients
72. Occasionally forms pus with a bluish tinge

For each of the features listed below, choose whether it is characteristic of primary syphilis, secondary syphilis, tertiary syphilis, all of these stages, or none of these.

    A. Primary syphilis
    B. Secondary syphilis
    C. Tertiary syphilis
    D. All of these
    E. None of these

73. A generalized skin eruption typically occurs
74. The syphilitic gumma is the histologic hallmark
75. Obliterative endarteritis is the histologic hallmark
76. Treponemes are extremely difficult to demonstrate in lesions
77. Tabes dorsalis develops
78. Charcot's joints develop
79. Hutchinson's teeth develop

For each of the characteristics listed below, choose whether it describes *Candida albicans, Mucor, Aspergillus fumigatus, Cryptococcus neoformans*, or none of these.

    A. *Candida albicans*
    B. *Mucor*
    C. *Aspergillus fumigatus*
    D. *Cryptococcus neoformans*
    E. None of these

80. Most common cause of deep fungal infection
81. Typically forms pseudohyphae
82. Rarely, if ever, causes disease in immunocompetent individuals
83. India ink preps aid in identification
84. Most frequent clinical manifestation is meningitis
85. Causes hypersensitivity pneumonitis without lung infection
86. Causes oral infection in infants who are bottle-fed

For each of the features listed below, choose whether it is characteristic of blastomycosis, coccidioidomycosis, histoplasmosis, all of these, or none of these.

    A. Blastomycosis
    B. Coccidioidomycosis
    C. Histoplasmosis
    D. All of these
    E. None of these

87. Most prevalent in the southwest of the United States
88. Acquired from inhalation of contaminated soil
89. Causative fungus grows in tissue as a yeast form
90. Commonly produces asymptomatic primary disease
91. Commonly produces skin involvement in disseminated disease
92. Causes granulomatous lung disease
93. Occasionally causes sclerosing mediastinitis

For each of the features listed below, choose whether it is characteristic of malaria, babesiosis, Chagas' disease, all of these, or none of these.

    A. Malaria
    B. Babesiosis
    C. Chagas' disease
    D. All of these
    E. None of these

94. Mosquitos transmit the disease
95. Pigment is typically found in phagocytes
96. Sickle cell hemoglobin limits parasitemia
97. Myocarditis is common in adult infection
98. Progressive brain dysfunction occurs in the late stage disease

For each of the characteristics listed below, choose whether it describes infection by *Ascaris lumbricoides*, hookworm, Strongyloides, pinworm, or none of these.

    A. *Ascaris lumbricoides*
    B. Hookworm
    C. Strongyloides
    D. Pinworm
    E. None of these

99. Causes childhood night itch
100. Typically invades striated muscle
101. Diagnosed by duodenal aspiration
102. Causes mechanical obstruction of GI tract
103. Causes disease by sucking blood

4

INFECTIOUS DISEASES

ANSWERS

1. (B) In a world of extensive opportunities for tourism, infection by gastrointestinal pathogens causing "traveler's diarrhea" is a major nemesis. This disturbing and sometimes debilitating problem can be caused by a variety of infectious agents, including viruses, bacteria, and protozoa. Among the best known causes of "traveler's diarrhea" are parvoviruses, *Giardia lamblia*, *E. coli*, and Shigella species. *Campylobacter jejuni*, although a major gastrointestinal pathogen and a source of traveler's diarrhea, is primarily a cause of domestic diarrhea in the United States and not necessarily associated with travel abroad *(pp. 281, 318, 322, 323, 364).*

2. (D) Chlamydial urethritis and cervicitis caused by *C. trachomatis* are now two of the most common forms of chlamydial diseases in the United States. In the female, chlamydial infection is an increasingly more common cause of pelvic inflammatory disease. In the male, it causes nongonorrheal urethritis and may extend to produce acute epididymitis. Genital elephantiasis and rectal strictures are two of the more unusual sequelae of lymphogranuloma venereum, a venerally transmitted disease caused by three of the eight known serotypes of *C. trachomatis*. Lymphogranuloma venereum should not be confused with granuloma inguinale, a venereal disease caused by the bacterium *Calymmatobacterium donovani*. Condylomata lata are not produced by chlamydia; they are the characteristic papular lesions found on the penis or vulva in secondary syphilis, a disease caused by *Treponema pallidum* *(pp. 292–295, 337).*

3. (E) Ulcerated lesions characteristically occur on the penis in a number of venereal infections, including herpes genitalis infection, syphilis, chancroid, and granuloma inguinale. Obviously then, among patients with an ulcerated penile lesion, bacteriologic, serologic, or immunohistochemical testing may be required to make a diagnosis. However, gonorrhea, the most common venereal disease in the United States, does not produce a penile ulcer. In the male, gonococcal infection produces a mucopurulent exudate from the anterior urethra and meatus. The meatus becomes hyperemic, edematous, and obviously inflamed, but does not ulcerate *(pp. 284, 310, 336, 339, 340).*

4. (A) For obvious reasons, veterinarians are among those at greatest risk of developing infections from organisms that are harbored by domestic animals. Brucelli are gram-negative intracellular coccobacilli that originate in livestock and dogs. Most infections arise from animal contact; thus veterinarians and meat packers are at greatest risk. Leptospirae are zoonotic bacteria that infect both wild and domestic animals (principally dogs). Infection usually occurs from contact with animals or contaminated soil, and veterinarians, farmers, and trappers are among those at highest risk. Toxoplasmosis, caused by the protozoan *Toxoplasma gondii*, is most often contracted from domestic cats, which are the definitive host of this parasite. Glanders may occur as either an acute febrile illness or a chronic granulomatous disease. It is caused by *Pseudomonas mallei*, a gram-negative bacillus that is harbored by horses, mules, and donkeys. Although *Listeria monocytogenes*, the gram-positive bacillus that causes listeriosis, is harbored by many mammals and fowl, it is principally an opportunistic agent in human disease. Its chief victims are pregnant women and their fetuses, the elderly, the sick, or the immunosuppressed. Thus, in contrast to the other zoonotic agents discussed above, Listeria do not normally pose an increased threat of infection to the veterinarian *(pp. 328, 330–332, 373–374).*

5. (B) Trichomoniasis is a common venereal parasitic infection caused by the flagellate *Trichomonas vaginalis*. Infection occurs most commonly in the vagina of the postpubertal female and in the male urethra. The affected mucosa is typically erythematous and edematous; it is sometimes spotted with small blisters or granules, and its appearance is referred to as "strawberry mucosa." Raspberry tongue is associated with scarlet fever and refers to the tongue's bright red color and edematous papillae in the early stage of the disease dominated by pharyngitis and tonsillitis. Strawberry gallbladder refers to the gross appearance of the gallbladder mucosa in cholesterolosis. In this condition, the gallbladder mucosa is diffusely erythematous and studded with small yellow "seeds," which are actually collections of cholesterol-laden macrophages in the lamina propria. The anchovy paste abscess occurs in amebiasis with liver involvement. The contents of amebic abscesses in the liver made up of hemorrhage and digested liver cell debris appear grossly as a chocolate-colored pasty material resembling "anchovy paste" *(pp. 307, 363, 365, 951).*

6. (**C**) Mumps is an acute contagious disease caused by a single-stranded RNA paramyxovirus. It most commonly occurs in children, but may occur in adults. Reoviruses are a family of double-stranded RNA viruses, whose major pathogenic species is the rotavirus, the agent responsible for most childhood diarrhea. The mumps virus principally involves the parotid gland, producing the characteristic inflammation and swelling. Other glandular organs, principally the pancreas and the testes, are often affected as well. Mumps pancreatitis tends to be mild and self-limited. In contrast to mumps parotitis, which is most often bilateral, mumps orchitis in adults is most frequently unilateral and therefore rarely leads to male sterility. Like other RNA viruses, mumps virus does not produce characteristic cell inclusions by which it can be identified microscopically (*p. 281*).

7. (**B**) The acquired immune deficiency syndrome (AIDS) is a devastating and lethal disease of unknown etiology that has recently become epidemic. In addition to male homosexuals, those at particular risk include hemophiliacs receiving multiple transfusions or factor VIII concentrate, Haitians, and drug addicts. The disease is characterized by a loss of cellular immunity due to a depletion of T-*helper* cells. T-suppressor cells remain normal or increased in number. Affected individuals become vulnerable to infection by a large number of opportunistic agents and, uniquely, to a rapidly progressive form of Kaposi's sarcoma. Heretofore, Kaposi's sarcoma occurred predominantly in elderly males and characteristically had an indolent course. AIDS also imposes a significantly increased risk of developing malignant lymphoma (not leukemia), but death usually occurs from overwhelming infection rather than superimposed malignancy (*p. 292*).

8. (**C**) Body lice are the principal vectors of transmission of the organisms causing relapsing fever and typhus fever. Relapsing fever is caused by a zoonotic bacterium known as *Borrelia recurrentis*; it is transmitted from man to man by body lice and has no known animal reservoir. Epidemic typhus is caused by *Rickettsia prowazekii*, which, like all Rickettsiae, is a small, bacteria-like obligate intracellular parasite. It is transmitted from man to man by human head and body lice. Bubonic plague, caused by *Yersinia pestis*, is transmitted to man by fleas from infected rodents. Q fever, a Rickettsial infection, is transmitted to man by the respiratory route from infected animals and requires no arthropod vector (*pp. 297, 299, 328–329, 333*).

9. (**A**) Ticks transmit numerous infectious diseases, including Lyme disease, Rocky Mountain spotted fever, and babesiosis. Lyme disease, an inflammatory disease characterized by skin rash and migratory polyarthritis, is believed to be caused by a Treponema-like spirochete. Rocky Mountain spotted fever is a Rickettsial disease, whereas babesiosis is caused by a protozoan that is a close relative of the plasmodia. Although these diseases are caused by disparate classes of organisms, they are all transmitted to man by ticks. Chagas' disease, in contrast, is caused by an intracellular protozoan (a trypanosome) and is transmitted from man to man or from animals to man by "kissing bugs" (triatomidae or reduviid bugs) (*pp. 296, 334, 369, 370*).

10. (**A**) Infectious diseases caused by organisms that typically invade vessel walls are usually characterized by hemorrhage and thrombosis and are thus particularly destructive. *Pseudomonas aeruginosa*, aspergillus species, and Rickettsial organisms are prototypic examples of organisms that readily invade vessels. Plasmodia, the protozoal organisms that cause malaria, typically induce thromboses of small vessels, but they do not do so by direct vascular invasion. Rather, they produce changes in the infected erythrocyte membranes that increase red cell stickiness and induce clumping. Plugging of small vessels results, and tissue hypoxia or ischemic necrosis is produced (*pp. 295, 313, 355, 367*).

11. (**E**) Gonorrhea is the most common reportable communicable disease in the United States. Although it usually produces acute exudative and purulent inflammation, infection can be asymptomatic. In the female it is the most common cause of pelvic inflammatory disease. Spread into the peritoneum can result in perihepatitis, producing stabbing right upper quadrant pain known as the Fitz-Hugh–Curtis syndrome. Gonococcal bacteremia may result in gonococcal arthritis produced either by seeding of joints by organisms or as a result of immunologically mediated processes in the absence of culturable organisms. The frequency of gonococcemia and arthritis in women is on the rise (*pp. 309–310*).

12. (**A**) Wound infections comprise the primary source of disease produced by *Clostridium tetani*, *Corynebacterium diphtheriae*, and *Clostridium perfringens*. *Clostridium tetani* is an anaerobic organism that thrives in the devitalized tissue of penetrating wounds and produces a powerful neurotoxin that causes convulsive contractions of voluntary muscles that characterize tetanus. Diphtheria used to occur primarily as a communicable childhood upper respiratory tract infection with systemic manifestation resulting from exotoxin production by the causative agent, *Corynebacterium diphtheriae*. At present, vaccination has made diphtheria a rare childhood disease, and most infection now occurs from the neglected skin wounds in adults. Gas gangrene is a severe form of necrotizing anaerobic infection caused by the gas-producing *Clostridium perfringens*. The infection is most frequently the result of invasion of traumatic surgical wounds. Botulism is a severe par-

alyzing illness caused by the powerful neurotoxin produced by *Clostridium botulinum*. Although botulism can be caused by wound infection, this occurs only rarely. By far the most common cause of botulism is ingestion of contaminated foods containing the preformed botulinum neurotoxin *(pp. 317, 324–326)*.

13. (E) Although a granulomatous response is commonly associated with mycobacteria, spirochetes, fungi, and parasites, several bacterial organisms also elicit granulomatous responses in the host. Principal among these are *Brucella suis*, *Pseudomonas mallei*, *Francisella tularensis*, and *Yersinia pestis*. Thus, the respective infectious diseases caused by these organisms—brucellosis, glanders, tularemia, and plague—are typically associated with granulomas in affected organs *(pp. 328–332)*.

14. (B) Amebiasis is a protozoal disease caused by *Entamoeba histolytica*. Infection is primarily limited to the lumen of the colon, but systemic spread of the organism may occur. Although amebiasis is a well-known cause of dysentery, infection far more commonly produces an asymptomatic carrier state, which is principally responsible for transmission of the disease. The colitis produced most often affects the cecum and ascending colon but occasionally involves the sigmoid, rectum, or appendix. The organisms produce mucosal ulcerations with a classic flask-shaped contour when viewed in tissue sections (a narrow neck and a broad base). In contrast to idiopathic ulcerative colitis, the colonic mucosa between ulcerations is characteristically normal in amebiasis and does not show pseudopolyp formation *(pp. 362–363)*.

15. (D) Tapeworm infection is usually contracted by ingestion of undercooked meat or fish containing encysted larvae. Schistosomiasis, a trematode infection, is transmitted by water contact with the free-swimming, four-tailed cercarial forms of the organism released by infected snails. They burrow quickly through the skin, maturing into young worms. Liver fluke infection is acquired by eating contaminated watercress containing the metacercarial form of the parasite. Filariasis, a group of roundworm infections, is transmitted to man by insect bites *(pp. 381, 384, 386, 388)*.

16. (True); 17. (False); 18. (True); 19. (True); 20. (False)

(16) Infectious mononucleosis is a benign lymphoproliferative disease caused by the Epstein-Barr virus, a member of the herpes family and the same virus that is suspected to cause the malignant lymphoproliferative disease known as African Burkitt's lymphoma.

(17) After an initial replicative phase within the salivary epithelial glands, the Epstein-Barr virus infects the B lymphocytes in lymphoid tissues. Since B cells possess surface receptors for the virus, they are the primary target of infection. Infected B cells display viral-directed antigens on their surface that are recognized by T cells and stimulate multiplication of the latter. The activated T lymphocytes appear in the peripheral blood as atypical mononuclear cells (mononucleosis cells) but represent response to the infection rather than virally-transformed cells.

(18) The diagnosis of infectious mononucleosis can be difficult, because the disease may mimic other disorders both clinically and pathologically. The microscopic changes produced in the liver resemble those of viral hepatitis with mononuclear inflammation of the portal tracts and focal hepatocellular necrosis. **(19)** Affected lymph nodes have markedly expanded paracortical (T cell) zones that occasionally contain large binucleate cells resembling Reed-Sternberg cells. Thus, a histologic appearance resembling Hodgkin's disease is produced. **(20)** Clinically, the acute exudative pharyngitis that may occur in infectious mononucleosis resembles streptococcal infection, but bacterial cultures will be negative *(pp. 288–289)*.

21. (C); 22. (A); 23. (A); 24. (B); 25. (B); 26. (B); 27. (A)

(21) Streptococci and staphylococci are two of the most common and versatile human bacterial pathogens. Impetigo, a common superficial infection of the skin characterized by erosive lesions covered by honey-colored crust, can be caused by either streptococci or staphylococci *(pp. 305, 307)*.

(22) Erysipelas is a disorder characterized by a rapidly spreading edematous and erythematous cutaneous infection, usually on the face. It is caused by group A beta hemolytic streptococci *(p. 307)*.

(23) Erythema nodosum, the most common type of panniculitis, is commonly associated with beta hemolytic streptococcal infection. Erythema nodosum may occur in association with other infectious diseases, such as tuberculosis, leprosy, coccidioidomycosis, or histoplasmosis, but is not associated with staphylococcal infection *(p. 1288)*.

(24) Carbuncles are deep-seated suppurative lesions of the skin and subcutaneous tissues that spread laterally beneath the deep subcutaneous fascia and then erupt onto the skin surface, forming multiple adjacent skin sinuses. They typically appear on the upper back and posterior neck and are caused by staphylococcal infection *(p. 304)*.

(25 and 26) Food poisoning and the toxic shock syndrome are two examples of diseases caused by staphylococcal toxin production. Staphylococcal food poisoning results from the ingestion of a preformed enterotoxin without invasive staphylococcal enterocolitis. The toxic shock syndrome is caused by unique toxins produced by staphylococci that propagate in blood-soaked vaginal tampons during menstruation. In contrast to staphylococci, streptococci are not known to produce exotoxins; they commonly produce disease by suppurative spreading infection or via the complications of a host hypersensitivity response (p. 305).

(27) Poststreptococcal glomerulonephritis is a fairly common renal glomerular disease that is produced by streptococcal-antistreptococcal immune complexes (pp. 305, 1007–1009).

28. (C); 29. (A); 30. (D); 31. (A); 32. (C)

(28) Leprosy is an indolent, chronic debilitating disease caused by *Mycobacterium leprae*. Infection typically takes one of two forms, lepromatous leprosy or tuberculoid leprosy, depending upon the response of the host. The causative agent has never been successfully cultured in vitro from patients with either form of the disease.

(29) Large numbers of organisms are typically demonstrable in the lesions of lepromatous leprosy, the form of disease characterized by a poor cellular immune response to the invading organism. In contrast, tuberculoid leprosy is characterized by a brisk cellular immune response with granuloma formation and a paucity of demonstrable organisms.

(30) Although patients with lepromatous leprosy fail to produce an adequate cellular immune response, they often have a *polyclonal* hypergammaglobulinemia thought to be due to the dearth of T-suppressor cells together with massive lepra antigen exposure. Monoclonal hypergammaglobulinemia is associated with neoplastic rather than reactive proliferations of plasma cells and is not a feature of leprosy.

(31) With the production of large amounts of anti-lepra antibody in lepromatous leprosy, antigen-antibody complexes often form, producing immune complex–mediated disorders such as erythema nodosum or vasculitis.

(32) Regardless of the type of host response and subsequent form of disease, leprosy typically involves the peripheral nerves and the skin (pp. 347–348).

33. (A); 34. (D); 35. (C); 36. (B); 37. (B)

(33) The actinomycetales are a fungus-like bacteria closely related to mycobacteria. Nocardia and Actinomyces are the most important human pathogens in this group of organisms. Unlike actinomycetes, which are not opportunistic and infect healthy individuals, nocardia primarily infect patients who are immunosuppressed or chronically ill.

(34) There is no evidence of person-to-person spread in either nocardiosis or actinomycosis; all infections appear to be derived endogenously.

(35) Both organisms characteristically produce abscesses in the tissues they affect. Nocardia most often involve the lung and typically cause single or chronic necrotizing walled-off abscesses. Actinomycosis most frequently involves the cervicofacial soft tissues, forming abscesses that lead to sinus formation. Abdominal actinomycosis resulting from invasion of the intestinal mucosa and bowel wall penetration typically forms a localized peritoneal abscess. Similarly,

thoracic actinomycosis causes lung abscesses or empyemas.

(36) A distinguishing feature of the actinomycotic abscess is its content of grossly visible yellowish colonies called "sulfur granules." These are composed of intertwined radiating filaments of bacteria.

(37) A further distinguishing feature between nocardiosis and actinomycosis is the culture requirements of the causative organism. Unlike nocardia, which are aerobes similar to *Mycobacterium tuberculosis*, actinomycetes are strict anaerobes that are difficult to culture (pp. 349–350).

38. (D); 39. (C); 40. (B); 41. (C); 42. (E); 43. (A); 44. (A)

(38) Viral diseases of the respiratory tract are the most common and least preventable of all human infectious diseases. Among the myriad species and serotypes responsible, adenovirus, influenza virus, Coxsackie virus, and rhinovirus are among the most important. Rhinovirus is the major cause of the common cold. Although it is the cause of the single most frequent infectious disease, it seldom produces serious sequelae.

(39 and 40) Coxsackie viruses produce many patterns of disease besides upper respiratory tract infections. Coxsackie B virus can cause the Guillain-Barré syndrome and myocarditis. Coxsackie A strain may cause herpangina, a blistering inflammation of the pharynx.

(40) Influenza viruses are the leading causes of lower respiratory tract infection ("flu"). In addition, they may cause serious extrapulmonary complications such as Reye's syndrome in aspirin-treated children (see Chapter 9, Question 2).

(42) Also of particular importance among viral respiratory pathogens affecting infants and children are the parainfluenza and respiratory syncytial viruses, which produce croup (lethal bronchiolitis) or pneumonia. Adenovirus may also cause croup but does so infrequently.

(43) Adenoviruses produce a number of febrile respiratory syndromes of varying severity but are also commonly associated with eye infections, particularly acute conjunctivitis. The more severe adenovirus-induced keratoconjunctivitis may occur in sharp outbreaks related to inadequately chlorinated swimming pools.

(44) Among the major respiratory viruses, only adenovirus produces characteristic inclusion bodies that are diagnostic by light microscopy. Other viral agents that produce characteristic inclusion bodies and may involve the respiratory tract include the herpesvirus and rubeola (measles virus) (pp. 278–280).

45. (A); 46. (D); 47. (A); 48. (A); 49. (B); 50. (E); 51. (A); 52. (C); 53. (D)

(45) Measles, German measles, and chickenpox are

three common viral infections of childhood with varying acute and chronic consequences. Measles, like mumps, is caused by a paramyxovirus. German measles is caused by a single-stranded DNA virus of the togavirus family; chickenpox is caused by varicella zoster, a double-stranded DNA herpesvirus.

(**46**) All of these diseases are highly contagious by droplet aspiration and hence spread rapidly among unimmunized children and nonimmune adults.

(**47**) Measles infection produces several unique clinical and pathologic features. The earliest diagnostic sign is the appearance of small blistering, ulcerating lesions, known as Koplik's spots, on the cheek mucosa near the opening of Stensen's ducts. Their appearance may precede the skin rash. (**48**) A pathognomonic histologic feature of measles is the Warthin-Finkeldey cells found in involved lymphoid organs. These multinucleated giant cells characteristically contain eosinophilic nuclear and intracytoplasmic inclusion bodies. (**51**) Another unique and sometimes life-threatening complication of measles infection is an interstitial pneumonia characterized by the abundance of giant cells for which it is named ("giant cell" pneumonia).

(**49**) In contrast to measles or chickenpox, German measles is a relatively mild childhood infection with few if any serious sequelae. Its major importance is its ability to produce congenital malformations in the offspring of affected mothers, a feature not associated with either measles or chickenpox.

(**50**) Although skin lesions occur in all three of these systemic viral diseases, none are pustular in character. Measles and German measles produce a maculopapular rash, and chickenpox characteristically causes macular lesions that rapidly progress to a vesicular stage without forming pustules.

(**52 and 53**) Although recovery from all three of these childhood infections confers life-long immunity to reinfection, only varicella zoster causes latent disease. Following the production of chickenpox, the virus may remain latent for years in the sensory dorsal root ganglia. With advancing age or immunosuppression, the virus may become reactivated and cause a localized vesicular eruption in the distribution of the corresponding dermatomes, known as "shingles" (*pp. 282–283, 285–286*).

54. (A); 55. (E); 56. (B); 57. (C); 58. (C)

(**54**) Yellow fever is an arthropod-borne hemorrhagic fever caused by a single-stranded RNA togavirus. The yellow fever virus characteristically produces severe hepatocellular damage with resultant jaundice, a feature that has given the disease its name (*p. 290*).

(**55**) Kawasaki's disease, also known as the mucocutaneous lymph node syndrome, is an acute febrile disease of as yet unknown etiology characterized by arteritis and lymphadenopathy. The syndrome may follow a viral upper respiratory tract infection, but thus far, attempts to isolate infective agents from Kawasaki patients have proved unsuccessful (*pp. 291–292*).

(**56**) Psittacosis is a disease caused by a chlamydial organism found in contaminated excreta from infected birds. Chlamydia are obligate intracellular organisms and produce intracytoplasmic inclusions ("elementary" bodies) in infected cells. Thus, elementary bodies can be identified in the alveolar cells of patients with this acute flu-like illness (*p. 293*)

(**57**) Legionnaire's disease is an acute, potentially fatal necrotizing pneumonia produced by a gram-negative bacterial pathogen that was recognized anew by microbiologists after the epidemic in Philadelphia in 1976 (*p. 313*).

(**58**) Bubonic plague is a periodically epidemic, systemic febrile disease caused by *Yersinia pestis*, a gram-negative bacillus. The disease is fortunately rare in the United States, but the organism is harbored by many wild animals, principally rodents, and occurs occasionally in the western United States where squirrels are the principal reservoir (*pp. 328–329*).

59. (A); 60. (C); 61. (D); 62. (B); 63. (E); 64. (D); 65. (E)

(**59**) Bacterial agents have evolved numerous clever ways of combating human biologic defense mechanisms. Some organisms, like the pneumococcus, are particularly resistant to engulfment by neutrophils by virtue of their slippery hydrophilic polysaccharide (*p. 300*).

(**60**) Others, like *Borrelia recurrentis*, the agent of relapsing fever, elude immunologic defense mechanisms by continuously changing their antigenic surface determinants. This genetically programmed variation in surface antigens allows each successive generation of organisms to survive while the preceding generations are immunologically exterminated (*pp. 300 and 333*).

(**61 and 64**) Granuloma-forming facultative intracellular bacteria such as *Mycobacterium tuberculosis* and *Brucella suis* have evolved mechanisms to escape destruction following ingestion by phagocytes. By unknown mechanisms, they interfere with the fusion of phagocytic vacuoles and lysosomes, thus forestalling the enzymatic reactions that would lead to their digestion (*pp. 300–301*).

(**62**) *Clostridia perfringens* is a prime example of an organism that digests the cells of its host before it can be digested. It produces a plethora of bacterial enzymes, including a lecithinase (alphatoxin) that disrupts the plasma membranes of both white blood cells and erythrocytes (*p. 301*).

(**63 and 65**) In contrast to the above, *Vibrio cholerae* and *Clostridium botulinum* are two examples of organisms that do not need to invade the tissues of their host to produce disease. These organisms produce powerful, selective exotoxins that drastically alter the physiologic functions of their target tissues (the intestinal epithelium and the cholinergic nerves respectively) without any tissue invasion or damage (p. 301).

66. (E); 67. (E); 68. (D); 69. (A); 70. (D); 71. (C); 72. (C)

(66) Gram-negative rods, together with the group D streptococci, now account for the majority of nosocomial and opportunistic bacterial infections. All of the gram-negative organisms have cell walls that contain lipopolysaccharide-protein complexes known as "endotoxins." The release of endotoxins from disintegrating bacteria is responsible for the dramatic systemic effects of gram-negative sepsis such as high fever, increased capillary permeability with shock, and disseminated intravascular coagulation (p. 301).

(67) All of the gram-negative bacilli grow best in the presence of oxygen and except for Enterobacter species are only facultatively anaerobic (p. 310).

(68 and 70) *Klebsiella pneumoniae* is a cause of respiratory and urinary tract infection. Klebsiella characteristically produces a bronchopneumonia distinguished by its tendency to produce multiple small abscesses and pleural involvement. Another characteristic feature of *Klebsiella pneumoniae* is the copious slimy mucopurulent exudate that oozes from the cut surface of the lung on gross pathologic examination (pp. 311–312).

(69) *Escherichia coli (E. coli)* is a common noninvasive commensal organism that inhabits the human intestine but can also cause a variety of human infections. *E. coli* is the most common cause of primary uncomplicated urinary tract infection. In addition, *E. coli* is a common cause of various suppurative intraabdominal processes such as acute cholecystitis, diverticulitis, and cholangitis (p. 311).

(71 and 72) In contrast to *E. coli, Pseudomonas aeruginosa* is of low virulence for normal individuals and usually causes nosocomial and opportunistic infections. It is the most common cause of skin infections and generalized sepsis in burn patients. Pigment-producing strains of *Pseudomonas aeruginosa* can be recognized at the bedside since they impart a bluish tinge to the purulent exudate they produce (p. 313).

73. (B); 74. (C); 75. (D); 76. (C); 77. (C); 78. (C); 79. (E)

(73) Syphilis is a venereal disease caused by *Treponema pallidum*. The untreated disease has three stages, each with its own unique features. Primary syphilis is manifest only by the painless chancre that occurs on the external genitalia at the site of treponemal invasion. Secondary syphilis appears following a latent period of two weeks to six months after the primary stage. It is characterized by a generalized skin eruption that disappears spontaneously in about four to 12 weeks.

(74) It is the tertiary stage of syphilis that appears years or decades later that has the most devastating consequences. During this final stage of disease, localized destructive lesions known as syphilitic gummas appear in virtually any tissue.

(75) Whatever the stage of the disease, the histologic hallmark of the syphilitic lesions is an obliterative endarteritis with plasma cell infiltrates. Swelling and proliferation of endothelial cells in affected arterioles and small arteries produces a characteristic concentric "onionskin" appearance and luminal narrowing.

(76) Treponemes are characteristically extremely difficult to demonstrate in the gummas of tertiary syphilis in contrast to the ease with which they are demonstrated in the lesions of primary and secondary syphilis.

(77) Central nervous system involvement is also characteristic of tertiary syphilis and may produce tabes dorsalis, a locomotor ataxia produced by degeneration of the posterior columns of the spinal cord or (78) a rapidly destructive arthritis of the knee joint known as "Charcot's joint," the result of sensory loss from the spinal cord.

(79) In contrast to the above characteristics of venereally transmitted *Treponema pallidum* infection in the adult, Hutchinson's teeth are one of the features that may result from congenital syphilis, contracted in utero from the mother (pp. 335–338).

80. (A); 81. (A); 82. (B); 83. (D); 84. (D); 85. (C); 86. (A)

(80) Among the few fungal species that infect human beings, *Candida albicans, Mucor, Aspergillus fumigatus,* and *Cryptococcus neoformans* are the most important. *Candida albicans* is the single most common form of human fungal disease. (81) The organism can be recognized by its formation of pseudohyphae, which represent concatenations of individual yeast forms.

(82) Although most fungal infection tends to occur in immunosuppressed or chronically debilitated patients, many fungal species are capable of causing disease in otherwise healthy individuals. Only mucormycosis seldom, if ever, occurs in healthy individuals and is most often encountered in patients with diabetes, acidosis, advanced malignancy, or some form of immunodeficiency. Examples of fungal infections occurring in healthy individuals are (1) vaginal candidiasis in women taking oral contraceptives; (2) colonizing aspergillosis (aspergilloma) occurring at the site of a previous lung abscess or infarct; and (3) cryptococcosis arising in a healthy individual exposed to contaminated bird excreta.

(83) *Cryptococcus neoformans* is a round budding yeast about the size of an erythrocyte that has a heavy gelantinous capsule and can be identified by a simple laboratory test known as an India ink prep. The carbon particles of the ink serve as a contrast medium that offsets the gelatinous capsule and permits ready identification of the organism. (84) In contrast to the

other fungi, *Cryptococcus neoformans* has a special affinity for the central nervous system. This organism frequently produces meningitis as a result of seeding from a primary focus in the lung, where the infection may be mild or asymptomatic. Thus, the most common form of cryptococcal infection to come to clinical attention is meningitis.

(85) Aspergillus is distinctive among the fungi in its ability to produce disease in the absence of true infection. In some sensitized individuals, inhalation of aspergillus spores leads to a florid hypersensitivity pneumonitis. This immunologically mediated lung disease, known as bronchopulmonary aspergillosis, can produce marked pulmonary pathology in the absence of actual colonization or infiltration of the lung by organisms.

(86) Oral thrush is the name by which candidiasis of the oral cavity is commonly known. Although it may occur in adults receiving broad-spectrum antibiotic therapy, it is most commonly encountered in neonates, especially those who are bottle-fed. In infants, the disease is usually self-limited and disappears when the normal microflora of the mouth develop (*pp. 352–356*).

87. (B); 88. (D); 89. (D); 90. (D); 91. (A); 92. (D); 93. (C)

(87) In the United States there are three major mycotic infections that occur in the normal host and establish systemic infection. They are caused by *Blastomyces dermatitidis, Coccidioides immitis,* and *Histoplasma capsulatum.* In contrast to blastomycosis and histoplasmosis, which occur most frequently in the midwestern United States, particularly in the Mississippi-Ohio River basins, coccidioidomycosis is most prevalent in the southwestern United States, especially in the San Joaquin Valley of California.

(88) The fungal agent in each of these diseases is dimorphic. These fungi grow in nature as mycelium (mold)-bearing infectious spores, which are aerosolized from contaminated soil and inhaled. (89) In the host, the fungi evolve to a yeast-like phase, the pathogenic form of the organism.

(90) The diseases have many clinical as well as microbiologic features in common. Each of these infections may produce acute disease, chronic progressive disease, or no symptoms at all. In fact, asymptomatic disease is the most common outcome in all three of these disorders.

(91) In the systemic form of blastomycosis, the skin is commonly involved and may be the only site of active infection. Skin lesions typically consist of fleshy fungating ulcers that may be confused with cutaneous malignancies. Although coccidioidomycosis and histoplasmosis may cause cutaneous infection with dissemination, it is not common.

(92) The histologic hallmark of all of these fungal infections is granulomatous inflammation, and all may be counted among the causes of granulomatous lung disease. (93) Only histoplasmosis, however, is known to produce the condition known as sclerosing mediastinitis. This results from extension of the histoplasma infection from the mediastinal lymph nodes into the surrounding tissues, causing progressive scarring and contraction of mediastinal structures. This condition may appear as a mediastinal mass and can be confused with a malignancy such as lymphoma (*pp. 356–359*).

94. (A); 95. (A); 96. (A); 97. (C); 98. (E)

(94) Malaria, babesiosis, and Chagas' disease are protozoal diseases caused by Plasmodia species, Babesia species, and *Trypanosoma cruzi* respectively. Although all of these diseases are transmitted to man by insects, only malaria is transmitted by mosquitos. Babesiosis is transmitted by a tick, and Chagas' disease is transmitted by "kissing bugs" or reduviid bugs.

(95) The protozoal agents of both malaria and babesiosis characteristically invade red blood cells and may be difficult to differentiate from one another. A distinguishing feature of malaria, however, is the characteristic pigment found in the cells of the monocyte-phagocyte system. The pigment represents products of heme digestion that have been released into the bloodstream upon destruction of the infected erythrocytes. In babesiosis, pigment is not found in the cells of the monocyte-phagocyte system.

(96) Sickle cell hemoglobin has a protective effect in infection by Plasmodia, since it forces the parasite to leave the cell when sickling begins and since erythrocytes have a shortened life span in sickle cell disease.

(97) In contrast to malaria and babesiosis, Chagas' disease is produced by an organism that does not multiply within the bloodstream. The trypanosomes invade tissues to proliferate, and the subsequent tissue injury induces inflammation. The heart is the organ most frequently involved by parasitic invasion. Thus, acute myocarditis or chronic heart disease with progressive cardiac failure are characteristic of Chagas' disease.

(98) Progressive brain dysfunction is not a feature of any of these three diseases. It is characteristic of *African trypanosomiasis,* so-called "sleeping sickness" (*pp. 366–371*).

99. (D); 100. (E); 101. (C); 102. (A); 103. (B)

Worms are the largest human parasites and produce a number of distinctive diseases. Among the most common are ascariasis, hookworm disease, strongyloidiasis, and pinworm infection (enterobiasis).

(99) The pinworm, *Enterobius vermicularis,* causes the childhood "night itch" syndrome in children when the female worms migrate to the anal skin for egg laying during the night.

(**100**) The worm that typically invades striated muscle is *Trichinella spiralis*. Trichinosis is acquired by ingesting viable cysts present in meat that has been inadequately cooked.

(**101**) *Strongyloides stercoralis* is a roundworm that causes human disease principally by inhabiting the gut lumen, damaging the mucosa, and giving rise to the malabsorption syndrome. Since its eggs mature high in the intestine, duodenal aspiration or biopsy may be particularly helpful in diagnosing this form of helminth infection.

(**102**) *Ascaris lumbricoides* is another intestinal roundworm that tends to be a luminal dweller. In contrast to the malabsorption syndrome of strongyloidiasis, intestinal obstruction by worms tends to be more characteristic of ascariasis.

(**103**) Like strongyloidiasis, hookworm infection is acquired by larval penetration, migration to the lung via the blood, and finally intestinal luminal habitation after being coughed and swallowed by the host. Once in the small intestine, hookworms attach themselves to the mucosal villi and continuously suck blood from the underlying capillaries, causing chronic blood loss (*pp. 376–377*).

5

THE CARDIOVASCULAR SYSTEM

DIRECTIONS: For Questions 1 to 17, choose the ONE BEST answer to each question.

1. Myocardial hypertrophy is most accurately assessed by:

A. Left ventricular wall thickness
B. Histologic appearance of left ventricular myocardium
C. Weight of the heart
D. Measurement of the heart size by chest radiogram
E. None of these

2. Which of the following situations is the most common outcome of an acute myocardial infarction?

A. Sudden cardiac death
B. Recovery without complications
C. Left ventricular congestive failure
D. Cardiogenic shock
E. Cardiac arrhythmias

3. The most common cause of death from systemic hypertension is:

A. Stroke
B. Aortic aneurysm rupture
C. Heart failure
D. Renal failure
E. Berry aneurysm rupture

4. Major risk factors for myocardial infarction include all of the following EXCEPT:

A. Cigarette smoking
B. Hyperlipidemia
C. Systemic hypertension
D. Obesity
E. Diabetes mellitus

5. Immediate consequences of a first ischemic cardiac event include all of the following EXCEPT:

A. Angina pectoris
B. Sudden death without infarction
C. Transmural infarction
D. Cardiac rupture
E. No symptoms

6. Compared with the rest of the myocardium, the subendocardial region is at higher risk of ischemic injury for all of the following reasons EXCEPT:

A. The subendocardial muscle has a higher metabolic demand than the rest of the myocardium
B. The intermuscular vascular bed is compressed with the greatest force in this area
C. Vascular tone and capacity for dilatation are poor in this region
D. This region is less likely to have a collateral vascular supply
E. This region is most remote from the central coronary arterial supply

7. Therapeutic regimens currently employed with the aim of improving long-term survival following myocardial infarction include all of the following EXCEPT:

A. Treatment with hyaluronidase
B. Treatment with beta adrenergic blocking agents
C. Treatment with calcium channel blocking agents
D. Oral anticoagulant therapy
E. Aspirin administration

8. *Chronic* ischemic heart disease is characterized by all of the following EXCEPT:

A. Chronic angina pectoris
B. Myocardial atrophy
C. Severe stenosing coronary atherosclerosis
D. Diffuse, small myocardial scars
E. Evolution to congestive heart failure

9. Compensated hypertensive heart disease is associated with all of the following features EXCEPT:

A. Reduced contractility of myocardial fibers
B. Doubling of normal heart weight
C. Increased myocardial oxygen demand
D. Marked increase in cardiac silhouette by chest x-ray
E. Absence of clinical symptoms

10. Microscopic features of hypertensive heart disease include all of the following EXCEPT:

A. Increased diameter of myofibers
B. Increased size of myofiber nuclei
C. Hyperchromatism of myofiber nuclei

D. Increased number of capillaries between my-ofibers

E. Thickening of intramyocardial arterioles

11. Cardiac changes related to aging (senile changes of unknown etiology) include all of the following EXCEPT:

A. Calcific aortic stenosis
B. Mitral stenosis
C. Mitral anulus calcification
D. Cardiac amyloidosis
E. Brown atrophy of the heart

12. Common complications of prosthetic heart valves include all of the following EXCEPT:

A. Hemolytic anemia
B. Infective endocarditis
C. Mechanical malfunction of the prosthesis
D. Arrhythmias
E. Thromboembolism

13. Antibodies to streptococcal M proteins cross-react with all of the following tissue antigens EXCEPT:

A. Cardiac myofiber–smooth muscle antigens
B. Synovial cell antigens
C. Heart valve fibroblast antigens
D. Neuronal antigens in the central nervous system
E. Connective tissue antigens

14. All of the following statements about isolated aortic stenosis are true EXCEPT:

A. Most isolated aortic stenosis is rheumatic in origin

B. It is often associated with an underlying congenital valvular malformation
C. Asymptomatic left ventricular hypertrophy develops
D. Critical stenosis is not reached until ⅔ of the valve area is obstructed
E. Heart failure is the most common cause of death

15. Pathologic findings often associated with infective endocarditis include all of the following EXCEPT:

A. Lung abscesses
B. Acute splenitis
C. Glomerulonephritis
D. Linear hemorrhages in nail beds
E. Cerebral emboli

16. Infectious myocarditis is commonly caused by all of the following EXCEPT:

A. Coxsackie A virus
B. Trypanosoma (Chagas' disease)
C. Diphtheria bacillus
D. Staphylococcus
E. Meningococcus

17. Hypertrophic cardiomyopathy (idiopathic hypertrophic subaortic stenosis) is characterized by all of the following features EXCEPT:

A. A disproportionately enlarged ventricular septum
B. Aortic valve thickening
C. Myofiber disarray in the ventricular septum
D. Small left ventricular volume
E. Large left atrial volume

DIRECTIONS: For Questions 18 to 23, ONE or MORE of the completions given correctly finishes the incomplete statement. Choose:

A—if only *1,2, and 3* are correct
B—if only *1 and 3* are correct
C—if only *2 and 4* are correct
D—if only *4* is correct
E—if all are correct

18. Cardiac toxicity is known to be produced by which of the following chemotherapeutic agents?

1. Prednisone
2. Cyclophosphamide
3. Bleomycin
4. Adriamycin

A. 1,2,3   B. 1,3   C. 2,4   D. 4 Only   E. All

19. Causes of cor pulmonale include:

1. Pulmonary embolus
2. Pickwickian syndrome
3. Chronic lung disease
4. Congenital heart disease

A. 1,2,3   B. 1,3   C. 2,4   D. 4 Only   E. All

20. Which of the following histologic features are characteristic of normal cardiac muscle?

1. Intercalated discs
2. Peripherally located nuclei
3. Branching myofibers
4. Longitudinal striations

A. 1,2,3   B. 1,3   C. 2,4   D. 4 Only   E. All

21. Which of the following statements about cardiac myxomas is/are true?

1. They are the most common primary tumor of the heart

2. They occur most frequently in the left ventricle
3. They are often associated with syncopal attacks
4. They tend to be malignant in the pediatric age group

A. 1,2,3   B. 1,3   C. 2,4   D. 4 Only   E. All

22. Which of the following factors is/are known to exacerbate ischemic heart disease?

1. Pregnancy
2. Myocardial hypertrophy
3. Anemia
4. Tachycardia

A. 1,2,3   B. 1,3   C. 2,4   D. 4 Only   E. All

23. In a patient with myocardial hypertrophy, the diagnosis of hypertensive heart disease *cannot* be made if the individual has:

1. No prior history of hypertension
2. Idiopathic hypertrophic subaortic stenosis
3. Takayasu's arteritis
4. Aortic stenosis

A. 1,2,3   B. 1,3   C. 2,4   D. 4 Only   E. All

DIRECTIONS: For Questions 24 to 45, you are to decide whether EACH choice is TRUE or FALSE.

For each of the statements about myocardial infarction (MI) listed below, choose whether it is TRUE or FALSE.

24. In the United States, more than 3000 people suffer myocardial infarctions every day
25. Only a minority of cases are associated with widespread, severe coronary atherosclerosis
26. The incidence of MI is higher in whites than in blacks
27. The incidence of fatal MI in males decreases after age 65
28. Physical conditioning (exercise) is associated with a reduction in the rate of fatal MI

For each of the following statements about rheumatic fever (RF), choose whether it is TRUE or FALSE.

29. The disease is caused by systemic infection and tissue invasion by group A beta hemolytic streptococcus
30. Rheumatoid arthritis is a late complication of previously involved joint tissues
31. Rheumatic heart disease is a late complication of previously involved heart tissues
32. Rheumatic fever is more common in children than in adults
33. Culture-positive streptococcal pharyngitis is usually present at the onset of a rheumatic attack
34. Prompt antibiotic therapy of streptococcal pharyngitis is the major factor in the declining incidence of acute RF

35. Group A streptococcal infections of the skin are more likely to cause acute glomerulonephritis than acute RF
36. There is no correlation between the severity of the initial streptococcal infection and the likelihood of developing RF
37. An individual who has once had acute RF is more vulnerable to developing the disease again
38. In the absence of cardiac involvement, complete recovery without residual pathologic changes is the rule
39. Prophylactic long-term antistreptococcal therapy is required for patients who have had RF
40. Genetic predisposition is suggested by the high incidence of HLA-B27 antigens in affected individuals

For each of the following statements about carcinoid heart disease, choose whether it is TRUE or FALSE.

41. The disease is unlikely to develop in association with intestinal carcinoid tumors unless liver metastases are present
42. The disease mainly affects the left side of the heart
43. The characteristic lesion is an endocardial plaque rich in elastic fibers
44. The disease usually produces insufficiency of affected valves
45. The tumor product believed to induce the characteristic lesions is kallikrein

DIRECTIONS: For Questions 46 to 90, the set of lettered headings is followed by a list of numbered words or phrases. For each numbered word or phrase choose:
A—if the item is associated with (A) only
B—if the item is associated with (B) only
C—if the item is associated with *both* (A) and (B)
D—if the item is associated with *neither* (A) nor (B)

For each of the features listed below, decide whether it describes atherosclerotic aneurysm, syphilitic aneurysm, both, or neither.

   A. Atherosclerotic aneurysm
   B. Syphilitic aneurysm
   C. Both
   D. Neither

46. Marked dilatation of the aorta is NOT a common feature
47. The thoracic aorta is usually involved
48. Most fatalities occur from rupture
49. Cystic medial necrosis is the characteristic histopathologic change
50. Aggressive antihypertensive therapy is indicated

For each of the following statements, choose whether it describes acute bacterial endocarditis, subacute bacterial endocarditis, both, or neither.

   A. Acute bacterial endocarditis
   B. Subacute bacterial endocarditis
   C. Both
   D. Neither

51. Distinguished by a rapidly declining incidence rate
52. Produced by *Staphylococcus aureus* in the majority of cases
53. Characteristically occurs on an abnormal valve
54. Yields positive blood cultures in 90% of cases
55. Produces painful subcutaneous nodules in palms and soles (Osler's nodes)
56. Associated with chronic alcoholism
57. Associated with drug addiction

For each of the characteristics listed below, choose whether it describes rheumatic mitral valve disease, mitral valve prolapse (floppy valve syndrome), both, or neither.

   A. Rheumatic mitral valve disease
   B. Mitral valve prolapse (floppy valve syndrome)
   C. Both
   D. Neither

58. Occurs more commonly in women
59. Predisposes to bacterial endocarditis
60. Causes commissural fusion of valve cusps

61. Causes fibrosis and thickening of chordae tendineae
62. Associated with ventricular arrhythmias and sudden death
63. Eventually requires valve replacement in most cases

For each of the features listed below, choose whether it describes valvular heart disease producing regurgitation, stenosis, both of these, or neither of these.

   A. Valvular regurgitation
   B. Valvular stenosis
   C. Both
   D. Neither

64. Characterized by failure of the valve to open completely
65. Characterized by failure of the valve to close completely
66. Almost always due to abnormalities of the valve cusps alone
67. Produced by postinflammatory scarring (rheumatic heart disease)
68. Produced by infective endocarditis
69. Occasionally occurs in association with rheumatoid arthritis
70. Frequently produced by severe atherosclerosis

For each of the characteristics listed below, choose whether it describes subendocardial myocardial infarction, transmural myocardial infarction, both, or neither.

   A. Subendocardial infarction
   B. Transmural infarction
   C. Both
   D. Neither

71. Severe atherosclerosis of multiple extramyocardial coronary vessels is usually present
72. Stenosing atherosclerosis of penetrating intramyocardial arterial vessels is usually present
73. The distribution of the myocardial lesion correlates closely with pathologic findings in the corresponding vessel
74. Acute coronary thrombosis is present in most cases

75. Involvement is limited to the left ventricle in most cases
76. This lesion constitutes major findings at autopsy in most patients who suffer sudden cardiac death

For each of the following cardiac regions, choose whether it usually receives its blood supply from the left coronary artery, the right coronary artery, both, or neither.

    A. Left coronary artery
    B. Right coronary artery
    C. Both
    D. Neither

77. Interventricular septum
78. Anterior wall of the left ventricle
79. Posterior wall of the left ventricle
80. Mitral valve
81. Anterior wall of the right ventricle

82. Posterior wall of the right ventricle
83. Endothelium of the left lateral wall

For each of the following features, choose whether it is *commonly* associated with left-sided heart failure, with right-sided heart failure, both left and right heart failure, or neither.

    A. Left-sided heart failure
    B. Right-sided heart failure
    C. Both
    D. Neither

84. Caused by ischemic heart disease
85. Caused by valvular heart disease
86. Caused by chronic obstructive pulmonary disease
87. Produces pulmonary edema
88. Produces aldosterone-induced sodium retention
89. Produces prerenal azotemia
90. Produces centrilobular necrosis of liver

DIRECTIONS: Questions 91 to 131 are matching questions. For each numbered item, choose the most likely associated lettered item from those provided. Each numbered item has ONLY ONE answer. Within each group, each lettered item may be the answer to one, more than one, or none of the numbered items.

For each of the characteristics listed below, choose whether it corresponds to a transmural myocardial infarction less than 4 hours old, 4 to 24 hours old, 1 to 2 days old, 2 to 4 days old, 5 to 14 days old, or none of these.

    A. Less than 4 hours old
    B. 4 to 24 hours old
    C. 1 to 2 days old
    D. 2 to 4 days old
    E. 5 to 14 days old
    F. None of these

91. Peak serum levels of myocardial lactate dehydrogenase
92. Peak tissue infiltration by neutrophils
93. Normal appearance of myocardium on gross examination
94. Peak serum levels of creatine kinase
95. Formation of granulation tissue at the periphery of the infarct
96. Maximal coagulative necrosis
97. Predominance of macrophages in the inflammatory infiltrate

For each of the features of vasculitis listed below, choose whether it is characteristic of polyarteritis nodosa, giant cell arteritis, Kawasaki's disease, Buerger's disease, or none of these.

    A. Polyarteritis nodosa
    B. Giant cell arteritis
    C. Kawasaki's disease
    D. Buerger's disease
    E. None of these

98. Young children and infants are most often affected
99. The disease is rare under age 50
100. Cigarette smoking is an etiologic factor
101. Cardiac involvement is very common
102. Kidney involvement is very common
103. Gangrene of the extremities is often produced
104. Lymph node enlargement is an associated finding
105. Response to steroids alone is excellent

For each of the conditions listed below, choose the type of pericardial effusion it is most likely to produce.

    A. Serous effusion
    B. Serosanguineous effusion
    C. Chylous effusion

D. Cholesterol effusion
E. Serosuppurative effusion

106. Cardiopulmonary resuscitation
107. Myxedema
108. Congestive heart failure
109. Nephrotic syndrome
110. Mediastinal tumor

For each of the causes of ischemic heart disease listed below, choose the pathogenetic mechanism with which it is most closely related.

    A. Atherosclerotic narrowing of coronary arteries
    B. Vasospasm of coronary arteries
    C. Coronary osteal stenosis
    D. Coronary embolism
    E. Systemic hypotension
    F. Coronary artery thrombosis

111. Syphilitic (luetic) aortitis
112. Myocardial infarction associated with surgery
113. Prinzmetal's (variant) angina
114. Nonbacterial thrombotic endocarditis
115. Chronic ischemic heart disease
116. Rheumatoid arteritis
117. Stable angina pectoris

For each of the statements listed below, choose whether it describes stable angina only, unstable angina only, Prinzmetal's angina only, both stable and unstable angina, both unstable and Prinzmetal's angina, or all of these.

    A. Stable angina only
    B. Unstable angina only
    C. Prinzmetal's angina only
    D. A and B
    E. B and C
    F. All of these

118. Induced by exertion, relieved by rest
119. Most commonly accompanied by S-T segment elevation on EKG
120. Most commonly accompanied by S-T segment depression on EKG
121. Occurs at rest
122. Frequently associated with normal coronary artery angiographic findings
123. Frequently causes reversible injury to myocardial cells
124. Associated with very high risk of myocardial infarction

Match each of the therapeutic alternatives for treatment of acute myocardial infarction listed below with the most important rationale for its use.

    A. Reduction of myocardial oxygen demand
    B. Prevention of coronary thrombosis
    C. Coronary thrombolysis
    D. Reduction of coronary vasospasms
    E. Relief of pain
    F. None of these

125. Phenobarbital
126. Verapamil
127. Streptokinase
128. Morphine
129. Enforced activity restriction
130. Propranolol
131. Lidocaine

5

THE CARDIOVASCULAR SYSTEM

ANSWERS

1. (C) Heart weight is the most accurate reflection of myocardial hypertrophy. It is independent of such superimposed factors as cardiac dilatation in the failing heart, the contractile state of the ventricles that could cause variations in the ventricular wall thickness, or the histologic picture of the left ventricular myocardium. Measurement of heart size by cardiac silhouette on chest x-ray is the least accurate way to assess myocardial hypertrophy; a markedly hypertrophied heart may have a normal cardiac silhouette size. Only when the hypertrophied heart begins to fail and undergo dilatation will the cardiac silhouette increase in size.

Although the weight of the heart varies with the stature of the individual, the range of normal heart weight for the average female is 250 to 300 grams, and for the average male 300 to 350 grams (*p. 568*).

2. (E) Acute myocardial infarctions are seldom without complications. In fact, the initial ischemic event proves fatal in approximately ¼ of the patients. Of those who survive, only approximately 10 to 20% recover without complications. Over half of the survivors (60%) develop left ventricular congestive failure and pulmonary edema, but only 10 to 15% suffer frank cardiogenic shock. By far the most common complication of myocardial infarction is the appearance of cardiac arrhythmias. Ninety per cent of patients who survive an acute ischemic event develop arrhythmias, and it is believed that arrhythmias are responsible for many of the sudden deaths related to cardiac ischemia (*pp. 564–565*).

3. (C) Hypertensive heart disease is the second most common cause of cardiac death. Although the morbidity and mortality from hypertension and hypertensive heart disease have been declining, hypertension remains a major health problem. Although this positive trend has been attributed to effective treatment methods, the decline in mortality actually began before such therapy was widely used. At present, about 30 to 50% of patients with untreated systemic hypertension die of hypertensive heart disease, most commonly heart failure. The remainder usually succumb to stroke, hypertensive renal vascular disease, or vascular complications such as aneurysms. Rupture of berry aneurysms is frequently unrelated to systemic hypertension (*p. 567*).

4. (D) Epidemiological studies have shown that an increased risk of myocardial infarction is associated with numerous variable factors. Cigarette smoking increases the risk of myocardial infarction from 2 to 20 times over that of nonsmokers. Both present and past use of oral contraceptives has been shown to carry an increased risk of myocardial infarction in women. Current users have about a 3- to 4-fold greater risk of myocardial infarction than controls who never used oral contraceptives, whereas past users have twice the risk if the oral contraceptives were used for 5 years or more. There is also a clearcut association between systemic hypertension and susceptibility to ischemic heart disease and myocardial infarction. The higher the blood pressure, the greater the risk, with diastolic pressure being the most important predictive factor. Diastolic pressures greater than 105 mm. Hg are associated with a 4-fold risk of ischemic heart disease over that of individuals with diastolic pressures of 84 mm. Hg or less.

Numerous prospective studies in well-defined population groups have identified hyperlipidemia as a major risk factor predisposing to ischemic heart disease. Of particular significance is the level of low-density lipoproteins, which contain about 70% of the total plasma cholesterol and are strongly correlated with atherosclerosis. In contrast, the serum levels of high-density lipoproteins are inversely related to risk of ischemic heart disease. Diabetes mellitus is a clearcut risk factor for ischemic heart disease and is associated with an increase in atherosclerosis observed at autopsy and a 2-fold increase in the incidence of myocardial infarction as compared with nondiabetics.

Although obesity is not considered to be a *major* risk factor for myocardial infarction, it tends to exacerbate hyperlipidemia, hypertension, and diabetes mellitus when present and may act as a risk factor independent of other associations (*p. 508*).

5. (D) The immediate consequences of acute cardiac ischemia are varied and include (1) reversible ischemic injury producing classic substernal chest pain known as angina pectoris, (2) sudden death without infarction believed in most cases to be related to ischemia-induced arrhythmias, (3) irreversible transmural myocardial damage (transmural infarction), and (4) less commonly, no clinical symptomatology.

Asymptomatic ischemic heart disease is most commonly associated with diabetes mellitus, since diabetic neuropathy sometimes interferes with the sensory perception of ischemic pain.

Cardiac rupture rarely occurs as an immediate consequence of ischemic damage. It is an uncommon event that occurs many *days* (1 to 2 weeks) after an acute transmural infarction during the period of peak muscle necrosis, when weakening and thinning of the infarcted wall is most pronounced (*pp. 552, 555–560*).

6. (D) For several anatomic and physiologic reasons, the subendocardial region is the area of the heart at highest risk of myocardial infarction. It has a higher metabolic demand (oxygen requirement) than the outer zone of the myocardium and its contraction exerts a greater compressive force on the vascular bed. In addition, the intermuscular vessels of this region have a lower vascular tone, which limits their capacity for dilatation. Anatomically, the subendocardial region is the most remote from the central coronary arterial supply in the heart's modified end-arterial system. Any fall in pressure in the system, therefore, would affect the subendocardium first. There is no evidence, however, that the collateral vascular supply to this region is less abundant than that in peripheral zones of the myocardium (*pp. 553, 557*).

7. (A) There are two basic aims of therapy of acute myocardial infarction: (1) acute intervention to improve immediate survival and to reduce or limit the size of the infarction and (2) long-term intervention to improve survival during the year or two following the acute infarction. Clinical studies have shown that the long-term prognosis is improved by treatment with beta adrenergic blocking agents, calcium channel blocking agents (e.g., nifedipine, verapamil), oral anticoagulants, and antiplatelet drugs such as aspirin. Hyaluronidase, however, is a drug used in the immediate postinfarction period in an attempt to rescue the muscle at the edge of an infarct from irreversible injury. Its beneficial effect on myofiber recovery is believed to result from depolymerization of mucopolysaccharides in the ground substance of the myocardial interstitium. This, in turn, facilitates transport of substrates (nutrients) to injured myofibers at the edge of an infarct. Hyaluronidase would, however, have no place in long-term therapy (*p. 566*).

8. (A) Chronic ischemic heart disease is characterized by insidious ischemic atrophy of the myocardium from atherosclerotic narrowing of the coronary arteries. Histologically, diffuse, small myocardial scars are present amid atrophic myofibers. As more and more myofibers undergo ischemic atrophy, cardiac decompensation occurs, and congestive heart failure develops. Although some patients have anginal attacks or acute myocardial infarctions during the course of their disease, chronic ischemic heart disease is usually asymptomatic until heart failure becomes manifest. Thus, chronic continuing anginal pain is not usually a feature of this form of heart disease (*pp. 566–567*).

9. (D) Hypertensive heart disease is characteristically insidious in its onset. It develops over a period of time during which the heart undergoes hypertrophy in order to maintain a normal cardiac output in the face of increased peripheral resistance. During this period of compensation, the patient is usually free of clinical symptoms. Myocardial hypertrophy may lead to a doubling of the normal heart weight with significantly increased myocardial oxygen demand and decreased myofiber contractility. During the compensated phase of hypertensive heart disease, however, the size of the heart as measured by chest x-ray is not significantly increased. Only when the heart can no longer compensate and dilatation of the failing heart ensues does the cardiac silhouette on chest x-ray show a significant increase (*pp. 567–569*).

10. (D) The microscopic changes of myocardial hypertrophy and hypertensive heart disease are subtle and require close attention to the cytologic features of the myofibers. Characteristic features of hypertrophied myofibers include (1) increased cell diameter, (2) increased nuclear size, and (3) nuclear hyperchromatism. The intramyocardial arterioles, like arterioles elsewhere in the body, are thickened as a result of the hypertension, but there is no other alteration of the myocardial vascular bed. Although the myocardial oxygen demand is increased, there is no detectable change in the number or distribution of capillaries in the hypertensive heart (*p. 568*).

11. (B) A number of cardiac changes are associated with aging, although their etiologies remain largely unknown. Such senile changes include calcific aortic stenosis, a fibrotic and calcific deformity of the aortic valve in the elderly that in most cases is related to neither a congenitally deformed valve nor a healed infective endocarditis. Equally obscure in its etiology is calcification of the mitral annulus or deposition of amyloid in the geriatric heart. Brown atrophy refers to the organ shrinkage (atrophy) and lipofuscin accumulation that are sometimes seen in the heart and/or liver of elderly patients.

Mitral stenosis is usually the result of injury from rheumatic heart disease but may also occur as a consequence of healed infective endocarditis. It does not occur as a nonspecific concomitant of aging (*pp. 23, 200, 574, 578–579*).

12. (D) Diseased heart valves are frequently surgically excised and replaced by mechanical or bioprosthetic valves. Although valvular heart disease produces significant morbidity and mortality, prosthetic valves used in treatment are also associated with numerous complications and considerable risks.

Hemolytic anemia may develop from the mechanical destruction of erythrocytes passing through the prosthesis, especially one that is degraded from wear. Partial separation of the suture line anchoring the valve (dehiscence), besides occasionally causing mechanical problems, may cause hemolysis as blood is forced through the narrow channel of the dehiscence. The prosthesis may become septic, seeded by blood-borne bacteria. The resultant prosthesis-associated infective endocarditis is a serious complication and is often fatal. The prosthesis itself may cease to function properly for a number of mechanical reasons, the most common being: 1) the formation of a thrombus in a strategic area, impairing the function of a moving part, and 2) degradation of the materials from which the valve is constructed. Mechanical prostheses vary in their thrombogenic potential, but thromboembolic problems remain one of the most frequent causes of prosthesis-associated fatalities.

Whereas arrhythmias occasionally occur in the postoperative period, they are not commonly associated with prosthetic valves installed by an experienced cardiac surgeon (p. 571).

13. (B) Thus far, four distinct types of streptococcal antibodies have been identified that cross-react with four separate tissue targets: (1) cardiac smooth muscle antigens, (2) heart valve fibroblast antigens, (3) central nervous system neuronal antigens, and (4) connective tissue antigens. It is believed that these four antibodies are related to the tissue injury that produces the carditis, valvulitis, Sydenham's chorea, and subcutaneous rheumatoid nodule formation that characterize rheumatic fever. Although rheumatic arthritis occurs in over 90% of adults with rheumatic fever (less commonly in children), a streptococcal antibody cross-reacting with synovial cells has not been identified (see Question 30 and p. 572).

14. (A) Although aortic stenosis may occur in rheumatic heart disease, either alone or in combination with mitral valve involvement, most isolated calcific aortic stenoses are nonrheumatic in origin. Although the etiology is obscure in most cases, isolated aortic stenosis is often associated with a congenitally deformed (bicuspid) valve or advanced age. Left ventricular hypertrophy occurs with the obstruction to left ventricular outflow, but this is usually asymptomatic until the point of critical severity has been reached. Critical obstruction usually occurs when the valve orifice is constricted to two thirds of its original area. Once symptoms occur, the prognosis is poor. The average survival after onset of symptoms is 2 to 3 years, with heart failure being the most common cause of death (p. 578).

15. (A) Several pathologic conditions may be associated with infective endocarditis. These include secondary infection of other organs from bacteria that seed from the infected valve. The spleen is commonly involved in such a process (acute splenitis), as are the kidney and brain. Complications may also be produced by the formation of immune complexes producing an acute vasculitis. In the skin, immune complex–induced vasculitis produces small hemorrhages, which may also appear in the nail beds; in the kidney, glomerulonephritis may result. Septic emboli from the friable valvular vegetations may also produce nail bed hemorrhages or even microabscesses. Valvular vegetations often embolize to the brain and kidney as well, where they produce infarction and metastatic abscesses. Lung abscesses, however, are rarely associated with infective endocarditis, since the right side of the heart is so infrequently involved. Only in bacterial endocarditis associated with drug abuse are right heart valves typically affected and metastatic abscesses in the lung produced (pp. 583–584).

16. (D) A multitude of microorganisms may cause infectious endocarditis, including viruses, chlamydia, bacteria, fungi, and metazoans. Viruses are the most common cause of myocarditis, producing over half of all cases. Coxsackie A and B, ECHO, polio, and influenza viruses are the most frequently encountered viral agents. Among the causative bacterial agents are diphtheria bacillus, meningococcus, and leptospira. Although Chagas' disease is uncommon in the United States, trypanosoma is a common cause of myocarditis in endemic regions. Staphylococcus, although a common cause of endocarditis, rarely causes myocarditis (pp. 593–594).

17. (B) Hypertrophic cardiomyopathy, commonly known as idiopathic hypertrophic subaortic stenosis, is characterized by asymmetric ventricular septal hypertrophy. Microscopically, a characteristic pattern of myofiber disarray is seen in the involved portion of the septum. The thickened septal wall causes a reduction in the volume of the left ventricular cavity in 90% of the cases and a dilated left atrium in virtually every case. The aortic valve itself, however, is characteristically normal in this condition and does not contribute to the aortic outflow obstruction (pp. 597–599).

18. (C) Cause of damage to heart muscle is known to be produced by numerous chemical agents, including some that are used in the treatment of malignant tumors. Cyclophosphamide and adriamycin (doxorubicin), as well as daunorubicin, are common chemotherapeutic agents that have known cardiac toxicity. Neither prednisone nor bleomycin, however, is known to cause cardiac toxicity (pp. 601–602).

19. (A) Cor pulmonale, or pulmonary heart disease, refers to right ventricular enlargement occurring as a consequence of hypertension in the pulmonary vascular tree. The pulmonary hypertension may be primary or may result from pulmonary parenchymal disease with secondary vascular changes. Occasionally, pulmonary hypertension may be produced by inadequate function of the chest bellows (e.g., Pickwickian syndrome) or inadequate ventilatory drive from the respiratory centers in the brain. In addition, acute cor pulmonale may develop from massive pulmonary embolization. Since the definition of cor pulmonale is limited to right ventricular hypertrophy or dilatation secondary to disorders of lung structure or function, acquired or congenital heart diseases, even though they may involve the right heart, are not included in this disease complex (pp. 569–570).

20. (B) Cardiac muscle is a highly specialized form of striated muscle that can easily be distinguished from skeletal muscle on the basis of several unique histologic features. Cardiac muscle has a characteristic branching pattern of myofibers that are joined to one another by specialized structures known as intercoalated discs. This branching pattern contrasts with the regular parallel alignment of skeletal muscle cells, which connect not to each other but rather to the connective tissue of the muscle sheath or its tendinous insertion. Also unique to cardiac muscle is the central location of the nuclei within the muscle fibers. In skeletal muscle, the nuclei occupy a peripheral position. These differences notwithstanding, both types of striated muscle are characterized histologically by so-called "cross striations" of the cell cytoplasm, an illusion created by the alignment of the A band and I band of the myofibrils across the short axis of the cell. Striated muscle, in fact, is named for this feature. Longitudinal striations are characteristic of smooth, rather than striated, muscle (pp. 547–548).

21. (B) Cardiac myxomas are the most common primary tumor of the heart. They occur most frequently in the atria. When they occur in the left atrium, they are associated with intermittent ball valve obstruction of the mitral valve orifice and often produce syncopal attacks.

Cardiac myxomas are benign tumors in all age groups. Their major morbidity and mortality is associated with fragmentation and embolization or the above-mentioned ball valve obstruction that may lead to acute cardiac insufficiency and even sudden death (pp. 605–606).

22. (E) Ischemic heart disease may be produced by processes that create an imbalance between myocardial oxygen supply and myocardial oxygen demand. A diminished oxygen-carrying capacity of the blood (anemia) will reduce myocardial oxygen supply. Increased muscle mass (myocardial hypertrophy), increased contractile activity (tachycardia), or increased cardiac output states (pregnancy) will increase myocardial oxygen demand. All of these factors may be superimposed on coronary atherosclerosis and contribute significantly to the production of myocardial ischemia (p. 555).

23. (E) Two criteria must be met in order to make the diagnosis of hypertensive heart disease: a prior history of hypertension and left ventricular hypertrophy as an isolated finding. The diagnosis of hypertensive heart disease cannot be made in the presence of other cardiovascular abnormalities, which can themselves lead to increased left ventricular pressure or volume overload with subsequent compensatory hypertrophy (e.g., idiopathic hypertrophic subaortic stenosis; valvular disease that impedes left ventricular outflow, such as aortic stenosis; or disease of the aorta, such as Takayasu's arteritis). In Takayasu's arteritis, systemic hypertension may be produced by a primary effect on the aorta or a secondary effect on the renal artery. Although concomitant hypertension may occur in these disease processes, their presence precludes the diagnosis of hypertensive heart disease, which refers exclusively to cardiac hypertrophy resulting from primary systemic hypertension (p. 567).

24. (True); 25. (False); 26. (True); 27. (True); 28. (True)

(24) Myocardial infarction is the most important consequence of ischemic heart disease. It is, unfortunately, very common in the United States, where about 3400 individuals suffer a myocardial infarction each day.

(25) The vast majority of cases of myocardial infarction are associated with severe, widespread atherosclerosis of the coronary arteries. Thus the primary importance of coronary atherosclerosis in the pathogenesis of MI is evident.

(26) The incidence of MI is higher among whites than blacks, although blacks tend to die of MI at a younger age.

(27) The incidence of fatal MI rises steadily with increased age to a peak incidence in the 55- to 64-year-old age group. Most male deaths from MI occur between the ages of 35 and 64. Thereafter, the incidence of MI begins to decline.

(28) A number of variables are believed to influence the risk and/or outcome of MI. Coincident with the current interest in physical fitness, a number of studies have been carried out that suggest that regular physical conditioning reduces the rate of fatal MI. However, there is no sound evidence that exercise plays a role in the *prevention* of coronary atherosclerosis (pp. 556–557).

29. (False); 30. (False); 31. (True); 32. (True); 33. (False); 34. (True); 35. (True); 36. (False); 37. (True); 38. (True); 39. (True); 40. (False)

(29) Rheumatic fever is an inflammatory disease

process that is caused not by infection by group A beta hemolytic streptococcus but rather by the immunologic response to that organism. Thus, tissue damage in this disease is not the direct result of streptococcal sepsis but is produced by immunologically-mediated injury most likely occurring as the result of cross-reactivity between streptococcal antigens and native tissue antigens.

(30) Although the heart is the most common tissue damaged by this process, the large joints may also be affected, producing a migratory polyarthritis known as rheumatic arthritis (not rheumatoid arthritis). Rheumatic arthritis is a transitory process and always resolves without sequelae. Rheumatoid arthritis, on the other hand, is a chronic systemic inflammatory disease of unknown etiology that produces progressive crippling deformity of involved joints. There is no known etiologic connection between the two diseases, despite the similarity of their names.

(31) The most significant consequence of rheumatic fever is injury to the cardiac tissues. Although injury may be produced in any layer of the heart from epicardium to endocardium, it is rheumatic valvulitis that produces the most significant late complications. Injured valves undergo progressive fibrous scarring and permanent deformity.

(32) Although acute rheumatic fever is principally a disease of children, it does occur in adults and usually follows a pharyngeal infection with group A beta hemolytic streptococcus. (33) At the time of the rheumatic attack, throat cultures are usually negative. Evidence of immunologic response to streptococcal antigens in the form of antistreptolysin O (ASO), antihyaluronidase, antistreptokinase, or anti-NADase antibodies is present in 90 to 95% of patients, however.

(34) Prompt antibiotic therapy of streptococcal pharyngitis reduces the incidence of injurious immune responses and is the major factor responsible for the declining incidence of acute rheumatic fever.

(35) Streptococcal sepsis occurring through other portals of entry such as the skin (impetigo) is usually not followed by rheumatic fever. Streptococcal skin infections, like streptococcal infections elsewhere in the body, tend to induce an immune response that causes immune complex–mediated glomerulonephritis. In fact, acute rheumatic fever and acute poststreptococcal glomerulonephritis rarely occur together and do so only coincidentally. It is believed that the nephritogenic strains of streptococci lack the antigens to which the cross-reacting antibodies of rheumatic fever are directed.

(36) There is a strong correlation between the severity and duration of the initial streptococcal pharyngitis and the likelihood of developing subsequent rheumatic fever. (37) Furthermore, an individual who has once had an initial attack of rheumatic fever is more vulnerable to recurrence of the disease with subsequent bouts of streptococcal pharyngitis. If the initial attack of rheumatic fever produces carditis, subsequent attacks usually produce increasingly severe recurrences of this lesion. Even in the absence of reactivation, however, rheumatic carditis generally produces postinflammatory fibrocalcific valvular deformity as a late consequence. (38) In the absence of cardiac involvement, however, the patient often recovers completely from rheumatic fever and is spared recurrences or chronic sequelae. (39) In order to prevent recurrent attacks to which the rheumatic patient is more prone, long-term prophylactic antistreptococcal therapy is required.

(40) There is no evidence that genetic factors influence susceptibility to rheumatic fever. There is no sexual predominance in this disease nor is there a characteristic HLA profile in rheumatic fever (*pp. 571–576*).

41. (True); 42. (False); 43. (False); 44. (True); 45. (False)

(41) Involvement of the heart is one of the major histologic concomitants of the carcinoid syndrome. This syndrome is produced by carcinoid tumors (argentaffinomas) that release a variety of bioactive products into the blood stream. These substances include serotonin, kallikrein, histamine, and prostaglandins that produce the principal manifestations of the syndrome: (1) vasomotor disturbances (flushing of the skin), (2) intestinal hypermotility (diarrhea, cramps, and vomiting), and (3) bronchoconstriction (asthmalike symptoms of dyspnea and wheezing). The cardiac involvement of the carcinoid syndrome, like the syndrome itself, is unlikely to develop in association with intestinal carcinoid tumors unless liver metastases are present. Tumor products can then bypass the rapid polypeptide deamination that occurs in the liver, reach the systemic circulation, and produce the carcinoid syndrome and carcinoid heart disease. (42) The characteristic cardiac lesion associated with the syndrome occurs mainly on the right side of the heart and (43) consists of sclerotic, endocardial plaques that, unlike atherosclerotic plaques, do not contain elastic fibers. (44) Characteristically, the plaques occur on the pulmonary valve, although the tricuspid valve and mural endocardium may be involved. The affected valve leaflets become thickened and fused, producing valvular insufficiency. (45) Although the pathogenesis of these lesions is still uncertain, it is believed that they are most likely due to elevated serum levels of serotonin (*pp. 579–580*).

46. (D); 47. (B); 48. (C); 49. (D); 50. (D)

(46) The three major types of aortic aneurysms are atherosclerotic, syphilitic, and dissecting aneurysms. Only the latter fails in most cases to produce the

marked dilatation of the aorta that is the hallmark of atherosclerotic and syphilitic aneurysms. (**47**) Syphilitic aneurysms almost always involve the thoracic aorta, usually the ascending and transverse portions of the arch. Atherosclerotic aneurysms, in contrast, usually occur in the distal abdominal aorta, although they may occasionally involve the descending portion of the aortic arch. (**48**) Rupture of the dilated, weakened wall of an atherosclerotic or syphilitic aneurysm is a catastrophic, all too common event that constitutes the major cause of mortality associated with these lesions. Death from congestive heart failure is also common with syphilitic aneurysms that lead to dilatation and incompetency of the aortic valve or narrowing of the coronary ostia.

(**49**) Whereas arteriosclerosis and endarteritis of the vasa vasorum of the aorta are the major histopathologic changes in atherosclerotic and syphilitic aneurysms respectively, cystic medial necrosis is the hallmark of dissecting aneurysms of the aorta. This lesion causes weakening of the media of the aorta, allowing blood to dissect into the wall at a point of intimal tearing of the vessel. Intimal tears and extension of dissecting hemorrhage within the vessel wall once a tear has occurred are both believed to be consequences of hypertension. (**50**) Thus, aggressive antihypertensive therapy is often effective in limiting the extent of dissection in these aneurysms (*pp. 530–535*).

51. (D); 52. (A); 53. (B); 54. (C); 55. (B); 56. (A); 57. (A)

(**51**) Bacterial infective endocarditis (IE) is a life-threatening condition whose incidence has not diminished, despite the efforts of modern medicine. (**52**) Acute bacterial endocarditis, the form associated with abrupt onset and rapid valvular destruction, often occurs on normal cardiac valves and is commonly caused by *Staphylococcus aureus*. (**53**) Subacute bacterial endocarditis, in contrast, characteristically occurs on abnormal valves, either congenitally deformed valves or rheumatic valves. This form of infective endocarditis is often insidious in onset, and the most common causative organisms tend to be of relatively low virulence like *S. viridans*. (**54**) In both acute and subacute IE, the causative agent can be identified from blood cultures when repeated sufficiently often in 90% of cases.

(**55**) Osler's nodes are painful subcutaneous nodules that typically occur in subacute IE but are uncommon in acute IE.

(**56**) It is the acute form of infective endocarditis that is frequently associated with chronic alcoholism and drug addiction. The cardiac lesions in drug addiction are distinctive, however, because they tend to affect normal, right-sided heart valves, especially the tricuspid valve.

(**57**) Although the enterococcus may occasionally cause subacute bacterial endocarditis, it is not a common causative agent. *Streptococcus viridans* is by far the most common cause of subacute bacterial endocarditis and is second in frequency only to *Staphylococcus aureus* in causing acute bacterial endocarditis. Overall, enterococci can be cultured from only 5 to 7% of infective endocarditis cases (*pp. 580–584*).

58. (C); 59. (C); 60. (A); 61. (C); 62. (B); 63. (A)

(**58**) There is no sexual predominance in rheumatic carditis. Once the disorder occurs, however, women are more prone to the subsequent development of mitral stenosis than men. Mitral valve prolapse is primarily a disorder of females.

(**59**) Both rheumatic mitral valve disease and mitral valve prolapse predispose to bacterial endocarditis and require antibiotic prophylaxis for procedures known to induce bacteremias (e.g., dental extractions).

(**60**) One of the most characteristic gross pathologic features of rheumatic mitral valve disease is fibrous bridging across the valvular commissures (commissural fusion), producing the characteristic "fish-mouth" stenotic deformity. In mitral valve prolapse, individual leaflets are enlarged and may show myxoid degenerative changes that may become fibrotic at a later stage, but the commissures are not affected. (**61**) Fibrosis and thickening of chordae tendineae may occur in either disorder and are present in virtually every case of rheumatic mitral valve disease.

(**62**) Although myocarditis occurring during an acute attack of rheumatic fever may cause fatal arrhythmias, rheumatic mitral valve disease, the product of postinflammatory scarring, is only associated with rhythm disorders late in the clinical course. Mitral valve prolapse, in contrast, is occasionally associated with ventricular arrhythmias, particularly ventricular tachycardia and fibrillation, and even sudden death.

(**63**) Mitral stenosis from rheumatic valve disease is one of the most significant causes of late morbidity and mortality in rheumatic patients; thus most patients eventually require valve replacement. Although severe isolated mitral regurgitation may complicate mitral valve prolapse and require valvular replacement, overall this is quite uncommon. However, since isolated mitral regurgitation severe enough to require valvular replacement is itself uncommon, mitral valve prolapse has become the most common cause of this problem in some major medical centers (*pp. 571–578, 581*).

64. (B); 65. (A); 66. (B); 67. (C); 68. (A); 69. (A); 70. (D)

Valvular heart disease encompasses a number of disorders whose primary features are cardiac valvular damage and dysfunction. Although the causes are numerous and often produce fairly distinctive morphologic changes in the valves, the functional deficits produced tend to fall into only two categories: (1) valvular regurgitation and (2) valvular stenosis. In certain conditions, both regurgitation and stenosis may be present.

(64) Valvular stenosis is characterized by a failure of the valve to open completely, impeding flow through the valve. (65) Valvular regurgitation implies a failure of the valve to close completely, producing valvular insufficiency.

(66) Although valvular insufficiency may result from damage to either valve cusps or supporting structures, such as papillary muscles, annular rings, or chordae tendineae, valvular stenosis is almost always due to pathologic changes in the valve cusps.

(67) Both types of valvular dysfunction may occur in valves damaged by rheumatic heart disease, which characteristically produces fibrosis, distortion, and dysfunction of the valve cusps and of the supporting structures (chordae tendineae).

(68) Infectious endocarditis produces destructive lesions of the valves and supporting structures that can cause perforation of the valve leaflet, erosion of the free margins of the valve, or both. These anatomic changes destroy the competency of the valve and produce valvular regurgitation.

(69) Cardiac involvement by rheumatoid arthritis is associated with valvular regurgitation. In this condition, rheumatoid granulomas form in the mitral and aortic valve rings and in the myocardium. The granulomas cause fibrosis, thickening, and calcification of the affected valve leaflets and the attached chordae tendineae, which leads to valvular incompetence and regurgitation.

(70) Although atherosclerotic lesions may be found on heart valves, it is usually of no functional significance (pp. 570–571).

71. (C); 72. (D); 73. (D); 74. (B); 75. (C); 76. (D)

According to the extent of the ischemic damage, acute myocardial infarction may be divided into two basic patterns: subendocardial infarction or transmural infarction. Subendocardial infarction typically appears as multifocal areas of necrosis confined to the inner one third to one half of the left ventricular wall. Transmural infarction extends from the endocardium to the epicardium and by definition must involve an area of myocardium at least 2.5 cm. in greatest dimension. Occasionally, the patterns may overlap, and in some cases transmural infarcts begin with subendocardial necrosis that is extended by increasing severity or duration of ischemia.

(71) Regardless of the pattern, myocardial infarction is associated with severe multivessel stenotic atherosclerotic disease in the great majority of cases. (72) The atherosclerotic lesions of the coronary vessels are virtually always confined to the extramyocardial arterial segments. Intramyocardial arterial vessels are free of atherosclerotic changes in virtually all forms of ischemic heart disease.

(73) Morphologic studies fail to reveal a close correlation between the distribution of the myocardial lesion with pathologic changes in the corresponding coronary arterial vessel in either pattern of infarction.

(74) The reported incidence of occlusive coronary thrombosis varies from study to study. Overall, however, greater than half the cases of transmural myocardial infarction are associated with acute coronary thrombosis. Subendocardial infarction, in contrast, is associated with occlusive thrombus in less than 10% of cases.

(75) Virtually all subendocardial and transmural infarctions involve the left ventricle and are limited to the left ventricular wall in most cases. In only 15 to 30% of transmural infarction is the adjacent right ventricular wall involved. Isolated infarction of the right ventricle is extremely rare.

(76) Because morphologic evidence of myocardial necrosis is not present for hours after irreversible injury has occurred, morphologic diagnosis of early acute myocardial infarction is seldom possible in most patients who suffer sudden cardiac death (death within 24 hours of a cardiac event). Many cases of sudden cardiac death are believed to be related to arrhythmias and show no myocardial abnormalities by gross, histologic, or ultrastructural examination (pp. 558–564).

77. (C); 78. (A); 79. (B); 80. (D); 81. (C); 82. (B); 83. (D)

The most common pattern of coronary artery distribution is a right dominant pattern, in which the right coronary artery supplies the posterior descending arterial system. Thus the right coronary artery normally supplies (79 and 82) the posterior wall of both the right and left ventricles, the posterior half of the interventricular septum, and (81) the anterolateral wall of the right ventricle. (78) The left coronary artery normally supplies the anterior wall of the left ventricle, part of the anterior wall of the right ventricle, and the anterior half of the interventricular septum.

(80 and 83) The mitral valve is a thin, endothelium-covered, avascular structure that, like the endothelial lining of the chambers, receives its oxygen supply directly from the blood within the lumen and does not require coronary arterial supply (p. 548).

84. (A); 85. (A); 86. (B); 87. (A); 88. (C); 89. (C); 90. (C)

The right side of the heart receiving the systemic venous return and supplying the low-pressure pulmonary vascular system and the left side of the heart receiving the pulmonary venous return and supplying the high pressure systemic arterial system comprise two separate anatomic and functional systems. Failure of one of these systems can be related to either decreased myocardial contractility and/or an increased work load imposed upon it.

(**84**) Because the left ventricle comprises the bulk of the cardiac muscle, ischemic heart disease has a profound effect on left ventricular function and is most frequently associated with left-sided heart failure. (**85**) Valvular heart disease commonly involves the mitral and aortic valves and therefore is also most often associated with left-sided heart failure.

(**86**) Chronic obstructive pulmonary disease causes secondary abnormalities in the pulmonary vasculature that impose an increased work load on the right side of the heart and may cause right-sided heart failure. (**87**) Pulmonary edema is most commonly the result of left heart failure and increased back pressure in the pulmonary venous system.

(**88**) Aldosterone-induced sodium retention is produced by both left-sided and right-sided heart failure. Left-sided failure leads to decreased cardiac output and a reduction in renal perfusion, whereas right-sided failure leads to congestion and hypoxia of the kidneys from increased venous pressure. In both of these conditions, the angiotensin-aldosterone system is activated, leading to sodium and fluid retention. (**89**) The decreased renal blood flow and renal hypoxia induced by either left-sided or right-sided heart failure can, in addition, lead to impaired excretion of nitrogenous waste products and produce prerenal azotemia.

(**90**) Centrilobular necrosis of the liver can result from either passive congestion in the centrilobular area or ischemia associated with reduced arterial flow. Thus centrilobular necrosis is a common concomitant of both left-sided and right-sided heart failure (*pp. 548–551*).

91. (D); 92. (C); 93. (A); 94. (B); 95. (E); 96. (C); 97. (E)

The histopathologic changes associated with an acute myocardial infarction evolve in a relatively predictable progression. This reproducible sequence of histologic changes makes it possible to estimate the age of the infarction. (**93**) During the first few hours after an ischemic event, the myocardium appears grossly and histologically normal. Coagulative necrosis cannot be seen by routine histologic staining or by histochemical stains for the first 4 to 8 hours. (**92 and 96**) Histologically, coagulative necrosis of the myocardium and neutrophilic infiltration of the infarcted area are maximal 24 to 48 hours after the ischemic event. (**93**) Toward the end of the first week, the formation of granulation tissue begins at the periphery of the infarcted area. (**97**) Digestive resorption of the necrotic muscle by macrophages is maximal at this time and is reflected histologically by the predominance of macrophages in the inflammatory cell infiltrate.

(**94**) Clinically, the diagnosis of acute myocardial infarction can best be made on the basis of temporal patterns of specific serum enzyme elevations. Alterations of serum enzyme levels are the most sensitive and reliable indicators of myocardial infarction. (**95**) The myocardial isozyme of creatine phosphokinase (CPK-MB) appears in the serum shortly after myocardial damage and reaches its peak approximately 19 hours after infarction. (**91**) The myocardial isozyme of lactate dehydrogenase (LDH) is apparent in the serum about 12 hours post infarction but reaches peak levels in 48 to 72 hours. The elevation in this isozyme is found to be about 90% sensitive and 95% specific for acute myocardial infarction. It usually persists for up to 6 days after the ischemic event (*pp. 559–563*).

98. (C); 99. (B); 100. (D); 101. (C); 102. (A); 103. (D); 104. (C); 105. (B)

(**98, 101, and 104**) Although the vasculitides are a diverse group of disorders producing vascular inflammation and necrosis, they tend to fall into a set of distinctive clinicopathologic syndromes. Kawasaki's disease, for example, is a distinctive disorder of young children and infants manifested by fever, conjunctival and oral erythema and erosion, skin rash, and enlargement of lymph nodes. A severe vasculitis primarily involving the heart (coronary arteries) is the major pathologic feature and major cause of mortality.

(**99 and 105**) Giant cell arteritis, in contrast, is a condition that rarely occurs in individuals under the age of 50 (average age 70) and most commonly involves the temporal artery. The disease may be difficult to diagnose and can cause visual impairment if untreated, but the therapeutic response to steroids is excellent.

(**100 and 103**) Buerger's disease is a distinctive vasculitic syndrome, apparently etiologically related to cigarette smoking, that causes thrombosis and occlusion of the intermediate and small arteries and veins of the extremities. Vascular insufficiency that often leads to severe pain and gangrene of the extremities is produced.

(**102**) Polyarteritis nodosa is the prototypic systemic vasculitis that may affect any artery of medium or small size in any organ or system of the body. In contrast to the other disorders mentioned above, the kidneys are commonly (85%) involved by polyarteritis nodosa. In fact, kidney involvement with renal failure is the most common cause of death in this disorder. This disease most often affects young adults and can be effectively treated in 80% of cases by corticosteroids and cyclophosphamide administration (supportive evidence of an immunologic origin for this disorder) (*pp. 520–522, 524–527*).

106. (B); 107. (D); 108. (A); 109. (A); 110. (C)

The character of a pericardial effusion is often an indication of its etiology. (**106**) Cardiopulmonary resuscitation produces cardiac trauma and acute inflammation that characteristically produce a serosanguineous effusion. Myxedema, which commonly but not invariably produces hypercholesterolemia, is the most common form of nonidiopathic cholesterol pericardial effusion. (**108**) Congestive heart failure with its increased hydrostatic pressure is the most common cause of a serous pericardial effusion. (**109**) Serous pericardial effusion may also be caused by hypoproteinemic states and decreased serum oncotic pressure. Hypoproteinemia may be produced by increased renal losses (e.g., the nephrotic syndrome), decreased hepatic production (e.g., cirrhosis), or decreased protein intake (e.g., malnutrition). (**110**) Mediastinal tumor with lymphatic infiltration and blockage characteristically causes a chylous effusion in the pericardium (*p. 603*).

111. (C); 112. (E); 113. (B); 114. (D); 115. (A); 116. (F); 117. (A)

(**111**) Syphilis causes an obliterative endarteritis of the vasa vasorum of the aorta. Consequently, ischemic destruction of the aortic wall produces fibrous scarring of the media. These medial scars often form around the ostia of vessels branching off the aortic trunk, including the coronary arteries. The coronary ostia are frequently drastically narrowed and coronary insufficiency can result (*pp. 531–532*).

(**112**) Ischemic myocardial damage associated with a surgical procedure is most often caused by an intraoperative or perioperative drop in systemic blood pressure. An abrupt reduction in coronary perfusion in a patient with some degree of fixed coronary narrowing is the most important hemodynamic cause of myocardial infarction and is the most significant factor in surgery-related myocardial ischemia (*p. 553*).

(**113**) Prinzmetal's (variant) angina is a form of angina that classically occurs at rest when myocardial oxygen *demand* is low. Thus, it is believed that coronary vasospasm and a reduction in oxygen *supply* produce Prinzmetal's angina (*p. 555*).

(**114**) Nonbacterial thrombotic endocarditis is characterized by the formation of sterile fibrin thrombi on the leaflets of the involved valves, usually the mitral or aortic valves. The small, bland vegetations sometimes embolize to the coronary arteries and produce myocardial infarction. This disorder often occurs in association with chronic debilitating disease such as cancer (especially mucin-producing adenocarcinomas) (*p. 585*).

(**115**) Chronic ischemic heart disease is defined by slow, progressive atherosclerotic narrowing of the coronary arteries. This gradual diminution in the myocardial blood supply leads to diffuse ischemic atrophy and interstitial fibrosis of the myocardium. Often large areas of scarring from previous episodes of infarction are present as well (*pp. 566–567*).

(**116**) Rheumatoid arteritis is an acute necrotizing vasculitis of immunologic origin. Small and medium-sized arteries as well as the aorta are prime targets for this process. The immunologically mediated damage to the vessel wall leads to secondary luminal thrombosis. Myocardial infarction may result when coronary arteries are involved (*pp. 528, 1352*).

(**117**) Stable angina pectoris is characterized by severe chest pain produced by an increase in myocardial oxygen demand (e.g., exercise) in the face of limited arterial flow. Atherosclerotic narrowing of the coronary vessels is the major cause of reduced arterial flow (and oxygen supply) in this disorder, although superimposed coronary vasospasm may be a secondary contributing factor (*p. 555*).

118. (A); 119. (C); 120. (D); 121. (E); 122. (C); 123. (F); 124. (B)

(**118 and 121**) Stable angina is characteristically induced by exertion and relieved by rest. In contrast to stable angina, unstable angina and Prinzmetal's angina often occur at rest.

(**119 and 120**) Most commonly, only Prinzmetal's angina is associated with S-T segment elevations on EKG. Stable angina and unstable angina typically produce S-T segment depressions corresponding to subendocardial ischemia in the left ventricle.

(**122**) Angiography may reveal normal coronary arteries in patients with Prinzmetal's angina, since this disorder is caused mainly by spasm of the vessels and not architectural distortion from atherosclerosis. Stable and unstable angina, however, are nearly always associated with severe atherosclerotic narrowing of the coronary arteries, readily visualized by angiography.

(**123**) All forms of anginal pain are caused by myocardial ischemia, which falls short of producing infarction. Thus the myocardial injury that occurs during a transient anginal attack is usually reversible. The myocardial cells will recover if the balance of oxygen supply and demand are restored relatively quickly.

(**124**) The development of unstable angina, characterized by either prolonged pain, onset of pain at rest in a patient with stable angina, or an increased intensity of exertional anginal pain, is an ominous sign portending myocardial infarction and has thus been dubbed "pre-infarction angina" (*pp. 555–556*).

125. (A); 126. (D); 127. (C); 128. (E); 129. (A); 130. (A); 131. (F)

(**125**) Phenobarbital or diazepam is often used in the initial management of acute myocardial infarction to sedate the patient, relieve anxiety, and thereby reduce stress-related increase in cardiac work load.

(**126**) Verapamil is a calcium channel blocker that produces vasodilatation and is especially useful in reducing the vasospastic component of an acute ischemic event. It also has negative inotropic and chronotropic effects on the heart, which help to reduce myocardial work.

(**127**) Streptokinase is used primarily for its fibrinolytic effects. It may be infused directly into the coronary arteries or into the systemic circulation to lyse coronary thrombi.

(**128**) Although morphine has sedative and sympatholytic effects that may be beneficial in initial treatment, the most important reason for its use is for prompt relief of the severe pain of acute myocardial infarction.

(**129**) Restriction of the patient's physical activities is of primary importance in reducing the work of the heart and minimizing its oxygen demand.

(**130**) Propranolol is a beta adrenergic blocking agent that reduces heart rate, contractility, and blood pressure. All of these effects tend to reduce oxygen consumption by the myocardium.

(**131**) Lidocaine is a local anesthetic that stabilizes neuronal membranes and prevents the initiation and conduction of nerve impulses. The drug also increases the electrical stimulation threshold of the myocardium during diastole. It is sometimes used intravenously in the management of acute myocardial infarction to control life-threatening arrhythmias of ventricular origin (*pp. 564–566*).

6

THE RESPIRATORY SYSTEM

DIRECTIONS: For Questions 1 to 11, choose the ONE BEST answer to each question.

1. Clara cells:

A. Make mucus
B. Make surfactant
C. Make immunoglobulins
D. Have cilia
E. Make bronchiolar lining protein

2. All of the following commonly contribute to atelectasis in the seriously ill postoperative patient EXCEPT:

A. Respiratory distress syndrome
B. Diaphragmatic elevation
C. Voluntary suppression of coughing
D. Excessive bronchial secretions
E. Limitation of respiratory movements

3. Diffuse alveolar damage (adult respiratory distress syndrome) is the major pattern of pulmonary damage produced by all of the following EXCEPT:

A. Oxygen toxicity
B. Narcotic overdose
C. Septic shock
D. Cardiopulmonary bypass surgery
E. Legionnaire's disease

4. All of the following features are commonly associated with chronic bronchitis EXCEPT:

A. Hypertrophy of bronchial mucus glands
B. Productive cough
C. Severe dyspnea
D. Increased airways resistance
E. Frequent infections

5. Complications of necrotizing bronchopneumonia include all of the following EXCEPT:

A. Chronic bronchitis
B. Bronchiectasis
C. Pleural fibrosis
D. Metastatic abscess formation
E. Permanent lobar solidification

6. All of the following factors commonly predispose to bacterial pneumonias EXCEPT:

A. Viral respiratory tract infections
B. Cigarette smoking
C. Congestive heart failure
D. Bacterial urinary tract infection
E. General anesthesia

7. Aspiration of gastric contents produces any of the following types of pulmonary injury EXCEPT:

A. Adult respiratory distress syndrome
B. Lipoid pneumonia
C. Lung abscess
D. Empyema
E. Loeffler's syndrome

8. Known causes of diffuse interstitial fibrosis include all of the following EXCEPT:

A. Sarcoidosis
B. Asbestos
C. Rheumatoid arthritis
D. Cigarette smoke
E. Bleomycin

9. Eosinophilic infiltrates characterize all of the following disorders EXCEPT:

A. Pneumocystis infection
B. Loeffler's syndrome
C. Allergic bronchopulmonary aspergillosis
D. Bronchial asthma
E. Pigeon breeders' lung

10. All of the following statements about diffuse alveolar damage (adult respiratory distress syndrome) are true EXCEPT:

A. Complement activity initiates the process
B. Type I pneumocytes sustain a greater degree of injury than type II cells
C. Interstitial infiltrates on chest x-ray generally precede the onset of dyspnea
D. The overall mortality rate is about 50%
E. It is the underlying cause of most diffuse interstitial fibrotic lung disease

11. Cigarette smoke contributes to the pathogenesis of *emphysema* by all of the following mechanisms EXCEPT:

A. Attracts neutrophils into the lung
B. Stimulates release of neutrophil elastase
C. Inhibits the ability of pulmonary leukocytes to clear bacteria
D. Directly inhibits alpha-1-antitrypsin (α1-AT) activity
E. Stimulates macrophages to liberate free radicals that inhibit α1-AT

DIRECTIONS: For Questions 12 to 16, ONE or MORE of the completions given correctly finishes the incomplete statement. Choose:

A— if only *1,2, and 3* are correct
B—if only *1 and 3* are correct
C—if only *2 and 4* are correct
D—if only *4* is correct
E—if *all* are correct

12. Primary pulmonary hypertension:

1. Occurs most commonly in elderly women
2. Is often associated with Raynaud's phenomenon
3. Is usually associated with chronic obstructive lung disease
4. Produces atherosclerosis of the pulmonary arteries

   A. 1,2,3   B. 1,3   C. 2,4   D. 4 Only   E. All

13. An air bronchogram or a chest x-ray in a 15-year-old girl who has suffered from repeated pulmonary infections all her life show bilateral bronchiectasis. Which of the following disorders is this patient likely to have?

1. Cystic fibrosis
2. IgA immunodeficiency
3. Kartagener's syndrome
4. Congenital bronchiectasis

   A. 1,2,3   B. 1,3   C. 2,4   D. 4 Only   E. All

14. A patient with large cell non-Hodgkin's lymphoma being treated with systemic chemotherapy develops diffuse pulmonary infiltrates. An open lung biopsy is *likely* to reveal:

1. *Pneumocystis carinii* infection
2. A drug reaction
3. Cytomegalovirus infection
4. Lymphomatous infiltrates
   A. 1,2,3   B. 1,3   C. 2,4   D. 4 Only   E. All

15. Vasculitis in the lungs commonly occurs in:

1. Wegener's granulomatosis
2. Rheumatoid arthritis
3. The Churg-Strauss syndrome
4. Systemic lupus erythematosus

   A. 1,2,3   B. 1,3   C. 2,4   D. 4 Only   E. All

16. Mesothelioma:

1. Often resembles an adenocarcinoma histologically
2. Often resembles a sarcoma histologically
3. Is causally related to asbestos exposure
4. Is causally related to cigarette smoke
   A. 1,2,3   B. 1,3   C. 2,4   D. 4 Only   E. All

DIRECTIONS: For Questions 17 to 35, you are to decide whether EACH choice is TRUE or FALSE.

For each of the following statements about pulmonary emboli, choose whether it is TRUE or FALSE.

17. They are associated with the use of birth control pills
18. The most common source of emboli is the pelvic veins
19. They are usually readily apparent on chest x-ray
20. They usually resolve completely without treatment
21. Infarction of the lung rarely occurs when the bronchial arterial supply is adequate
22. The mortality rate for patients treated for this disorder is less than 10%
23. Unresolved pulmonary emboli eventually lead to diffuse interstitial fibrosis (honeycomb lung)

For each of the following statements about bronchial asthma, choose whether it is TRUE or FALSE.

24. Most bronchial asthma is mediated by an immune response producing IgE
25. In nearly all patients with asthma, the airways are hyperreactive to bronchoconstrictor agents
26. Infection-induced asthma is usually caused by gram-positive cocci
27. Aspirin-sensitive asthma is caused by the formation of immune complexes
28. Eosinophils containing Curschmann's spirals are a characteristic histologic finding

For each of the following statements about pulmonary tuberculosis, choose whether it is TRUE or FALSE.

29. The primary focus of infection is most commonly located in the apex of the upper lobe
30. Pneumonia occurs with initial infection in immunodeficient individuals
31. Most initial infections produce fever and cough
32. Reactivation of the primary infection occurs eventually in the majority of untreated individuals
33. Miliary dissemination throughout the body is likely to occur if a tuberculous lesion extends into a pulmonary artery
34. With the most severe tuberculous infections, granulomas frequently fail to form
35. Most patients newly developing a floridly positive PPD (purified protein derivative) skin test require antituberculous chemotherapy

DIRECTIONS: For Questions 36 to 48, the set of lettered headings is followed by a list of numbered words or phrases. For each numbered word or phrase choose:

A—if the item is associated with (A) only
B—if the item is associated with (B) only
C—if the item is associated with *both* (A) and (B)
D—if the item is associated with *neither* (A) nor (B)

36. Bronchiectasis in the adult is most often associated with:

A. Bronchial obstruction
B. Bronchial infection
C. Both
D. Neither

For each of the characteristics listed below, choose whether it describes bronchogenic cysts, pulmonary cysts, both, or neither.

A. Bronchogenic cysts
B. Pulmonary cysts
C. Both
D. Neither
37. Usually occur singly
38. Usually occur in a peripheral location
39. Rarely communicate with a main bronchus

40. Frequently become infected
41. Occasionally contain adenocarcinoma

For each of the characteristics listed below, choose whether it describes Goodpasture's syndrome, idiopathic pulmonary hemosiderosis, both, or neither.

A. Goodpasture's syndrome
B. Idiopathic pulmonary hemosiderosis
C. Both
D. Neither

42. Striking male predominance
43. Associated with interstitial nephritis
44. Usually occurs in children
45. Characterized by necrotizing hemorrhagic interstitial pneumonitis
46. Characterized by pulmonary vasculitis
47. Caused by anti–basement membrane antibodies
48. Often improves without treatment

DIRECTIONS: Questions 49 to 70 are matching questions. For each numbered item, choose the most likely associated item from those provided. Each numbered item has ONLY ONE answer. Within each group, each lettered item may be the answer to one, more than one, or none of the numbered items.

For each of the characteristics listed below, choose whether it describes centriacinar (centrilobular) emphysema, panaciner (panlobular) emphysema, irregular emphysema, interstitial emphysema, or none of these.

    A. Centriacinar (centrilobular) emphysema
    B. Panacinar (panlobular) emphysema
    C. Irregular emphysema
    D. Interstitial emphysema
    E. None of these
49. Associated with alpha-1-antitrypsin deficiency
50. Occurs most commonly in cigarette smokers
51. Occurs in residual lung after lobectomy
52. Occurs in children with whooping cough
53. Does not produce bullae

For each of the microorganisms listed below, choose the pattern of pulmonary injury with which it is most commonly associated: diffuse alveolar damage, lobar pneumonia, necrotizing bronchopneumonia, lung abscess, or none of these.

    A. Diffuse alveolar damage
    B. Lobar pneumonia
    C. Necrotizing bronchopneumonia
    D. Lung abscess
    E. None of these
54. Cytomegalovirus
55. *Staphylococcus aureus*

56. *Streptococcus pneumoniae* (pneumococcus)
57. Bacteroides
58. Microfilariae
59. Thermophilic bacteria
60. *Mycobacterium tuberculosis*
61. *Mycoplasma pneumoniae*
62. Klebsiella pneumoniae
63. Legionella

For each of the characteristics listed below, choose which type of bronchogenic carcinoma it describes: squamous cell carcinoma, adenocarcinoma, small ("oat") cell carcinoma, or none of these.

    A. Squamous cell carcinoma
    B. Adenocarcinoma
    C. Small ("oat") cell carcinoma
    D. None of these

64. Most common histologic type of lung cancer
65. Occurs with equal frequency in males and females
66. Usually occurs in the periphery of the lung
67. Etiologically unrelated to cigarette smoking
68. Elaborates parathyroid hormone more frequently than any other lung cancer
69. Produces the syndrome of inappropriate antidiuretic hormone secretion more frequently than any other lung cancer
70. Is not usually treated by surgery

6

THE RESPIRATORY SYSTEM

ANSWERS

1. (E) Clara cells are specialized secretory cells found only in bronchioles. They secrete a protein, poor in mucus, that covers the bronchiolar surface. The proteinaceous secretion coats the ciliated cells that make up the majority of the bronchiolar surface area. Clara cells themselves have no cilia. Because they lack mucin, bronchiolar secretions differ from those of bronchi, which are largely composed of mucosubstances produced by epithelial goblet cells and mucosal mucus glands. Bronchiolar secretions are also distinct from those of the alveoli; they lack the surfactant that is the distinctive product of the alveolar type II pneumocytes. Although bronchiolar secretions are characteristically rich in immunoglobulins, these are not produced by the Clara cells. Like immunoglobulins produced elsewhere in the body, those found in the bronchiolar secretions are made by immunocompetent cells of the B lymphocyte series. These immunocompetent cells reside in or beneath the bronchiolar epithelium and contribute their products to the water-protein layer coating the bronchiolar surface (*p. 706*).

2. (A) Atelectasis in seriously ill postoperative patients is frequently multifactorial. The compressive form of atelectasis may result from elevated diaphragms secondary to abdominal distention. Compressive atelectasis also occurs in this setting because of patients' voluntary suppression of coughing and/or limitation of respiratory movements due to pain. Furthermore, with increased bronchial secretions elicited by general anesthetics, the obstructive form of atelectasis often occurs in postoperative patients.

Although the respiratory distress syndrome (adult hyaline membrane disease) may complicate the postoperative course of a seriously ill patient who has suffered a hypotensive episode intra- or postoperatively, the process does not cause atelectasis. On the contrary, hyaline membranes distend the alveolar spaces, reduce compliance and elasticity, and prevent the lung from collapsing. Indeed, the principal gross pathologic features of the lungs in adult hyaline membrane disease are their rubbery consistency and refusal to collapse upon standing (*pp. 709–710*).

3. (E) Diffuse alveolar damage (DAD) is the pathologic equivalent of the adult respiratory distress syndrome. It is a pattern of pulmonary injury characterized by alveolar congestion, edema, and interstitial inflammation. Fibrin deposition and necrosis of alveolar epithelial cells result in the formation of "hyaline membranes" in the air spaces. DAD is characteristic of injury caused by: (1) oxygen toxicity; (2) narcotic overdose; (3) shock associated with sepsis, trauma, hemorrhagic pancreatitis, burns, or complicated surgery, especially cardiac surgery involving extracorporeal cardiac bypass pumps; (4) inhalation of toxins and irritant gases; (5) aspiration of gastric contents; (6) hypersensitivity reactions to organic solvents and drugs; and (7) diffuse pulmonary infections, most commonly viral.

Although Legionnaire's disease has been associated with diffuse alveolar damage, the process is usually superimposed on the necrotizing bronchopneumonia that is the classic pattern of injury in Legionnaire's disease. In most cases, DAD is probably a superimposed complication of oxygen therapy (*p. 714*).

4. (C) Chronic bronchitis is defined clinically as a condition causing persistent cough with sputum production for at least 3 months in at least 2 consecutive years. Histologically, the condition is characterized by hypertrophy of the tracheal and bronchial submucosal glands and goblet cell hyperplasia of the bronchial epithelium. One of the earliest manifestations of the disease is an alteration in the resistance of the small airways measurable by a closing volume test. Such tests have shown that small airway dysfunction is present in young smokers *before* the development of clinical symptoms of respiratory obstruction. Chronic bronchitis predisposes to frequent pulmonary infections that in turn play a secondary role in maintaining or exacerbating the condition. In contrast to patients with pulmonary emphysema, patients with chronic bronchitis do not suffer from severe dyspnea. In long-standing cases of chronic bronchitis, dyspnea on exertion eventually develops but is never as marked as in patients with other forms of chronic obstructive pulmonary disease (*pp. 725–726*).

5. (A) Necrotizing organisms are by definition capable of tissue destruction. They elaborate extracellular enzymes, which allow them to penetrate and destroy normal structures. Additional tissue injury is produced by the liberation of lysozomal enzymes from neutrophils attracted to the site of infection. Thus, the consequences of necrotizing bronchopneumonia can be quite severe. The process may permanently damage airways and result in a postinfective bronchiectasis. Spread to the pleural cavities with resultant empyema formation may organize to form a ring of pleural fibrosis around the involved lung. Penetration of venous structures and lymphatics by the organism leads to systemic bacteremia and metastatic abscess formation. Organization of the exudate and scarring of the damaged lung may lead to permanent solidification of the lung parenchyma. Chronic bronchitis, however, is *not* a consequence of bronchopneumonia. It is caused by chronic irritation of airways by inhaled substances (usually cigarette smoke) with microbiologic infections playing only a secondary role in its pathogenesis *(pp. 734–735)*.

6. (D) Conditions that predispose to bacterial pneumonias are those that impair the natural defense mechanisms of the lung or the resistance of the host in general. Injury to the mucociliary apparatus is one of the most common predisposing factors, since it is produced by both viral respiratory tract infections and cigarette smoke. Another of the common predispositions to bronchopneumonia is pulmonary congestion and edema occurring in patients with congestive heart failure, although the exact mechanism by which this interferes with pulmonary bacterial clearance is not known. A third important predisposing factor is the loss or suppression of the cough reflex occurring from general anesthesia, coma, neuromuscular disorders, drugs, or chest pain.

Bacterial infections elsewhere in the body such as the urinary tract do not usually lead to bacterial bronchopneumonia unless some *other* predisposing factor is present. If, for instance, a bacteremia from a urinary tract infection occurs in a patient with pulmonary edema or bronchial obstruction with accumulation of secretions, the development of bronchopneumonia would be likely *(pp. 732–733)*.

7. (E) Diverse types of pulmonary injury may result from aspiration of regurgitated gastric contents. The specific pattern of injury is dependent upon the nature of the aspirated material. Aspiration of hydrochloric acid produces a pattern of diffuse alveolar damage and results in the clinical syndrome of adult respiratory distress. If the regurgitated material has a high lipid content (e.g., mineral oil or ice cream), alveolar macrophages ingesting the lipids fill the alveolar spaces. The resultant pattern of foamy macrophages and acute inflammation in alveolar spaces is known as lipoid pneumonia. Aspiration of infected material is most commonly associated with acute alcoholism, coma, anesthesia, sinusitis, gingival dental sepsis, and debilitation; lung abscess formation may result. Anaerobic organisms normally found in the oral cavity (Bacteroides, Fusobacterium, and Peptococcus species) are the most common causative agents. Likewise, aspiration of bacteria-laden material may result in an infection that extends to the pleural cavity, resulting in empyema.

Loeffler's syndrome is unrelated to aspiration injury. It is an immunologically mediated allergic reaction (commonly to Ascaris and Strongyloides parasites) that produces peripheral and pulmonary eosinophilia *(pp. 714, 734, 738, 748)*.

8. (D) The condition known as diffuse interstitial fibrosis of the lung includes a heterogeneous group of diseases, all of which lead to increased interstitial collagen deposition in the alveolar walls. Although the etiologies are diverse, the disorders tend to produce similar clinical signs, symptoms, x-ray alterations, and pathophysiologic changes that justify their consideration as a group. Among the known causes of diffuse interstitial fibrosis of the lung are sarcoidosis, asbestosis, collagen vascular diseases such as rheumatoid arthritis, and of diffuse alveolar damage (end-stage) of any etiology, including Bleomycin toxicity. Although cigarette smoke is associated with a multitude of pulmonary diseases, including chronic bronchitis, emphysema, and bronchogenic carcinoma, it is not known to be associated with diffuse interstitial fibrosis *(pp. 747–748)*.

9. (A) A number of pathologic entities of the lung are characterized primarily by infiltration with eosinophils and are often accompanied by eosinophilia in the blood. These disorders run the gamut from benign transitory disease to chronic debilitating conditions. Whatever their clinical course or primary etiology, these disorders are all believed to be immunologically mediated. Loeffler's syndrome is a transient benign condition causing simple interstitial eosinophilia in the lung and is thought to result from an allergic reaction (Type I immune response) to parasitic agents. Allergic bronchopulmonary aspergillosis is an example of a chronic pulmonary eosinophilic syndrome; it is caused by hypersensitivity to Aspergillus antigens. Bronchial asthma is a classic example of a Type I immunologic response in the lung—usually to environmental antigens—causing bronchoconstriction. In bronchial asthma, the walls of the affected airways are infiltrated by eosinophils. (See Questions 24 to 28.) Pigeon breeders' lung is an example of a hypersensitivity pneumonitis caused by an allergic response to inhaled proteins from serum, excreta, or feathers of birds. In the acute phase of the disease, pigeon breeders' lung, like other forms of hypersensitivity pulmonary disease, is characterized pathologically by inflammatory infiltrates that include numerous eosinophils.

Although pulmonary eosinophilia is associated with a number of parasitic, fungal, and bacterial infections in the lung, it is not produced by the protozoan *Pneumocystis carinii*. This particular protozoan characteristically produces a pattern of diffuse alveolar damage in the lung *(p. 748)*.

10. (C) Although many diverse conditions may produce diffuse alveolar damage (DAD), one factor that most of them have in common is their propensity to activate the complement system. Complement activation is now believed to be the process that initiates the endothelial damage characteristic of DAD. Complement activation induces leukocyte aggregation and activation in the lung with the liberation of oxygen free radicals that injure both endothelial and alveolar epithelial cells. Of the two epithelial cell types, the type I pneumocyte is the more sensitive to injury and sustains the greater degree of damage in DAD. Because they are more hardy and replicate more readily, type II pneumocytes replace the destroyed type I cells during the reparative phases of DAD. Although the process does not necessarily progress in all patients and may be successfully treated with reversal of the underlying disease process and respiratory support therapy, the overall mortality for this syndrome is still about 50%. Many cases go on to chronic disease, however, and produce diffuse interstitial fibrosis of the lung. In fact, diffuse alveolar damage is the underlying cause of most interstitial fibrotic lung diseases. One of the clinical features peculiar to diffuse alveolar damage is the onset of rather profound symptomatology with severe dyspnea and tachypnea before any evidence of pulmonary pathology is seen on chest x-ray. Thus, early in the course of the disease, patients may have acute respiratory distress with a normal chest x-ray *(pp. 714–717)*.

11. (C) Emphysema is a chronic obstructive lung disease characterized by the destruction of alveolar walls. The damage is caused by enzymatic digestion of alveolar structural elements, principally elastic tissue. Neutrophils and macrophages produce elastases that initiate the injury. These cells are attracted to the lung and stimulated to release their proteases by cigarette smoke. Counterbalancing anti-elastase activity provided by α1-AT is concomitantly reduced by cigarette smoke, which directly inhibits the enzyme and also stimulates macrophages to produce free radicals that further reduce the enzyme's activity.

Although cigarette smoke does compromise the ability of pulmonary leukocytes to clear bacteria and thus increases susceptibility to infection, infection is not known to contribute to the pathogenesis of emphysema. It does, however, contribute to the pathogenesis of another obstructive lung disease of smokers, chronic bronchitis (see Question 4 and *pp. 721–722, 725*).

12. (C) Primary pulmonary hypertension is a disease process characterized by increased resistance in the pulmonary vascular tree in the absence of any known cause of increased pulmonary pressure (chronic lung disease, recurrent pulmonary emboli, or antecedent heart disease). The disease occurs most commonly in *young* women and is often associated with Raynaud's phenomenon. These two facts lend support to the

concept that primary pulmonary hypertension is a form of autoimmune collagen vascular disease, since both Raynaud's phenomenon and pulmonary hypertension occur in such disorders as scleroderma, systemic lupus erythematosus, and rheumatoid arthritis. At present, the underlying cause of primary pulmonary hypertension remains unknown. Yet, by definition, it is *not* associated with any form of chronic obstructive or interstitial lung disease, which are themselves known to produce pulmonary hypertension (secondary pulmonary hypertension). Whether primary or secondary, however, pulmonary hypertension produces identical changes in the pulmonary vascular tree. The increased pressures in the pulmonary arteries produce atheromatous lesions that, although not as severe, are indistinguishable from those of systemic atherosclerosis. Smaller arterial branches and arterioles show intimal thickening, medial hypertrophy, and varying amounts of intramural and adventitial fibrosis *(pp. 713–714)*.

13. (A) In children and young adults, bronchiectasis is usually the result of a congenital or hereditary condition, since bronchiectasis following necrotizing pneumonias complicating childhood diseases such as measles, whooping cough, and influenza is no longer common in the United States. Therefore, cystic fibrosis, immunodeficiency states, immotile cilia syndromes (e.g., Kartagener's syndrome), or congenital bronchiectasis are all associated with bronchiectasis in the pediatric and young adult age group. These conditions are associated with bronchial mucus plugging (obstruction), increased susceptibility to bronchial infection, or both. In cystic fibrosis, the characteristic thick tenacious bronchial secretions obstruct bronchi and frequently become infected with necrotizing bacterial organisms. With IgA immunodeficiency, the lung is robbed of one of its most important natural defense mechanisms against microbial invasion. Thus, heightened susceptibility to repeated bacterial infection results and is associated with localized or diffuse bronchiectasis. The immotile cilia syndromes result from structurally abnormal, dyskinetic, or akinetic cilia. In Kartagener's syndrome, this defect occurs in association with infertility and situs inversus.

Congenital bronchiectasis is caused by a defect in the development of bronchi. Although it is certainly a cause of bronchiectasis in the young, it usually affects either a lobe or an entire lung but is not usually diffuse (bilateral) *(p. 729)*.

14. (A) Patients with lymphoma who are being treated with systemic chemotherapy and are immunosuppressed may develop rapidly fatal pulmonary infections unless accurate diagnosis is made and immediate treatment is instituted. Frequently, however, pulmonary infiltrates on chest x-ray in such individuals reflect pulmonary damage from noninfectious causes, and an open lung biopsy is required to differentiate among the possible etiologies. Infection by the protozoan *Pneumocystis carinii* is relatively common among immunosuppressed patients, although it rarely, if ever, occurs in immunocompetent individuals. Viral infections are also common causes of pulmonary infiltrates in the immunosuppressed individual, and cytomegalovirus is frequently responsible. Numerous chemotherapeutic drugs are associated with the unpredictable production of diffuse alveolar damage in the lung. This produces a radiologic picture of diffuse pulmonary infiltrates that is often indistinguishable from infection.

Although large cell lymphomas may themselves infiltrate the lung, this occurs *uncommonly*. Moreover, lymphomatous infiltration usually produces *focal* rather than diffuse pulmonary infiltrates on chest x-ray.

The correct diagnosis is of emergent importance in cases such as the one described. Antibiotics would have no effect on drug reactions or lymphomatous infiltrates. Conversely, additional chemotherapy (and further immunosuppression) would be contraindicated in the case of infection or drug reaction but required if the infiltrate were of lymphomatous origin (*pp. 366, 737, 743*).

15. (B) Vasculitis in the lung, although uncommon, occurs in certain well-defined syndromes. Wegener's granulomatosis and the Churg-Strauss syndrome (allergic granulomatosis and angitis) are two conditions that are characterized primarily by pulmonary vasculitis. Wegener's granulomatosis produces the classic triad of (1) necrotizing granulomas of the upper and lower respiratory tract, (2) focal necrotizing vasculitis of the lungs, and (3) necrotizing glomerulitis. Unlike Wegener's granulomatosis, the Churg-Strauss syndrome lacks respiratory tract granulomas and glomerulonephritis. The Churg-Strauss syndrome is strongly associated with bronchial asthma and eosinophilia and only rarely involves the kidneys.

Rheumatoid arthritis and systemic lupus erythematosus may indeed involve the lung and usually produce an interstitial pneumonitis, but these entities rarely if ever produce pulmonary vasculitis (*pp. 522–524, 748–749*).

16. (A) Mesotheliomas are uncommon tumors that arise from either the viscera or the parietal pleura. They can present diagnostic difficulties because they manifest several different histologic patterns. The tubular pattern resembles adenocarcinoma histologically and can be difficult to differentiate from a peripheral bronchogenic adenocarcinoma that has secondarily involved the pleura. In addition, mesotheliomas may exhibit a spindle cell growth pattern and resemble a sarcoma. Mesotheliomas are causally related to heavy asbestos exposure, and the lifetime risk of developing this tumor in heavily exposed individuals is as high as 7 to 10%. Cigarette smoking

does not seem to be causally related to mesothelioma, since asbestos workers who smoke appear to be at no greater risk than their nonsmoking cohorts. However, asbestos workers who smoke are at much greater risk of developing *bronchogenic carcinoma* than nonsmoking asbestos workers (*pp. 760–761*).

17. (True); 18. (False); 19. (False); 20. (True); 21. (True); 22. (True); 23. (False)

Pulmonary emboli are by far the most common cause of occlusion of the pulmonary artery by blood clot, since *in situ* thrombosis is rare. (**17**) Pulmonary embolism usually occurs in patients suffering from some underlying disease (e.g., cardiac disease or cancer) or in those immobilized for long periods of time. However, young women who use oral contraceptive steroids, who are nearing parturition, or who have just given birth are also at increased risk of pulmonary embolism. (**18**) The most common source of emboli is the deep veins of the lower extremities.

(**19**) Unfortunately, pulmonary emboli are quite elusive on chest x-ray. If infarction has occurred, a wedge-shaped infiltrate may appear on the chest x-ray 12 to 36 hours later. In the absence of infarction, however, the chest x-ray of a patient with pulmonary embolism may be entirely normal. (**20**) Happily, most emboli resolve completely after the initial acute insult without medical treatment. The embolus initially contracts like all thrombi and is subsequently reduced in size by the serum thrombolytic activity. Total lysis of the clot usually ensues.

(**21**) Because of its dual blood supply, the lung undergoes infarction from pulmonary emboli only if the bronchial arterial supply is also compromised. Thus, pulmonary infarction tends to occur in elderly patients with severe systemic atherosclerosis. Overall, less than 10% of pulmonary emboli actually cause infarction.

(**22**) Although pulmonary embolus is a common and potentially lethal disorder causing more than 50,000 deaths in the United States each year, the overall mortality rate in patients treated for pulmonary embolism is less than 10%. In the presence of an underlying predisposing disease process, however, patients who have suffered one pulmonary embolus have a 25% chance of developing a second.

(**23**) Unresolved multiple small pulmonary emboli may eventually lead to pulmonary hypertension and pulmonary vascular sclerosis with cor pulmonale but do not cause interstitial fibrosis in the lungs (*pp. 711–713*).

24. (True); 25 (True); 26. (True); 27. (False); 28. (False)

Bronchial asthma is a chronic obstructive pulmonary disease characterized by irritability of the tracheobronchial tree, producing paroxysmal episodes of bronchospasm with severe dyspnea. Asthma has been divided into three basic types according to the precipitating factor and the pathogenetic mechanism:

(1) extrinsic or atopic asthma triggered by environmental antigens (dust, pollen, foods, and so forth); (2) intrinsic or idiosyncratic asthma precipitated by respiratory tract infection but not clearly associated with a hypersensitivity immune response; and (3) mixed pattern asthma, which has some properties of both the intrinsic and extrinsic types. (24) Most bronchial asthma is the extrinsic type, which is mediated by an immune response to an environmental antigen that leads to the production of IgE. On exposure to the antigen, presensitized IgE-coated mast cells and basophils release a host of chemical mediators that cause bronchoconstriction, increase venular permeability, and increase bronchial secretions. (25) No matter what the type of asthma—extrinsic, intrinsic, or mixed—the airways are hyperreactive to bronchoconstrictor agents. Indeed, the hyperreactivity of the airways to nonspecific irritants and bronchoconstrictor agents is an important feature of patients with asthma of any type.

(26) Although hypersensitivity to microbial antigens may possibly play a role in triggering the intrinsic type of asthma produced by some respiratory tract infections, the organism involved is usually a virus. Gram-positive cocci are more commonly associated with bronchopneumonia than with bronchial asthma.

(27) Aspirin-sensitive asthma, in contrast to other types of asthma, is thought to be related to aspirin's inhibition of the cyclooxygenase pathway of arachidonic acid metabolism without affecting the lipooxygenase route. Thus, the elaboration of the bronchoconstrictor leukotriences is favored, and asthma ensues. The pathogenetic mechanism of aspirin-sensitive asthma does not appear to involve an immunologic response of any sort; no antibodies or immune complexes are formed.

(28) Histologically, the most striking feature in bronchial asthma is the occlusion of bronchi and bronchioles by thick mucus plugs that contain whorls of shed epithelium known as Curschmann's spirals. Within the bronchiole, numerous eosinophils are also present that contain characteristic inclusions known as Charcot-Leyden crystals (*pp. 727–729*).

29. (False); 30. (True); 31. (False); 32. (False); 33. (False); 34. (True); 35. (True)

The lungs are by far the most common site of infection by *Mycobacterium tuberculosis*. (29) The initial pulmonary infection has a characteristic pattern of involvement. This pattern, called the Ghon complex, consists of a focus of caseating granuloma formation in the pulmonary parenchyma plus involvement of the lymph nodes draining that area. The location of the parenchymal focus is characteristically either just above or just below the interlobar fissure between the upper and lower lobes. This is the region of the lung in which air flow is the greatest and, consequently, where the greatest number of organisms is likely to be carried. The apices of the lung are the sites of highest oxygen tension, and it is here that a *secondary* focus of reactivated tuberculosis is most likely to occur. (30) In the absence of normal immunologic responses to the organism, however, this common pattern of involvement is not likely. Instead, the organism tends to produce a diffuse necrotizing bronchopneumonia.

(31) Most primary tuberculosis is asymptomatic. It is only in the secondary form of the disease (chronic pulmonary tuberculosis) that symptoms are usually produced. (32) Most cases of secondary pulmonary tuberculosis develop from reactivation of an old, sometimes subclinical primary infection. Fortunately, however, reactivation occurs in no more than 5 to 10% of cases of untreated primary infection.

(33) Once reactivation has occurred, the subsequent course of the disease is somewhat unpredictable. Widespread hematogenous dissemination may occur with the erosion of caseous lesions into vascular structures. With erosion into the pulmonary artery, miliary spread throughout the lungs would occur. Systemic dissemination, however, would occur with erosion into a pulmonary *vein*. (34) In addition to the unpredictable pattern of spread of the disease, the pattern of host response may be unpredictable. Although granuloma formation is usually the hallmark of host response to the mycobacteria, in the most severe tuberculous infections this response can be overwhelmed, and granulomas may fail to form altogether. (35) Since the consequences of secondary pulmonary tuberculosis may be severe, eradication of the primary disease is warranted. Any patient who has recently developed a floridly positive PPD skin test (indicating recent infection) requires antituberculous chemotherapy for at least 1 year (*pp. 341–346, 739–741*).

36. (C) Bronchiectasis is a condition characterized by abnormal dilatation of bronchi and bronchioles and manifested clinically by cough, fever, and production of copious amounts of foul-smelling, purulent sputum. In the adult, this condition is most often the result of both bronchial obstruction and secondary necrotizing bronchial infection. Common causes of obstruction are tumor, foreign bodies, and occasionally mucus impaction. Once obstructed, the bronchus becomes filled with mucus, which may become infected. Infection then produces bronchial wall inflammation, weakening, and dilatation. In addition, endobronchial obliteration may result from extensive bronchiolitis and bronchiolar damage. Atelectasis developing distal to the obliteration may, in turn, lead to further bronchiectasis in the lung adjacent to the areas of collapse (*pp. 729–730*).

37. (A); 38. (B); 39. (B); 40. (C); 41. (D)

Congenital cysts of the lung are of two basic types: bronchogenic and pulmonary. The two types have numerous contrasting features. (37) Bronchogenic cysts usually occur singly and are generally central in location, although they may occur anywhere in the lung. (38) Pulmonary cysts are generally multiple, often bilateral, and usually peripheral in location. (38) Unlike bronchogenic cysts, pulmonary cysts rarely communicate with a main bronchus. (40) Because they are basically sacs filled with proteinaceous secretion, both types of cysts are prime sites for the development of infection, which may lead to abscess formation. (41) Although the cysts are lined by a glandular type of epithelium, neither of these two types of congenital cysts is associated with neoplastic transformation (p. 709).

42. (A); 43. (D); 44. (B); 45. (C); 46. (D); 47. (A); 48. (B)

Goodpasture's syndrome and idiopathic pulmonary hemosiderosis are two distinctive interstitial diseases of the lung that both produce intrapulmonary hemorrhage as their major manifestation. (42 and 43) Goodpasture's syndrome is characterized by the simultaneous development of a necrotizing hemorrhagic interstitial pneumonitis and rapidly progressing glomerulonephritis (not interstitial nephritis). The syndrome has a striking predominance among males usually in the second or third decade of life. (47) Although the underlying cause is still unknown, it is clear that Goodpasture's syndrome is mediated by the production of antibodies directed against the capillary basement membrane in glomeruli and alveolar septae.

(44) Idiopathic pulmonary hemosiderosis is an uncommon pulmonary hemorrhagic syndrome of unknown etiology and pathogenesis. Unlike Goodpasture's syndrome, it has no striking male sexual predominance and tends to occur in children and younger adults.

(45) Although both of these disorders are characterized by necrotizing hemorrhagic interstitial pneumonitis, (46) neither produces vasculitis. Vasculitis-associated hemorrhage constitutes a separate and distinctive category of pulmonary hemorrhagic syndromes, which includes polyarteritis nodosa and Wegener's granulomatosis.

(48) In contrast to Goodpasture's syndrome, which is a devastating disease process requiring treatment with immunosuppressant chemotherapy and plasmapheresis, idiopathic pulmonary hemosiderosis often improves without treatment. The course of idiopathic pulmonary hemosiderosis in any given patient is unpredictable. Some patients develop progressive disease with interstitial fibrosis and others die suddenly of massive pulmonary hemorrhage (pp. 745–746).

49. (B); 50. (A); 51. (E); 52. (D); 53. (D)

Emphysema is one of the four conditions (with chronic bronchitis, bronchial asthma, and bronchiectasis) that are known as chronic obstructive pulmo-

nary diseases. Emphysema is defined by the American Thoracic Society as a condition "characterized by abnormal permanent enlargement of the air spaces distal to the terminal bronchioles, accompanied by destruction of their walls." Some types of emphysema have been defined on the basis of their particular pathologic and clinical patterns. (49) One of the most clinically distinctive types is panacinar (panlobular) emphysema. This type is associated with alpha-1-antitrypsin deficiency and is characterized pathologically by uniform enlargement of the acini from the level of the respiratory bronchioles to the terminal alveolar sacs. (50) Centriacinar (centrilobular) emphysema, in contrast, is the type that occurs most commonly in cigarette smokers. As its name implies, centriacinar emphysema is characterized by enlargement of the central or proximal structures of the acini (the respiratory bronchioles) with sparing of the distal alveoli.

(51) Although hyperinflation of the residual lung occurs after surgical removal of the lobe, the process does not involve any pulmonary parenchymal destruction and cannot be classified as an emphysematous process even though it is known by the unfortunate term of "compensatory emphysema." (52) Likewise, it should be recognized that interstitial emphysema is a process wholly separate from and unrelated to pulmonary emphysema as defined above. Interstitial emphysema refers to the entrance of air into the connective tissue stroma of the lungs, mediastinum, or subcutaneous tissue, most commonly resulting from tears in the alveolar walls. Usually alveolar tears occur when pressures in the alveolar sacs are sharply increased by a combination of coughing plus some bronchiolar obstruction such as occurs in children with whooping cough. (53) Thus, since it is not a form of pulmonary emphysema or chronic obstructive pulmonary disease, interstitial edema would not be associated with bullous disease. Any of the subtypes of pulmonary emphysema may form bullae or blebs when extensive alveolar destruction has occurred. The class of emphysema most commonly associated with bulla formation is irregular emphysema, a type almost invariably associated with pulmonary scarring (pp. 717–724).

54. (A); 55. (C); 56. (B); 57. (D); 58. (E); 59. (E); 60. (E); 61. (A); 62. (C); 63. (C)

Although not totally predictable in every case, specific microorganisms tend to produce characteristic patterns of pulmonary injury. (54 and 61) Diffuse alveolar damage is a pattern of injury most commonly seen in viral and mycoplasma pneumonias. (56) Bronchopneumonia involving an entire lobe (lobar pneumonia) is most commonly caused by *Streptococcus pneumoniae* (pneumococcus) but may be caused by other non-necrotizing bacteria. (55, 62, 63) Necrotizing bronchopneumonia is characteristic of such virulent organisms as *Staphylococcus aureua, Klebsiella pneumoniae*, and Legionella. Although any necrotizing bronchopneumonia may go on to abscess formation, this is a relatively infrequent complication. **(57)** Bacteroides species and other anaerobic organisms, however, are more commonly associated with lung abscess formation than with any other pattern of pulmonary injury. Pulmonary abscesses from anaerobic organisms are usually the result of aspiration.

(59) Thermophilic bacteria, such as those that infect heated water reservoirs in humidifiers or air conditioners, are of low virulence and do not cause direct pulmonary injury. Instead, thermophilic bacteria elicit a hypersensitivity immune response (both type I and type IV immune reactions). A hypersensitivity pneumonitis results that is characterized by an interstitial inflammatory infiltrate of mononuclear cells and eosinophils and scattered, noncaseated granulomata. **(60)** *Mycobacterium tuberculosis* is an organism of low virulence that in the immunocompetent host elicits a type IV immune response, producing granulomata that are the hallmark of this type of infection.

(58) Microfilariae produce a distinctive reaction in the lung characterized by patchy interstitial and intra-alveolar inflammatory infiltrates comprised predominantly of eosinophils. Thus the disease is known as tropical pulmonary eosinophilia *(pp. 733–740, 744, 748)*.

64. (A); 65. (B); 66. (B); 67. (D); 68 (A); 69. (C); 70. (C)

In industrialized nations, bronchogenic carcinoma is the most common visceral malignancy and accounts for the highest number of cancer deaths. **(64)** Among the histologic types of lung cancer, squamous cell carcinoma is the most common, accounting for 35 to 50% of all bronchogenic malignancies. Although there are no squamous cells in the normal lung, squamous cell carcinoma tends to arise from the large airways, which have undergone squamous metaplasia, become dysplastic, and have finally progressed to frank neoplasia.

(65) Unlike squamous cell carcinoma or small cell carcinoma, which both occur more frequently in men, adenocarcinoma of the lung occurs with equal frequency in males and females. **(66)** Since adenocarcinoma usually occurs in a peripheral location, it differs even further from squamous and small cell carcinomas, which tend to occur centrally in the lung. **(67)** Although adenocarcinoma is less frequently associated with a history of cigarette smoking than squamous cell or oat cell carcinomas, none of the major forms of bronchogenic carcinoma can be said to be etiologically unrelated to cigarette smoking.

(68) Bronchogenic carcinomas occasionally produce and secrete hormones that are not responsive to normal feedback regulatory mechanisms. One of the most characteristic ectopic hormonal syndromes associated with a specific tumor type is the production of parathyroid hormone by squamous cell carcinoma of the lung. The other major histologic types of bronchogenic carcinoma rarely, if ever, produce parathyroid hormone. **(69)** Small cell carcinoma of the lung, in contrast, is the most common type of malignancy to be associated with the syndrome of inappropriate antidiuretic hormone production.

(70) Small cell carcinoma of the lung is the only type of lung tumor for which surgical resection is ineffective. In fact, this diagnosis usually precludes attempts at operative treatment. For the other histologic types, early diagnosis with lobectomy or pneumonectomy is the best chance for cure of the disease. Unfortunately, most bronchogenic carcinoma is discovered in clinically advanced stages, accounting for the overall poor prognosis of the disease *(pp. 750–755)*.

7

THE HEMATOPOIETIC AND LYMPHOID SYSTEMS

DIRECTIONS: For Questions 1 to 6, choose the ONE BEST answer to each question.

1. Manifestations of hereditary spherocytosis include all of the following EXCEPT:

A. Mild jaundice
B. Hemoglobinuria
C. Splenomegaly
D. Cholelithiasis
E. Reduced plasma haptoglobin levels

2. Features of megaloblastic anemia include all of the following EXCEPT:

A. Hypersegmented neutrophils
B. Giant platelets   a.s.
C. Increased intramedullary hemolysis
D. Increased extramedullary hemolysis
E. Epithelial atypia of the gastric mucosa

3. Systemic lupus erythematosus (SLE) predisposes to the development of all the following hematologic disorders EXCEPT:

A. Microangiopathic hemolytic anemia
B. Pernicious anemia
C. Warm antibody autoimmune hemolytic anemia
D. Idiopathic thrombocytopenic purpura
E. Immunoblastic sarcoma of B cells

4. All of the following are known causes of aplastic anemia EXCEPT:

A. Whole body irradiation
B. Infectious mononucleosis
C. Paroxysmal nocturnal hemoglobinuria
D. Chloramphenicol
E. Metastatic carcinoma

5. All of the following statements about disseminated intravascular coagulation are true EXCEPT:

A. The disorder is characterized by widespread thromboses
B. The disorder is characterized by widespread hemorrhages
C. It most often presents as a primary (idiopathic) condition
D. The brain is the organ most often involved
E. The disorder is associated with mucin-secreting adenocarcinomas

6. Multiple myeloma is associated with all of the following features EXCEPT:

A. Hypercalcemia
B. Renal failure
C. Amyloidosis
D. Increased susceptibility to viral infections
E. Rouleau formation on peripheral smear

DIRECTIONS: For Questions 7 to 15, ONE or MORE of the completions given correctly finishes the incomplete statement. Choose:

A—if only *1, 2, and 3* are correct
B—if only *1 and 3* are correct
C—if only *2 and 4* are correct
D—if only *4* is correct
E—if all are correct

7. Osmotic fragility characterizes the erythrocytes in:

1. Fanconi's syndrome
2. Sickle cell anemia
3. Glucose-6-phosphate dehydrogenase (G6PD) deficiency
4. Hereditary spherocytosis

A. 1,2,3   B. 1,3   C. 2,4   D. 4 Only   E. All

8. Hematologic disorders occurring mainly in populations in the Middle East (Mediterranean region) include:

1. Glucose-6-phosphate dehydrogenase (G6PD) deficiency
2. Thalassemia major
3. Alpha-chain disease
4. Factor IX deficiency (Christmas disease)

    A. 1,2,3 B. 1,3 C. 2,4 D. 4 Only E. All

9. Microangiopathic hemolytic anemia is encountered in:

1. Thrombotic thrombocytopenic purpura
2. The hemolytic-uremic syndrome
3. Malignant hypertension
4. Prosthetic heart valves

    A. 1,2,3 B. 1,3 C. 2,4 D. 4 Only E. All

10. Iron deficiency anemia:

1. Is associated with colon cancer
2. Is associated with lung cancer
3. Commonly occurs after gastrectomy
4. Commonly produces mild leukopenia

    A. 1,2,3 B. 1,3 C. 2,4 D. 4 Only E. All

11. Polycythemia vera:

1. Is an X-linked recessive disorder
2. Is associated with high levels of erythropoietin
3. Produces abnormalities in the red cell series only
4. Predisposes to myelofibrosis

    A. 1,2,3 B. 1,3 C. 2,4 D. 4 Only E. All

12. Viral hepatitis predisposes to which of the following hematologic disorders?

1. Idiopathic thrombocytopenic purpura
2. Aplastic anemia
3. Erythropoietic depression
4. Autoimmune hemolytic anemia

    A. 1,2,3 B. 1,3 C. 2,4 D. 4 Only E. All

13. Increased blood viscosity (hyperviscosity syndrome) is a major complication of which of the following disorders?

1. Polycythemia vera
2. IgA myeloma
3. Sickle cell anemia
4. Waldenström's macroglobulinemia

    A. 1,2,3 B. 1,3 C. 2,4 D. 4 Only E. All

14. Nodular lymphomas:

1. Are common in the pediatric age group
2. Have a better prognosis than diffuse lymphomas
3. Occur much more frequently in males than females
4. Are always composed of B lymphocytes

    A. 1,2,3 B. 1,3 C. 2,4 D. 4 Only E. All

15. Which of the following features is/are characteristic of myeloid metaplasia with myelofibrosis?

1. Giant platelets
2. Teardrop-shaped red cells
3. Elevated leukocyte alkaline phosphatase levels
4. Massive splenomegaly

    A. 1,2,3 B. 1,3 C. 2,4 D. 4 Only E. All

DIRECTIONS: For Questions 16 to 22, you are to decide whether EACH choice is TRUE or FALSE.

For each of the following statements about Hodgkin's disease, choose whether it is TRUE or FALSE.

16. The Reed-Sternberg cell is the malignant component of the tumor
17. Mixed cellularity is the most common subtype
18. All subtypes of Hodgkin's disease spread by contiguity from one lymph node group to another

19. A leukemic phase is common in the lymphocyte-predominant subtype
20. The subtype of Hodgkin's disease is the most important prognostic indicator
21. In young adults, infectious mononucleosis poses an increased risk of developing Hodgkin's disease
22. Patients successfully treated for Hodgkin's disease have an increased risk of developing a non-Hodgkin's lymphoma

DIRECTIONS: For Questions 23 to 35, the set of lettered headings is followed by a list of numbered words or phrases. For each numbered word or phrase choose:

A—if the item is associated with (A) only
B—if the item is associated with (B) only
C—if the item is associated with *both* (A) and (B)
D—if the item is associated with *neither* (A) nor (B)

For each of the features listed below, choose whether it is characteristic of warm antibody autoimmune hemolytic anemia (AHA), cold agglutinin AHA, both, or neither.

A. Warm antibody autoimmune hemolytic anemia
B. Cold agglutinin autoimmune hemolytic anemia
C. Both
D. Neither

23. Antibodies to red cells are usually monoclonal IgG
24. Antibodies to red cells are usually monoclonal IgM
25. The disorder is often caused by drugs
26. The disorder occurs in association with lymphoma
27. Splenomegaly is commonly produced
28. Complement-mediated intravascular hemolysis is commonly produced

For each of the statements listed below, choose whether it describes acute lymphocytic leukemia (ALL), acute myelogenous leukemia (AML), both, or neither.

A. Acute lymphocytic leukemia (ALL)
B. Acute myelogenous leukemia (AML)
C. Both
D. Neither

29. The disease most commonly occurs in the elderly
30. Leukemic cells usually contain the enzyme terminal deoxynucleotidyl transferase (TdT)
31. Leukemic cells are characterized by a unique chromosomal abnormality known as the Philadelphia chromosome
32. Leukemic cells commonly contain Auer rods
33. Bone marrow is characteristically replaced by a uniform population of primitive cells
34. Patients treated for Hodgkin's disease with chemotherapy and irradiation are at increased risk of developing the disease
35. Prominent lymphadenopathy is characteristically present

DIRECTIONS: Questions 36 to 81 are matching questions. For each numbered item, choose the most likely associated lettered item from those provided. Each numbered item has ONLY ONE answer. Within each group, each lettered item may be the answer to one, more than one, or none of the numbered items.

For each of the following features of hemolytic anemia, choose whether it is characteristic of beta-thalassemia, paroxysmal nocturnal hemoglobinuria (PNH), sickle cell anemia, glucose-6-phosphate dehydrogenase (G6PD) deficiency, or none of these.

A. Beta-thalassemia
B. Paroxysmal nocturnal hemoglobinuria (PNH)
C. Sickle cell anemia
D. Glucose-6-phosphate dehydrogenase (G6PD) deficiency
E. None of these

36. Antimalarial drugs cause hemolytic crises
37. Splenic hypofunction predisposes to infections

38. Ingestion of fava beans causes hemolytic crises
39. Heinz bodies appear within red cells
40. Hypoxia causes hemolytic crises
41. Platelets are abnormal
42. Granulocytes are abnormal
43. Transformation to acute myelogenous leukemia occasionally occurs
44. Usually leads to death before age 20
45. Red cell precursors are characteristically destroyed within the marrow
46. Expansion of the erythron within the bone marrow is *not* a feature of the disease
47. Autoantibodies to red cells contribute to the hemolysis

For each of the conditions or situations associated with hemorrhagic diatheses listed below, choose whether the major cause is vascular fragility, thrombocytopenia, defective platelet function, a clotting factor defect, or disseminated intravascular coagulation (DIC).

    A. Vascular fragility
    B. Thrombocytopenia
    C. Defective platelet function
    D. Clotting factor defect
    E. Disseminated intravascular coagulation (DIC)

48. Cushing's syndrome
49. Uremia
50. von Willebrand's disease
51. Massive transfusions
52. Henoch-Schonlein purpura
53. Rickettsial infection
54. Promyelogenous leukemia

For each of the drugs and chemicals listed below, choose whether the hematologic defect with which it is associated is autoimmune hemolytic anemia (AHA), aplastic anemia, neutropenia, all of these, or none of these.

    A. Drug-related autoimmune hemolytic anemia
    B. Drug-related aplastic anemia
    C. Drug-related neutropenia
    D. All of these
    E. None of these

55. Penicillin
56. Alpha-methyldopa
57. Thiouracil
58. Quinidine
59. Benzene
60. Aminopyrine
61. Phenacetin

For each of the diseases listed below, choose whether it is characterized by increased circulating numbers of neutrophils, lymphocytes, eosinophils, or none of these.

    A. Elevated neutrophil count
    B. Elevated lymphocyte count
    C. Elevated eosinophil count
    D. None of these

62. Tuberculosis
63. Bronchial asthma
64. Infectious mononucleosis
65. Myocardial infarction
66. Eosinophilic granuloma

For each of the features listed below, choose which type of nonHodgkin's lymphoma (Rappaport classification) it describes: well-differentiated lymphocytic lymphoma (WDLL), poorly-differentiated lymphocytic lymphoma (PDLL), histiocytic lymphoma (HL), lymphoblastic lymphoma, or none of these.

    A. Well-differentiated lymphocytic lymphoma (WDLL)
    B. Poorly-differentiated lymphocytic lymphoma (PDLL)
    C. Histiocytic lymphoma (HL)
    D. Lymphoblastic lymphoma
    E. None of these

67. Young adults are most commonly affected
68. Chronic lymphocytic leukemia is histologically identical
69. A "starry sky" histologic pattern is characteristic
70. The tumor occurs only in nodular form
71. Origin in extranodal sites is frequent
72. Prolonged survival is the rule
73. The tumor is usually composed of T lymphocytes
74. Leukemic dissemination is extremely uncommon
75. Frequently associated with a previous history of an autoimmune disorder
76. Tumor cells are characterized by convoluted "chicken footprint" nuclei

For each of the features listed below, choose whether it is characteristic of the Letterer-Siwe syndrome, Hand-Schüller-Christian disease, eosinophilic granuloma, all of these, or none of these.

    A. Letterer-Siwe syndrome
    B. Hand-Schüller-Christian disease
    C. Eosinophilic granuloma
    D. All of these
    E. None of these

77. Diabetes insipidus is frequently produced
78. The disease commonly occurs before the age of 3
79. The mortality rate is 100%
80. Infiltrating histiocytes contain pentalaminar inclusion bodies
81. Skin rash is characteristically absent

7

THE HEMATOPOIETIC AND LYMPHOID SYSTEMS

ANSWERS

1. (B) Hereditary spherocytosis is an autosomal dominant disorder characterized by a structural defect in the skeleton of the red cell membrane. The structural abnormality results in spherically-shaped cells that are less deformable and hence more vulnerable to splenic sequestration and destruction than normal erythrocytes. The premature destruction of red cells produces a chronic hemolytic anemia with accumulation of hemoglobin breakdown products and a concomitant increase in erythropoiesis in the bone marrow. The extravascular hemolysis produces a mild jaundice with unconjugated hyperbilirubinemia. Moderate splenic enlargement resulting from the congestion of the cords of Billroth is characteristic of hereditary spherocytosis. Pigment (bilirubin) gallstones are also found in many patients.

Haptoglobin, a serum glycoprotein whose physiologic function is to bind free hemoglobin in the serum and prevent its urinary loss, is characteristically reduced in hereditary spherocytosis since some hemoglobin invariably escapes from the phagocytic cells in the spleen. In contrast to intravascular hemolytic processes, the amount of hemoglobin released into the serum is small, and haptoglobin is reduced but not depleted. Depletion of haptoglobin and subsequent excretion of hemoglobin through the kidneys (hemoglobinuria) are characteristic of most forms of intravascular hemolysis but in general do not occur in hereditary spherocytosis (*pp. 616–617*).

2. (B) Megaloblastic anemias resulting from either vitamin B_{12} or folate deficiency are characterized by defective DNA synthesis in all hematopoietic cells. This defective synthesis leads to the production of abnormal red cells and leukocytes and a decrease in the production of all cell lines. Asynchrony between the nuclear and cytoplasmic maturation develops during hematopoiesis, resulting in macrocytic erythrocytes, giant neutrophils with hypersegmented nuclei, and large bizarre megakaryocytes. Defective erythropoiesis leads to increased intramedullary hemolysis of the abnormal precursors. Increased extramedullary hemolysis of defective red cells occurs as well, augmented by a poorly characterized plasma factor produced in this disease. Although the impact on the hematopoietic system is most profound, the acquired defect in DNA synthesis affects all rapidly proliferating cells in the body. Therefore, the intestinal mucosa (especially the gastric epithelium) also suffers from nuclear-cytoplasmic asynchrony and develops megaloblastic cytologic changes.

Although giant megakaryocytes are seen in megaloblastic anemia as mentioned above, giant platelets are *not* a feature of this disease. Instead, giant platelets usually occur either in the absence of the spleen or in myeloproliferative disorders such as myeloid metaplasia (*pp. 630–633*).

3. (B) Systemic lupus erythematosus (SLE) predisposes to a number of hematologic disorders. The necrotizing arteritis and arteriolitis that occur in SLE can produce a microangiopathic hemolytic anemia. The production of autoantibodies in SLE may result in a warm antibody autoimmune hemolytic anemia. Chronic idiopathic thrombocytopenic purpura, a disorder characterized by immune-mediated destruction of platelets, is sometimes associated with other immunologic disorders such as SLE. Immunoblastic sarcoma of B cells, a lymphoma believed to arise from transformed interfollicular B cells, is frequently (30% of cases) associated with a prior history of an immunologic disorder such as SLE.

Pernicious anemia is an autoimmune disease producing gastric mucosal injury. Although there is a significant association between pernicious anemia and autoimmune diseases affecting the thyroid and adrenal glands, there is no clear association between pernicious anemia and SLE (*pp. 628, 630, 633, 646, 664*).

4. (E) Aplastic anemia is a condition caused by a hematopoietic stem cell defect and characterized by bone marrow failure involving all cell lines. Although the condition may occasionally be primary and idiopathic or hereditary (Fanconi's anemia), it most often occurs as a result of stem cell injury from a variety of chemical agents, physical agents, infections, or other stem cell disorders. Whole body irradiation is the prototypic cause of injury by physical agents. Infections that are known to induce aplastic anemia are largely, if not exclusively, viral in origin and include infectious mononucleosis, dengue fever, and viral hepatitis. Paroxysmal nocturnal hemoglobinuria is a disorder of stem cells that causes a hemolytic anemia (see Questions 41 to 43) and sometimes evolves into aplastic anemia. Chloramphenicol is one of a long list of drugs that can cause aplastic anemia but is curiously the only one that is known to do so in either a dose-related or an idiosyncratic manner.

Metastatic carcinoma in the bone marrow may produce pancytopenia but is considered a form of myelophthisic anemia rather than aplastic anemia. Myelophthisic anemias are produced by space-occupying lesions that destroy significant amounts of normal marrow and, in contrast to aplastic anemias, are not associated with stem cell defects (*pp. 638–639*).

5. (C) Disseminated intravascular coagulation (DIC) is an acquired thrombohemorrhagic disorder characterized by activation of the coagulation cascades. The result is widespread thrombosis and hemorrhage (a consequence of depletion of the elements required for homeostasis). Although any organ can be affected, the brain is most often involved. DIC occurs in association with several disorders, especially sepsis, major trauma, obstetric conditions, and malignancy. Mucin-secreting adenocarcinomas are frequently associated with DIC, since they release a variety of thromboplastic substances including tissue factors, proteolytic enzymes, and mucin, all of which are thrombogenic. It is important to recognize that DIC is, in fact, always secondary to some other underlying condition and does not occur as a primary idiopathic process (*pp. 649–651*).

6. (D) Multiple myeloma is a neoplastic proliferation of plasma cells that are differentiated enough to secrete immunoglobulins or their components. These tumors have numerous distinctive manifestations resulting from their patterns of growth and secretory activity. Typically, multiple myeloma forms osteolytic lesions in bones that have a characteristic "punched-out" appearance on radiographs. The bony destruction frequently leads to hypercalcemia. Renal failure is common in patients with multiple myeloma and is a frequent cause of death in this disease. The most significant factor leading to renal failure is the toxic effect of filtered immunoglobin light chains (Bence-Jones proteins) on the renal tubular epithelium, although infiltration of the interstitium by tumor cells also occurs. Amyloidosis of immunologic origin occurs in about 10% of patients with multiple myeloma and may also contribute to renal failure. Coating of erythrocytes with circulating immunoglobulins causes a rouleau formation characteristically seen on peripheral smear.

Although susceptibility to infection is a common complication of multiple myeloma and the leading cause of death, it is due to the severe depression of normal immunoglobulin production in this disease.

Cellular immunity, however, is relatively unaffected. Therefore, increased susceptibility to viral infections is not prominent, whereas recurrent infections with encapsulated bacteria pose a major clinical problem (*pp. 689–692*).

7. (D) Osmotic fragility is a property of the red cells in hereditary spherocytosis and forms the basis of a common laboratory test used in confirming the diagnosis of this disease.

In the hereditary form of aplastic anemia, known as Fanconi's anemia, red cell production is drastically reduced, but the structural properties of the erythrocytes in this disease are not known to be abnormal. In sickle cell anemia, erythrocytes characteristically undergo structural deformation in environments of lowered oxygen tension but are not osmotically fragile. Therefore, common diagnostic tests for sickle cell anemia are based on mixing a blood sample with an oxygen-consuming reagent such as metabisulfite to induce sickling. Red cells in G6PD deficiency are characterized by their sensitivity to oxidative injury and will undergo hemolysis when exposed to oxidant drugs; however, they are not osmotically fragile (*pp. 616–620, 639*).

8. (A) A number of hematologic disorders occur largely in populations in the Mediterranean area or in patients of Middle Eastern extraction. Principal among these are two hereditary hemolytic anemias: a severe form of G6PD deficiency and beta-thalassemia (thalassemia major). The Mediterranean form of G6PD deficiency is characterized by impaired synthesis of this enzyme. The resultant abnormalities in glutathione metabolism impair the ability of the red cells to protect themselves against oxidative injuries and lead to hemolysis. Beta-thalassemia is a defect in the production of beta-globin chains that in combination with alpha chains make up the major adult human hemoglobin. The inability to produce normal hemoglobin leads to a severe, transfusion-dependent anemia.

Alpha-chain disease is a third disorder that occurs most commonly in Mediterranean populations. It is a form of IgA-producing monoclonal gammopathy characterized by massive infiltration of the intestinal mucosa with lymphocytes, plasmacytes, and histiocytes. The infiltrate also produces a severe malabsorption syndrome, a prominent feature of this disorder. Furthermore, transformation into an immunoblastic sarcoma of B cells occasionally occurs.

Christmas disease or hemophilia B is a rare but severe coagulopathy resulting from a deficiency of Factor IX. This disease has no increased incidence among Mediterranean populations (*pp. 617–618, 624, 649, 693*).

9. (E) Hemolysis due to narrowing or obstruction in the microvasculature is called microangiopathic hemolytic anemia. The disorder is always secondary to some vascular lesion that physically traumatizes and fragments red cells. Microangiopathic hemolytic anemia is encountered in thrombotic thrombocytopenic purpura, a disorder characterized by widespread platelet microthrombi in arterioles, capillaries, and venules. In the hemolytic-uremic syndrome, glomerular capillaries and afferent arterioles are occluded by microthrombi that constitute the source of red cell injury. In malignant hypertension, red cells are damaged while passing through the markedly narrowed arterioles. Prosthetic heart valves occasionally create turbulent blood flow and abnormal pressure gradients, which lead to red cell injury (pp. 629–630, 1046–1049).

10. (B) Although dietary deficiency is the most common cause of iron deficiency anemia world-wide, chronic blood loss is by far the most common cause of this disorder in the Western world. Chronic blood loss often occurs in benign or malignant diseases of the gastrointestinal tract, which cause bleeding into the lumen and subsequent loss of blood in the stool. In fact, patients with colon cancer may first present to the clinician with symptoms of iron deficiency anemia. With the exception of malignancies of the female genital tract and urinary tract, hemorrhage produced by other malignancies usually occurs within the tissues and does not lead to iron loss. Gastrectomy is commonly associated with iron deficiency anemia since gastric acid is important to iron absorption. Furthermore, gastrectomy reduces transit time through the duodenum, the principal site of iron absorption. Iron deficiency affects only red cell hemoglobin production and does not produce abnormalities in any of the other hematopoietic cell lines. Leukopenia, therefore, is not a feature of iron deficiency anemia (pp. 636–637).

11. (D) Polycythemia vera is believed to be a neoplastic monoclonal proliferation of myeloid stem cells. It characteristically produces a striking elevation in the total red cell mass. The etiology of the disorder is as yet unknown, and there is no well-defined mode of genetic transmission. A distinctive feature of this disorder is suppression of erythropoietin by the proliferation of abnormal red cells. Since the abnormal stem cells of polycythemia vera require only very small amounts of erythropoietin for their proliferation and differentiation, only the normal erythropoietic precursors are suppressed by the drop in erythropoietin production. Although the predominant manifestation of polycythemia vera is excessive proliferation of the erythroid series, the granulocytic and megakaryocytic cell lines are also affected to a lesser degree. In fact, the concomitant elevation in the granulocyte and platelet count is supportive evidence that polycythemia vera is indeed a disorder of pluripotent myeloid stem cells. The disease has a variable course, but a significant number of patients develop myelofibrosis after a period of years. Much less commonly, transformation to chronic myelogenous leukemia occurs (pp. 641–642).

12. (A) Viral hepatitis predisposes to a number of hematologic disorders, some of which have more severe consequences than the hepatitis itself. Idiopathic thrombocytopenic purpura, aplastic anemia, and a depression of red cell production are all associated with viral hepatitis. Idiopathic thrombocytopenic purpura occurring in association with viral hepatitis is an acute self-limited form of this disease. In contrast, aplastic anemia occurring in association with viral hepatitis has an extremely grave prognosis. The anemia associated with diffuse liver diseases of any form, including those of viral etiology, is attributed to bone marrow failure, but the exact pathogenetic mechanisms are still obscure. Although cold agglutinin autoimmune hemolytic anemia occasionally occurs in its acute form following a viral infection such as infectious mononucleosis or influenza, it is not known to be associated with infections by the hepatotropic viruses (pp. 628–629, 639, 640, 645).

13. (E) Circulatory impairment, particularly in the central nervous system and retina, yielding symptoms such as headache, dizziness, or visual impairment results from increased serum viscosity. A hyperviscosity syndrome is a common consequence of hematologic disorders that significantly increase either numbers of cellular elements or serum protein levels. Thus, hyperviscosity frequently complicates plasma cell dyscrasias and monoclonal gammopathies such as IgA myeloma and Waldenström's macroglobulinemia. It is also responsible for the major symptomatic manifestations of polycythemia vera. In sickle cell anemia, increased blood viscosity is caused by the inelasticity of sickled red cells. Hyperviscosity in turn contributes to the relative hypoxia that favors further sickling of red cells upstream, eventually leading to complete vascular occlusion and infarction (pp. 620, 642, 691, 692).

14. (C) Irrespective of their cellular morphology, non-Hodgkin's lymphomas that inhibit a nodular growth pattern have several notable similarities. They are always composed of neoplastic B cells, and their nodularity is a recapitulation of lymphoid follicle formation. Overall, nodular lymphomas have a much better prognosis than their diffuse counterpart. Their age and sex distribution also contrasts significantly with those of diffuse lymphomas. Unlike diffuse lymphomas, which occur with significant frequency in children and adolescents, nodular lymphomas are extremely rare in individuals under 20 years of age. Furthermore, nodular lymphomas occur with equal frequency in males and females, whereas diffuse lymphomas are much more common in males (pp. 658–659).

15. (E) Myeloid metaplasia with myelofibrosis is a myeloproliferative syndrome characterized by fibrous replacement of the bone marrow and extramedullary hematopoiesis. The spleen is the major site of the extramedullary hematopoiesis (myeloid metaplasia) and is usually markedly enlarged, weighing up to 4000 grams. The blood elements produced in this disease have numerous abnormalities. Particularly characteristic are teardrop-shaped erythrocytes and giant platelets. Since myeloblasts, myelocytes, and metamyelocytes typically constitute a small fraction of the white cell population on the peripheral smear in myelofibrosis, the disease can sometimes be difficult to differentiate from chronic myelogenous leukemia. In myeloid metaplasia, however, leukocyte alkaline phosphatase levels are often elevated, whereas in chronic myelogenous leukemia they are characteristically low (pp. 686–688). *The reaction consistent*

16. (True); 17. (False); 18. (True); 19. (False); 20. (False); 21. (True); 22. (True)

Hodgkin's disease has long been classified separately from the non-Hodgkin's lymphomas on the basis of its numerous unique features. **(16)** Hodgkin's disease is characterized by a proliferation of giant neoplastic B cells known as Reed-Sternberg (R-S) cells. The R-S cell is the only malignant element in Hodgkin's disease. In each of the histologic subtypes of Hodgkin's disease, R-S cells are associated with a variable number of other leukocytes, but these so-called "background cells" are reactive rather than neoplastic in nature.

(17) The most common subtype of Hodgkin's disease is nodular sclerosis, representing about 40% of cases. Mixed cellularity Hodgkin's disease is second in frequency.

(18) No matter what the subtype, Hodgkin's disease almost always spreads by contiguity from one chain of lymph nodes to the adjacent group, a feature rarely associated with non-Hodgkin's lymphoma.

(19) In further contrast to most non-Hodgkin's lymphomas, Hodgkin's disease (of any type) rarely manifests a leukemic state.

(20) Although the subtypes of Hodgkin's disease, based on the relative numbers of Reed-Sternberg cells and background cells, are associated with differences in clinical behavior, they are far less important than clinical staging as indicators of prognosis.

(21) Although the pathogenesis of Hodgkin's disease is still obscure, it has been suggested that it may represent a consequence of delayed infection with a common viral agent. Usually cited in support of this hypothesis is the resemblance of the Reed-Sternberg cell to a virally transformed cell and the increased incidence (2- to 3-fold) of Hodgkin's disease in young adults with infectious mononucleosis.

(22) Although the modern aggressive modes of therapy have largely obliterated the prognostic differences between the various subtypes of Hodgkin's disease and significantly improved survival, it appears that this has not happened without a cost. Long-term survivors of combined chemotherapy and radiotherapy have a significantly increased risk of developing a non-Hodgkin's lymphoma or an acute leukemia (pp. 670–674).

23. (D); 24. (B); 25. (A); 26. (C); 27. (A); 28. (D)

Autoimmune hemolytic anemias are characterized by the production of anti–red cell antibodies that either directly cause hemolysis or indirectly lead to increased red cell destruction. The type of antibody produced determines to a large extent the nature of the resultant disorder and forms the basis of the classification of the immunohemolytic disorders.

(23 and 24) In cold agglutinin autoimmune hemolytic anemia (AHA), the antibodies produced are primarily monoclonal IgM. Although the antibodies in warm antibody AHA are usually IgG, they do not appear to be of monoclonal origin.

(25) Warm antibody AHA often occurs in association with drugs. The drug acts as a hapten in inducing an immune response to red cells (e.g., penicillin, quinidine, and phenacetin) or may directly initiate the production of antibodies that are directed against intrinsic red cell antigens like the Rh blood group antigens (e.g., alphamethyldopa). **(26)** In contrast to drug-associated AHA, lymphoma-associated AHA may be of either the warm antibody or cold agglutinin type.

(27) In warm antibody AHA, antibody-coated red cells or red cells coated with drug-induced immune complexes are susceptible to splenic sequestration and destruction. Thus, splenomegaly is a common feature of warm antibody AHA. In cold agglutinin AHA, the liver sequesters most of the affected red cells, and splenomegaly is uncommon. The reason for this phenomenon is as yet poorly understood.

(28) The hemolysis in both warm antibody AHA and cold agglutinin AHA is extravascular. Only in cold hemolysin AHA, a third major class of autoimmune hemolytic anemia, does intravascular hemolysis occur. In this disorder, autoantibodies bind to red cells at low temperature and induce complement-mediated hemolysis when the temperature is elevated (pp. 628–629).

29. (D); 30. (A); 31. (D); 32. (B); 33. (C); 34. (B); 35. (A)

Acute leukemias are dramatic neoplastic proliferations of white blood cell precursors producing abnormal numbers and forms of immature white cells in the circulating blood. Although they have some common features, acute leukemias of lymphocytic origin differ from those of granulocytic origin in both pathologic and clinical behavior.

(29) Both acute lymphocytic leukemia (ALL) acute myelogenous leukemia (AML) are pred in the young. ALL is the most frequen' children under 15 years of age, whereas A mainly in young adults (the 15–39-year

– (**30 and 33**) By routine histologic examination, ALL and AML may be difficult to distinguish from one another, since both are composed of a uniform population of undifferentiated blast elements. Therefore, special enzymatic and histochemical marker studies are beneficial in determining the cell of origin in acute leukemias. Helpful in this regard is the enzyme terminal deoxynucleotidyl transferase (TdT), presumed to be a marker of primitive lymphoid cells. It is present in the majority of cases of ALL but lacking in AML.

(**31**) The Philadelphia chromosome, usually representing a reciprocal translocation from a long arm of chromosome 22 to chromosome 9, is present in about 95% of patients with *chronic* myelogenous leukemia but is not a feature characteristic of AML or ALL.

(**32**) Auer rods are needle-like inclusions in the cytoplasm of myelocytes formed from abnormal azurophilic granules and can commonly be identified in myeloblasts or promyelocytes in AML.

(**34**) Patients treated with chemotherapy and radiotherapy for Hodgkin's disease are at increased risk of developing AML and non-Hodgkin's lymphomas. ALL, however, does not occur with increased frequency in these patients (see Question 22).

(**35**) Although lymph nodes are known to be enlarged in all forms of leukemia, there is a marked difference in the degree of lymph node enlargement in lymphocytic and myelogenous leukemias. In keeping with their origin from lymphoid tissue, lymphocytic leukemias are associated with the most striking degree of lymph node involvement. The lymph nodes are somewhat enlarged in about half of patients with AML but are rarely as conspicuous as in patients with ALL *(pp. 676–685)*.

36. (**D**); **37.** (**C**); **38.** (**D**); **39.** (**D**); **40.** (**C**); **41.** (**B**); **42.** (**B**); **43.** (**B**); **44.** (**A**); **45.** (**A**); **46.** (**D**); **47.** (**E**)

Beta-thalassemia, paroxysmal nocturnal hemoglobinuria (PNH), sickle cell anemia, and glucose-6-phosphate dehydrogenase (G6PD) deficiency are all major forms of hemolytic anemias. The unique pathogenetic defect in each disorder produces characteristic features.

(**36**) G6PD deficiency produces derangements in the hexose monophosphate shunt and glutathione metabolism. Since glutathione is essential to red cell protection against oxidant injury, oxidant substances such as the antimalarial drugs trigger red cell injury and hemolysis in affected individuals. (**38**) Unique to this disorder are the hemolytic crises induced by ingestion of fava beans, which in some individuals are metabolized to a highly oxidant derivative. (**39**) Heinz bodies (precipitates of denatured hemoglobin) form within the red cells of G6PD-deficient individuals when oxidation of the sulfhydryl group of globin chains occurs. Heinz bodies contribute to the demise of the red cell in two ways: (1) They render the red cell membrane to which they are attached less de-

formable and more prone to sequestration in the spleen, and (2) when they are "pitted" from the cell by splenic macrophages, the resultant loss of cell membrane produces spherocytes that are themselves more susceptible to splenic sequestration. (**46**) Unlike the other forms of hemolytic anemias that produce chronic red cell destruction, G6PD deficiency produces *intermittent* bouts of acute hemolysis. It does not, therefore, lead to prolonged stimulation of erythropoietic production with expansion of the erythron in the bone marrow.

(**37**) Sickle cell anemia classically produces a unique if somewhat poorly understood depression of splenic function, even while the spleen is enlarged early in the course of the disease. The resultant splenic hypofunction predisposes to blood-borne infections, especially to those caused by Salmonella and pneumococci. Later in the course of the disease, the spleen may actually undergo autoinfarction as a result of repeated bouts of sickling in the sinuses, leading to thrombosis, hypoxic injury, and resultant scarring. Predisposition to bacterial infection is a major consequence of splenectomy (functional or otherwise) in any individual. (**40**) Since it is the deoxygenated form of sickle hemoglobin that undergoes polymerization and causes red cell deformation, hypoxia is the major stimulus to sickling and hemolytic crises.

(**41 and 42**) In contrast to thalassemia, sickle cell anemia, and G6PD deficiency, all disorders affecting red cell function only, paroxysmal nocturnal hemoglobinuria (PNH) is a disorder of myeloid stem cells that produces functional abnormalities in all hematopoietic cell lines. The cell membrane defect characteristic of PNH that renders red cells more sensitive to lysis by complement is also present in platelets and granulocytes. Additional functional abnormalities of platelets and granulocytes are manifested by the striking predisposition to intravascular thromboses and infection in individuals with PNH. (**43**) Supportive evidence that this unique form of hemolytic anemia is a stem cell disorder is its occasional transformation into other myeloid stem cell disorders such as acute myelogenous leukemia or aplastic anemia.

(**44**) Although the other forms of hemolytic anemia can be severe and debilitating, beta-thalassemia clearly has the worst prognosis. The disease produces such a profound, transfusion-dependent anemia that most patients die at an early age. Even with medical therapy, the average age at death is 17 years. (**45**) In this disorder, caused by a defect in the synthesis of beta-globin chains, red cell precursors are characteristically destroyed within the marrow. This occurs because the free alpha-globin chains form unstable intracellular aggregates that are injurious to the red cell precursors. In severely affected patients, it is estimated that 70 to 85% of the marrow normoblasts are destroyed *in situ*. This contrasts with the other forms of hemolytic anemia discussed above in which red cell destruction is primarily extramedullary.

(**47**) All four of these diseases are the result of an

intrinsic defect in the red cell. In contrast to autoimmune hemolytic anemias, which represent acquired defects of red cells and are often associated with autoantibodies to erythrocytes, these disorders are not associated with immunologic red cell destruction (*pp. 617–628*).

48. (A); 49. (C); 50. (D); 51. (B); 52. (A); 53. (A); 54. (E)

(48) Hemorrhagic disorders occur when an abnormality of vessel walls, platelets, coagulation factors, or a combination of these is present. In Cushing's syndrome, vascular fragility predisposing to skin hemorrhages results from the protein wasting effect of excessive corticosteroids.

(49) The hemorrhagic diathesis in uremia represents an acquired defect of platelet function. It is thought to occur as a consequence of impaired platelet membrane interaction with normal von Willebrand's factor.

(50) In von Willebrand's disease, on the other hand, von Willebrand's factor (the ristocetin cofactor of clotting factor VIII) is qualitatively or quantitatively defective. This component of the factor VIII complex is required for adhesion of platelets to subendothelial collagen; thus, a prolonged bleeding time and a marked tendency toward spontaneous bleeding occur in this disorder.

(51) Since blood stored for longer than 24 hours is virtually depleted of platelets, massive transfusions can produce a hemorrhagic diathesis simply by diluting platelets to thrombocytopenic levels. In the presence of a normal bone marrow, the effect is transient.

(52) Widespread weakening of vascular walls with resultant hemorrhage is a common feature of hypersensitivity vasculitides. Henoch-Schonlein purpura is a prototypic example of immune complex–mediated vascular damage with a resultant hemorrhagic diathesis.

(53) Direct damage to the vascular wall occurs in certain infections caused by organisms that have the ability to invade vessels. Rickettsial infections, for example, classically cause vascular damage and a hemorrhagic diathesis.

(54) Disseminated intravascular coagulation is a well-known complication of promyelogenous leukemia. In this disorder, the release of procoagulant substances from the granules of the neoplastic promyelocytes activates the coagulation cascade, producing disseminated coagulation and an attendant hemorrhagic diathesis (*pp. 643–644, 647–650, 997*).

55. (A); 56. (A); 57. (C); 58. (A); 59. (B); 60. (C); 61. (A)

Drugs and chemicals cause numerous hematologic problems. Although drug-related hematologic disorders are seldom completely predictable, many are repeatedly associated with particular drugs or drug classes. These hematologic effects are often among the most important complications of drug therapy.

(55) Penicillin is the prototype drug, which acts antigenically as a hapten. It combines with the red cell membrane, induces antibody production to the drug–red cell antigen complex, and produces a warm antibody autoimmune hemolytic anemia.

(56) Alphamethyldopa is also a prototype drug associated with autoimmune hemolytic anemia but, in contrast to penicillin, it directly initiates the production of antibodies against intrinsic red cell antigens.

(57) Thiouracil is one of a small number of drugs that are often associated with agranulocytosis, probably on the basis of decreased production and/or increased destruction of neutrophils. Thiouracil may also cause an immunologically-mediated destruction of mature neutrophils.

(58) Quinidine is another prototype drug responsible for the genesis of autoimmune hemolytic anemia. In contrast to both penicillin and alphamethyldopa, the drug serves as a hapten that binds to a plasma protein; the drug-protein complex, in turn, evokes antibody production. It is the attachment of the resultant complement-fixing immune complexes to the red cell membrane that is responsible for the red cell destruction. (61) Phenacetin is another drug associated with the induction of autoimmune hemolytic anemia by this same mechanism.

(59) Benzene is a well-known cause of acquired aplastic anemia. It is one of a number of toxic drugs that cause myeloid stem cell damage in a dose-related manner.

(60) Along with thiouracil and certain sulfonamides, aminopyrine is one of the drugs associated with immunologically-mediated agranulocytosis (*pp. 628–629, 638–639, 654*).

62. (B); 63. (C); 64. (B); 65. (A); 66. (D)

Reactive proliferations of white cells represent a normal host response to inflammatory stimuli. The relative degree of stimulation of each of the white cell series varies with the underlying cause. Certain inflammatory conditions classically stimulate one of the white cell lines much more than the others, a feature that can be helpful in diagnosis.

(62 and 64) An elevated lymphocyte count (lymphocytosis) is usually immunologic in origin. It often accompanies chronic inflammatory states with sustained immunologic stimulation such as tuberculosis. Lymphocytosis is also common in viral infections such as infectious mononucleosis, in which the primary host response is immunologic, and little acute inflammation is produced.

(63) Bronchial asthma is a prototypic example of a type I immune response with production of IgE that affixes to mast cells and stimulates mast cell degranulation upon exposure to the inciting antigen (see Chapter 6, Question 25). Mast cells then release their eosinophil chemotactic factor, and an eosinophilic leukocytosis occurs.

(65) Elevated neutrophil counts (polymorphonu-

clear leukocytosis) characteristically occur in association with acute inflammatory states such as those produced by bacterial infection or tissue necrosis. The muscle necrosis that accompanies acute myocardial infarction classically produces this response.

(66) Eosinophilic granuloma is a proliferative disorder of histiocytes of unknown etiology. Eosinophils are a variable though frequently prominent feature of the parenchymal lesions that usually involve the bone marrow. However, systemic elevation of eosinophils does not usually occur, and the standard hematologic tests tend to be nondiagnostic in this disease *(pp. 655, 695–696)*.

67. (D); 68. (A); 69. (D); 70. (E); 71. (C); 72. (A); 73. (D); 74. (C); 75. (E); 76. (D)
Malignant lymphomas are neoplastic proliferations of cells of the lymphoreticular system, most commonly lymphocytes. They commonly involve the lymph nodes, but occasionally extra-lymph nodal organs may give rise to lymphomas. Because of its exquisitely distinctive features (see Questions 16 to 22), Hodgkin's disease is classified separately. The non-Hodgkin's lymphomas constitute a much more heterologous group of disorders and have been classified according to several schemes based on differences in histologic appearance, clinical behavior, and more recently, immunologic origin. The Rappaport classification, based exclusively on morphology, is most widely used at present. *See pp. 658–662 for details.*

(67, 69, 73, 76) In contrast to the other types of non-Hodgkin's lymphoma, lymphoblastic lymphoma is largely a disease of adolescents and young adults. The tumor is composed of a remarkably homogeneous population of cells resembling lymphoblasts and always has a diffuse growth pattern. This lymphoma has a high mitotic rate, and consequently a "starry sky" pattern is produced by interspersed benign macrophages filled with nuclear remnants. Studies with monoclonal antibodies have shown that most of the tumor cells are of T lymphocyte lineage and express OKT10, a marker of primitive intrathymic T cells. Furthermore, the most characteristic clinical feature of the disease is a mediastinal mass (50 to 70% of cases) suggesting thymic origin. Another rather unique feature of this tumor is the convoluted (lobated) appearance of the tumor cells, which has been described as "chicken footprint" nuclei.

(68 and 72) Well-differentiated lymphocytic lymphoma (WDLL) is composed of a uniform population of small, round lymphocytes with little or no cytologic atypia. Histologically, these cells are indistinguishable from those of chronic lymphocytic leukemia. In fact, this type of lymphoma is believed to be the solid counterpart of chronic lymphocytic leukemia, and in about 40% of the cases it develops leukemic manifestations. Conversely, chronic lymphocytic leu-

kemia may involve the lymph nodes late in the course of the disease. In contrast to other types of non-Hodgkin's lymphoma, WDLL is a relatively indolent disease, and prolonged survival is the rule.

(70) It is of note that WDLL, like lymphoblastic lymphoma, occurs only in the diffuse form. However, none of the non-Hodgkin's lymphomas are known to occur only in the nodular form.

(71 and 74) Histiocytic lymphoma, a tumor characterized histologically by cells of large size that resemble histiocytes, is now known to be composed of neoplastic lymphocytes (B, T, or null cells) in the vast majority of cases. It is the type of non-Hodgkin's lymphoma that most often arises in extranodal sites; nearly one-third of large cell lymphomas present as localized extranodal tumors. In contrast to the other major types of non-Hodgkin's lymphoma, leukemic manifestations are distinctly uncommon in histiocytic lymphoma.

(75) Association with a previous history of an autoimmune disorder is common only with immunoblastic sarcoma of B cells (30% of the cases) *(pp. 658–662, 664)*.

77. (B); 78. (A); 79. (A); 80. (D); 81. (C)
(78 and 79) Proliferative disorders of histiocytes vary widely in their clinical and pathologic behavior. The Letterer-Siwe syndrome, also known as generalized histiocytosis, is an acute systemic proliferation of mature and immature histiocytes that has an aggressive clinical course. It typically occurs in infants and young children under the age of 3 and is sometimes present at birth. Although the course of the condition is variable, it invariably leads to death, and in general, the younger the age of the patient, the more rapid the course of the disease.

(77) In contrast to the devastating disease of the Letterer-Siwe syndrome, Hand-Schüller-Christian disease is relatively benign. It is characterized by histiocytic infiltrates in multiple tissues and is typically accompanied by a diffuse skin eruption. The classic triad of organ involvement in this disease is: (1) infiltration of the posterior pituitary stalk or hypothalamus leading to diabetes insipidus; (2) orbital involvement with exophthalmos; and (3) calvarial bone defects.

(80) In all of these syndromes of histiocytic proliferation, the infiltrating histiocytes contain unique rod-shaped cytoplasmic inclusions called pentalaminar bodies or HX bodies that can be seen by electron microscopic examination.

(81) In the Letterer-Siwe syndrome, a diffuse macropapular eczematous or purpuric skin rash is often present as mentioned above, and a seborrhea-like skin eruption is typically present in Hand-Schüller-Christian disease. Only in eosinophilic granuloma is skin involvement characteristically absent *(pp. 694–696)*.

8

THE GASTROINTESTINAL TRACT

DIRECTIONS: For Questions 1 to 11, choose the ONE BEST answer to each question.

1. Hiatal hernia is associated with all of the following pathologic lesions EXCEPT:

A. Esophageal webs
B. Acute esophagitis
C. Barrett's esophagus
D. Esophageal scarring
E. Esophageal tears

2. Abnormalities associated with achalasia include all of the following EXCEPT:

A. Incomplete relaxation of the lower esophageal sphincter
B. Lack of peristalsis in the esophagus
C. Loss of myenteric ganglion cells in the esophagus
D. Increased basal tone of the lower esophageal sphincter
E. Muscular hypertrophy of the lower esophageal sphincter

3. Cancer patients receiving medical treatment often develop esophagitis from all of the following EXCEPT:

A. Antibiotic toxicity
B. Viral infection
C. Chemotherapeutic agent toxicity
D. Radiation damage
E. Fungal infection

4. Esophageal disorders that are associated with pulmonary aspiration include all of the following EXCEPT:

A. Esophageal diverticula
B. Achalasia
C. Esophageal scleroderma
D. Uremic esophagitis
E. Esophageal carcinoma

5. The acute gastric ulcerations known as Cushing's ulcers occur in patients:

A. Ingesting exogenous corticosteroids
B. With severe sepsis
C. With brain tumors
D. With extensive burns
E. With Cushing's syndrome

6. All of the following statements about primary gastrointestinal tract lymphoma are true EXCEPT:

A. The stomach is the most common site of occurrence
B. Diffuse histiocytic (large cell) lymphoma is the most common histologic type
C. It occurs with increased frequency in individuals with inflammatory bowel disease
D. It is associated with an increased risk of gastric adenocarcinoma
E. The overall prognosis is worse than for carcinoma of the gastrointestinal tract

7. Mucosal ulceration is a characteristic histologic feature of all of the following causes of enterocolitis EXCEPT:

A. *Entamoeba histolytica* infection
B. Radiation to the bowel
C. *Candida albicans* infection
D. *Yersinia enterocolitica* infection
E. Rotavirus infection

8. All of the following statements about congenital megacolon (Hirschsprung's disease) are true EXCEPT:

A. Both Meissner's and Auerbach's plexuses fail to develop
B. Involvement of the entire colon is rare
C. The incidence is higher in patients with Down's syndrome
D. Massive dilatation of the affected bowel segment is characteristic
E. Surgical excision of the affected segment is curative

9. In the United States, the most likely cause of the form of enterocolitis pictured in Figure 8–1 is:

A. Ingestion of the infectious agent from an exogenous source
B. Reactivation of previous enteric infection
C. Blood-borne spread from another focus of infection in the body
D. Swallowing of organisms coughed up from a pulmonary source of infection
E. None of these

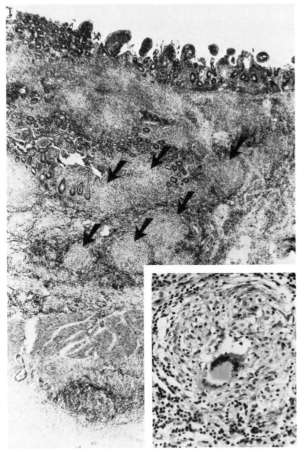

Figure 8–1

10. All of the following statements about small bowel neoplasms are true EXCEPT:

  A. They account for less than 10% of all gastrointestinal tumors
  B. Malignant tumors are more prevalent than benign tumors
  C. Adenomatous polyps are the most common type of benign tumor
  D. Large adenomas of the small bowel often undergo malignant transformation
  E. Malignant lymphoma of the small bowel occurs about as frequently as adenocarcinoma

11. All of the following statements about celiac sprue are true EXCEPT:

  A. It is associated with specific histocompatibility antigen (HLA) profiles
  B. The disorder is cured by a gluten-free diet
  C. Neurologic symptoms associated with long-standing disease are cured by administration of vitamin B
  D. The disease is characterized histologically by diffuse villous atrophy in the small bowel
  E. The disease is associated with an increased incidence of primary gastrointestinal lymphoma

DIRECTIONS: For Questions 12 to 20, ONE or MORE of the completions given correctly finishes the incomplete statement. Choose:

  A—if only *1,2, and 3* are correct
  B—if only *1 and 3* are correct
  C—if only *2 and 4* are correct
  D—if only *4* is correct
  E—if all of these are correct

12. The lower esophageal sphincter:

  1. Requires vagal innervation for relaxation
  2. Prevents reflux of gastric contents
  3. Closes after the swallowing reflex
  4. Relaxes in response to gastrin

  A. 1,2,3   B. 1,3   C. 2,4   D. 4 Only   E. All

13. Esophageal "webs":

  1. Are morphologically identical to lower esophageal "rings"
  2. Occur almost exclusively in men
  3. Are frequently associated with hypochlorhydria
  4. Are composed of constricting bands of subepithelial fibrosis (scar)

  A. 1,2,3   B. 1,3   C. 2,4   D. 4 Only   E. All

14. Which of the following factors is/are causally related to the development of reflux esophagitis?

  1. Lower esophageal sphincter incompetence
  2. Bile content of refluxed material
  3. Esophageal motility dysfunction
  4. Acid and pepsin content of refluxed material

  A. 1,2,3   B. 1,3   C. 2,4   D. 4 Only   E. All

15. Which of the following characteristics is/are likely to be found in a Barrett's esophagus?

  1. Pseudomembrane formation
  2. Metaplastic gastric parietal cells
  3. Nuclear inclusion bodies
  4. Adenocarcinoma of the esophagus

  A. 1,2,3   B. 1,3   C. 2,4   D. 4 Only   E. All

16. Which of the following factors stimulate(s) gastric acid secretion?

1. Gastric distention
2. Digested proteins in the small bowel
3. Histamine
4. Damage to the gastric mucosal barrier

    A. 1,2,3 B. 1,3 C. 2,4 D. 4 Only E. All

17. Which of the statements listed below describe angiodysplasia of the colon?

1. Multiple small arterial aneurysms are present in the submucosa
2. The sigmoid colon is most frequently involved
3. The disorder represents a congenital defect in the vascular media
4. Angiography is required for diagnosis

    A. 1,2,3 B. 1,3 C. 2,4 D. 4 Only E. All

18. Melanosis coli:

1. Is virtually always asymptomatic
2. Involves the small bowel in about 50% of cases
3. Is associated with chronic laxative abuse
4. Is associated with cutaneous malignant melanoma

    A. 1,2,3 B. 1,3 C. 2,4 D. 4 Only E. All

19. Pseudomembranous colitis is:

1. Caused by mucosal invasion by *Clostridium difficile*
2. Associated with clindamycin administration
3. Morphologically indistinguishable from uremia-associated colitis
4. Curable with vancomycin therapy

    A. 1,2,3 B. 1,3 C. 2,4 D. 4 Only E. All

20. Acute appendicitis is:

1. Mainly a disease of adolescents
2. Most commonly confused clinically with mesenteric lymphadenitis
3. Accompanied by luminal obstruction in most cases
4. Diagnosed histologically by massive lymphoid hyperplasia in the submucosa

    A. 1,2,3 B. 1,3 C. 2,4 D. 4 Only E. All

DIRECTIONS: For Questions 21 to 59, you are to decide whether EACH choice is TRUE or FALSE.

For each of the following statements about the *normal* esophagus, choose whether it is TRUE or FALSE.

21. The mucosa is composed of squamous epithelium that does not keratinize
22. The serosal surface is lined by a single layer of mesothelial cells
23. The wall of the upper third of the esophagus is composed of striated muscle
24. Esophageal sphincters are composed of hypertrophied segments of muscularis mucosae
25. The lumen narrows at the level of the bifurcation of the trachea

For each of the following statements about esophageal varices, choose whether it is TRUE or FALSE.

26. They occur in the majority of patients with alcoholic cirrhosis
27. They are rarely produced by biliary cirrhosis
28. They are a common cause of epigastric pain in alcoholic patients

29. The first episode of rupture leads to death in about half of the cases
30. Surgical ligation is highly effective in preventing second bleeding episodes

For each of the following statements about chronic peptic ulcer disease (CPUD), choose whether it is TRUE or FALSE.

31. Peptic ulcers occur most commonly in the gastric antrum
32. Peptic ulcers occur most often as solitary lesions
33. CPUD is increasing in incidence in most industrialized nations
34. CPUD does not develop in individuals with achlorhydria
35. Genetic predisposition is demonstrated only for duodenal peptic ulcer
36. Most patients with gastric peptic ulcer produce abnormally high levels of gastric acid
37. Most patients with gastric peptic ulcer also have chronic gastritis
38. Peptic ulcers are characteristically irregular in shape, with a shaggy base and beaded borders

For each of the following statements about diverticular disease of the colon, choose whether it is TRUE or FALSE.

39. In the United States, the disorder is found in about half of all autopsy cases

40. The disease is rare in patients under 30

41. Inflammation of diverticula (diverticulitis) almost always produces fever and leukocytosis

42. Perforation of diverticula usually initiates the inflammatory process

43. Histologically, diverticula appear as aneurysmic outpouchings of mural smooth muscle

44. High-fiber diets have been shown to prevent development of the disease

45. Surgical resection is required for most patients with acute inflammatory disease

For each of the following statements about carcinoma of the colon, choose whether it is TRUE or FALSE.

46. Colon cancer causes more deaths than any other form of cancer

47. The majority of colon cancers arise in the right colon

48. Cancers of the right colon tend to be more invasive than cancers of the left colon

49. The majority of colon cancers from any site are moderately differentiated adenocarcinomas

50. Most colon cancers produce carcinoembryonic antigen

51. Colon cancers that produce copious mucin have a better prognosis

52. Colon cancers associated with ulcerative colitis tend to be more invasive than other colon cancers

For each of the following statements about carcinoid tumors, choose whether it is TRUE or FALSE.

53. They occur in the lung more often than in the gastrointestinal tract

54. Their degree of histologic atypia (grade) usually correlates well with their metastatic potential

55. They can be identified positively by their cytoplasmic secretory granules

56. They constitute one of the causes of Cushing's syndrome

57. Those arising in the appendix rarely metastasize

58. Small bowel carcinoid tumors do not produce the carcinoid syndrome in the absence of liver metastasis

59. Gastrointestinal carcinoids are associated with an increased incidence of other malignant tumors of the GI tract

DIRECTIONS: For Questions 60 to 109, the set of lettered headings is followed by a list of numbered words or phrases. For each numbered word or phrase choose:

A—if the item is associated with (A) only
B—if the item is associated with (B) only
C—if the item is associated with *both* (A) and (B)
D—if the item is associated with *neither* (A) nor (B)

For each of the statements listed below, choose whether it describes esophageal carcinoma, gastric carcinoma, both, or neither.

A. Esophageal carcinoma
B. Gastric carcinoma
C. Both
D. Neither

60. Nearly all tumors are adenocarcinomas

61. The incidence is on the decline in the U.S.

62. Blacks are affected more than whites

63. The disease is epidemiologically related to cigarette smoking

64. The disease is epidemiologically related to preexistent chronic inflammatory states in the organ of origin

65. Epigastric pain typically develops as an early symptom

66. Metastases to the ovaries are called Krukenberg tumors

For each of the characteristics listed below, choose whether it describes acute gastritis, chronic gastritis, both, or neither.

A. Acute gastritis
B. Chronic gastritis
C. Both
D. Neither

67. Associated with alcohol consumption

68. Associated with cigarette smoking

69. Causally related to autoantibodies against gastric mucosal cells

70. Causally related to gastric mucosal hypoperfusion

71. Associated with nitrite ingestion

72. Productive of gastrointestinal bleeding

73. Associated with gastric peptic ulcers

74. Causally related to hypersecretion of acid

For each of the features listed below, choose whether it describes Menetrier's disease, the Zollinger-Ellison syndrome, both, or neither.

    A. Menetrier's disease
    B. Zollinger-Ellison syndrome
    C. Both
    D. Neither

75. Marked enlargement of gastric rugal folds is characteristic
76. Parietal and chief cell hyperplasia are common histologic features
77. Excessive protein loss is an associated complication
78. The risk of developing gastric lymphoma is increased
79. The risk of developing gastric carcinoma is increased
80. Pancreatic tumors are associated findings
81. Pheochromocytoma and medullary carcinoma of the thyroid are associated disorders

For each of the characteristics listed below, choose whether it describes hyperplastic gastric polyps, adenomatous gastric polyps, both, or neither.

    A. Hyperplastic gastric polyps
    B. Adenomatous gastric polyps
    C. Both
    D. Neither

82. Tend to be large (greater than 3.0 cm)
83. Usually occur in multiple numbers
84. Are commonly asymptomatic
85. Frequently undergo malignant transformation
86. Are often associated with carcinoma elsewhere in the stomach

For each of the features of inflammatory bowel disease listed below, choose whether it describes Crohn's disease, ulcerative colitis, both, or neither.

    A. Crohn's disease
    B. Ulcerative colitis
    C. Both
    D. Neither

87. Lesions occur at any level of the enteric tract
88. Organ systems other than the enteric tract are occasionally involved

89. The presence of granulomata is pathognomonic
90. Viral particles are usually found in diseased bowel
91. The disorder is associated with histocompatibility antigen HLA-B27
92. Affected bowel usually becomes thickened and narrowed
93. Toxic megacolon is an occasional complication
94. Distribution of lesions is generally discontinuous
95. Fissures and fistulas are characteristic
96. Incidence of gastrointestinal carcinoma is increased
97. Incidence of primary gastrointestinal lymphoma is increased

For each of the features listed below, choose whether it describes ischemic bowel disease producing transmural infarction, mucosal infarction, both, or neither.

    A. Transmural bowel infarction
    B. Mucosal bowel infarction
    C. Both
    D. Neither

98. Principally affects the small bowel
99. Results from venous thrombosis
100. Produced by arterial occlusion
101. Produced by atherosclerosis and hypotension
102. Produced by hypotension alone
103. Grossly appears hemorrhagic
104. Associated with a high mortality rate

For each of the characteristics listed below, choose whether it describes tropical sprue, Whipple's disease, both, or neither.

    A. Tropical sprue
    B. Whipple's disease
    C. Both
    D. Neither

105. The disorder has a strong female predominance
106. History of travel to an endemic area is essential to the diagnosis
107. Antibiotic therapy is usually curative
108. Systemic disease is occasionally present in addition to bowel involvement
109. Macrophages laden with rod-shaped bacteria are found in the small bowel mucosa

DIRECTIONS: Questions 110 to 141 are matching questions. For each numbered item, choose the most likely associated lettered item from those provided. Each numbered item has ONLY ONE answer. Within each group, each lettered item may be the answer to one, more than one, or none of the numbered items.

For each of the following statements about congenital gastrointestinal tract anomalies, choose whether it refers to the esophagus, stomach, small bowel, or large bowel.

    A. Esophagus
    B. Stomach
    C. Small bowel
    D. Large bowel

110. The most common location for congenital atresia
111. The most common location for a congenital stenosis
112. The most common location for congenital duplication
113. The most common location for congenital diverticula
114. The most common location for congenital absence of ganglion cells

For each of the characteristics listed below, choose whether it is characteristic of the gastric cardia, corpus (body), antrum, all of these regions, or none of these.

    A. Cardia
    B. Corpus (body)
    C. Antrum
    D. All of these
    E. None of these

115. Gastrin production
116. Pepsin secretion
117. Intrinsic factor production
118. Location of endocrine (enterochromaffin) cells
119. Location of goblet cells
120. Location of Paneth cells

For each of the features listed below, choose whether it is characteristic of the duodenum, jejunum, ileum, all of these segments of small bowel, or none of these.

    A. Duodenum
    B. Jejunum
    C. Ileum
    D. All of these
    E. None of these

121. Paneth cells
122. Peyer patches
123. Brunner's glands
124. Serotonin-secreting endocrine cells
125. Vitamin B_{12}–intrinsic factor absorption
126. Meckel's diverticula
127. Pancreatic rests

For each of the characteristics listed below, choose whether it describes salmonella enterocolitis, shigella enterocolitis, cholera, or none of these.

    A. Salmonella enterocolitis
    B. Shigella enterocolitis
    C. Cholera
    D. None of these

128. Shallow mucosal ulcers are typically produced
129. Submucosal lymphoid hyperplasia is a characteristic feature
130. Submucosal granulomas are a characteristic histologic feature
131. The causative organism does not invade the mucosal lining
132. The causative organism does not produce toxins
133. The large bowel is preferentially involved
134. The etiologic agent is a common cause of ulceroinflammatory proctitis in homosexual males

For each of the features of colonic polyps listed below, choose whether it describes the hyperplastic polyp, tubular adenoma, villous adenoma, or hamartomatous polyp.

    A. Hyperplastic polyp
    B. Tubular adenoma
    C. Villous adenoma
    D. Hamartomatous polyp

135. Most common type of colonic polyp
136. Largest sized colonic polyp overall
137. Greatest likelihood of harboring cancer
138. Typically occurs in familial polyposis
139. Typically occurs in the Peutz-Jeghers syndrome
140. Occasionally causes a protein-losing enteropathy
141. Characterized histologically by mucin-filled cysts lined by goblet cells

8

THE GASTROINTESTINAL TRACT

ANSWERS

1. (A) Hiatal hernia is a disorder in which the proximal portion of the stomach herniates through the diaphragmatic hiatus into the thorax. The competence of the lower esophageal sphincter is compromised, and reflux of gastric contents into the lower esophagus occurs. Thus, acute esophagitis is commonly produced (reflux esophagitis), which causes symptoms of retrosternal burning pain. In a small percentage of these patients, persistent reflux esophagitis leads to adenomatous metaplasia of the lower esophageal epithelium, a condition known as Barrett's esophagus. Much less commonly, postinflammatory esophageal scarring may result in severe cases. Small esophageal lacerations (Mallory-Weiss tears) have also been reported in association with underlying hiatal hernias that appear to potentiate abnormal esophageal dilatation in instances of increased intragastric pressure. Although hiatal hernia is twice as common in patients with lower esophageal ring as in the otherwise normal population, there is no increased incidence of hiatal hernia in patients with esophageal "webs" (pp. 799–800).

2. (E) Achalasia is an uncommon disorder of esophageal motility whose pathogenesis is still poorly understood. The disease appears to represent a group of functional abnormalities of the esophageal musculature. Primary among these defects is the failure of relaxation of the lower esophageal sphincter in advance of the propulsive peristaltic wave. In addition, diffuse esophageal spasm with aperistalsis and increased basal tone of the lower esophageal sphincter have also been noted. Although the etiology remains controversial, most studies show a loss of myenteric ganglion cells in the body of the esophagus. Muscular hypertrophy of the lower esophageal sphincter is not a feature of achalasia however. In fact, no histologic abnormalities of the esophageal musculature itself have been identified in this disorder (pp. 798–799).

3. (A) Esophagitis is a common problem among cancer patients and may result from a variety of factors. Cytotoxic chemotherapeutic drugs frequently cause esophageal damage and inflammation, as does therapeutic radiation. Furthermore, anticancer therapy produces immunologic deficiencies that predispose to viral and fungal infections of the esophagus. Although antibiotic therapy may be associated with fungal infections of the esophagus, direct toxic damage to the esophageal mucosa is rarely caused by antibiotics (p. 801).

4. (D) Esophageal disorders that lead to chronic regurgitation of ingested substances are often associated with pulmonary aspiration. Esophageal diverticula may become overdistended with food, leading directly to regurgitation and pulmonary aspiration. Esophageal diverticula are also associated with other disorders of esophageal motor function, including achalasia, hiatal hernia, and esophageal ring, which may themselves be primary causes of chronic regurgitation. When scleroderma (systemic sclerosis) involves the esophagus, it produces fibrosis of the submucosa and muscular wall, producing a narrowed esophagus with markedly abnormal motor function; chronic regurgitation is a common consequence. Esophageal carcinoma may lead to pulmonary aspiration through several mechanisms. Progressive dysphagia and obstruction may occur from intraluminal growth of fungating tumors, whereas infiltrating tumors may invade nerves and muscles, producing motor dysfunction. Furthermore, invasive esophageal carcinoma may occasionally produce a tracheal-esophageal fistula through which ingested material can be aspirated directly into the bronchial tree. Although uremic esophagitis is a common gastrointestinal manifestation of chronic renal failure, it does not produce obstruction or motor dysfunction of the esophagus and is not associated with aspiration pneumonia (pp. 799, 802, 806, 997).

5. (C) Focal acute gastric mucosal ulcerations are essentially a more severe form of acute erosive gastritis and are known to occur in a number of well-defined, biologically stressful situations. Those that occur in association with conditions that raise intracranial pressure, such as brain tumors, head trauma, or intracranial surgery, are known as Cushing's ulcers, after the great neurosurgeon Harvey Cushing, who described them. Increased intracranial pressure is believed to stimulate vagal nuclei, causing hypersecretion of gastric acid, a phenomenon that has only been documented with Cushing's ulcers. In addition, neurogenic or catecholamine-induced vasoconstriction with mucosal hypoperfusion and injury contributes to their pathogenesis.

Morphologically indistinguishable lesions are produced in other stressful conditions such as extensive burns (Curling's ulcers) and severe sepsis. Although Cushing's ulcers are not related to Cushing's syndrome (hyperadrenocorticism), acute gastric erosions are believed to occur in association with corticosteroid ingestion. Corticosteroids, as well as other agents including aspirin, ethanol, cigarette smoke, indomethacin, and phenylbutazone, are believed to be ulcerogenic to the gastric mucosa, although the evidence for this is controversial (pp. 813–814).

6. (E) The gastrointestinal tract is the most common site of primary extranodal lymphomas. The majority of primary gastrointestinal tract lymphomas arise in the stomach, and the most common histologic type is diffuse histiocytic (large cell) lymphoma. There is a well-known association of gastrointestinal lymphomas with inflammatory bowel disease (ulcerative colitis and Crohn's disease) as well as with gluten enteropathy (celiac disease or nontropical sprue). There is also an increased incidence of concomitant gastric adenocarcinoma, which often arises in close proximity to the gastric lymphoma. Overall, gastrointestinal lymphomas have a better prognosis than gastrointestinal carcinoma, and many are curable with surgical resection (p. 826).

7. (E) Mucosal ulceration in the affected portion of bowel is a feature characteristic of a number of infectious agents, including *Entamoeba histolytica* (a protozoan), *Candida albicans* (a fungus), and *Yersinia enterocolitica* (a gram-negative coccobacillus). Radiation enteritis can also produce mucosal ulceration that may mimic infectious enteritis. Only when specific causes of mucosal ulceration have been ruled out can the diagnosis of idiopathic ulceroinflammatory disease (ulcerative colitis or Crohn's disease) be made. Rotavirus is an important cause of viral gastroenteritis in infants and children. Although severe diarrhea may result, mucosal ulceration of the bowel is usually not observed (pp. 833–836).

8. (D) Hirschsprung's disease is a congenital anomaly of the colon caused by failure of development of both Meissner's and Auerbach's plexuses. Neuroblasts from the neural crest fail to complete their distal migration, leaving a portion of distal colon devoid of ganglion cells. In over 80% of cases, only the rectum or rectosigmoid colon is involved. Involvement of the entire colon is extremely rare. Hirschsprung's disease may occur as an isolated lesion but is often associated with other congenital anomalies. It is 10 times more common in patients with Down's syndrome than in the general population. The disorder can be cured by surgical excision of the affected segment, which is not usually dilated. It is the portion of normal colon proximal to the affected segment that becomes dilated with fecal material that cannot be moved through the narrowed, aganglionic segment that is incapable of peristalsis (pp. 855–856).

9. (D) The caseating granulomata within the bowel wall strongly suggest the diagnosis of gastrointestinal tuberculosis, although definitive diagnosis of this entity would require the identification of acid-fast bacilli within the lesions by histochemical stain or by microbial culture. In the United States, involvement of the gastrointestinal tract by a mycobacterial organism is most commonly a secondary consequence of primary pulmonary tuberculosis. Organisms from a primary pulmonary focus are coughed up and swallowed, thereby gaining access to the gastrointestinal tract. With the elimination of *Mycobacterium bovus* infection from contaminated cows, primary bovine tuberculosis of the gastrointestinal tract has been virtually eliminated in the United States. Thus, reactivation of a previous primary gastrointestinal infection is uncommon. Although any organ may be involved in systemic infection with *Mycobacterium tuberculosis*, blood-borne spread to the gastrointestinal tract is much less common than direct infection from swallowed contaminated mucus originating from a pulmonary focus as outlined above (pp. 341, 834–835).

10. (C) Neoplasms of the small intestine, whether benign or malignant, are rare entities. Altogether they account for only 3 to 6% of all gastrointestinal tumors. Benign tumors, of which the *leiomyoma* is the most common type, are even less common than malignant tumors in the small bowel. Of the benign tumors, however, adenomatous polyps are the most important. As in the large bowel, adenomatous polyps of large size often undergo malignant transformation to adenocarcinoma. In contrast to colonic adenocarcinoma, however, the incidence of adenocarcinoma of the small bowel is comparable to that of primary lymphoma in that site. Thus, reports vary as to whether adenocarcinoma or primary lymphoma is the most frequent form of malignancy in the small intestine (pp. 841–842).

11. (C) Celiac sprue (gluten-sensitive enteropathy or nontropical sprue) is a disorder of the small intestine that causes the malabsorption syndrome. It is known to have a genetic predisposition and is associated with HLA-B8 and HLA-DW3 histocompatibility antigens in the great majority of cases. The disorder responds dramatically to a gluten-free diet, and definitive diagnosis is based upon this characteristic. Histologically, the disorder is characterized by diffuse villous atrophy in the small intestine, although this feature is not pathognomonic for celiac sprue. Increased numbers of IgA-bearing lymphocytes and plasma cells are also present in the lamina propria. Furthermore, in some patients, antibodies to gluten fractions can be demonstrated in the serum. The disease is also associated with an increased incidence of primary gastrointestinal tract lymphomas as well as carcinomas.

One curious complication of long-term, untreated celiac sprue is the appearance of neuropathologic disorders, including cerebellar atrophy and patchy demyelination of the spinal cord. It was thought that these disorders were related to the malabsorption of B vitamins such as thiamine, riboflavin, and pyridoxine, which are important in neurophysiology. However, the neurologic complications of celiac sprue do not respond to the therapeutic administration of B vitamins (pp. 847–848).

12. **(A)** Although the lower esophageal sphincter mainly functions to prevent reflux of gastric contents into the esophagus, it opens at the proper time to allow the passage of food and fluid from the esophagus to the stomach. Relaxation of the lower esophageal sphincter requires vagal innervation and the transmission of vagal stimuli through Auerbach's plexus to the sphincter muscle. The sphincter opens in anticipation of the peristaltic wave and closes again after the swallowing reflex.

Rather than relaxing the sphincter, gastrin acts to increase the sphincter tone, maintaining sphincter competence and preventing reflux of the ingested material that stimulated the hormone's release (p. 797).

13. **(B)** Although they refer to luminal narrowing of the esophagus occurring at different levels, esophageal "webs" (upper esophagus) and esophageal rings (lower esophagus) are morphologically identical lesions. These lesions are composed of overhanging folds of esophageal mucosa, often circumferential, that constrict the lumen and produce dysphagia. Esophageal "webs" are found almost exclusively in women and are frequently associated with hypochlorhydria (the Plummer-Vinson syndrome). Although esophageal "webs" must be differentiated from esophageal strictures as a cause of obstruction and dysphagia, these delicate mucosal folds contrast dramatically with the postinjury subepithelial scar formation that characterizes esophageal strictures (p. 799).

14. **(E)** The most common cause of esophageal inflammation is reflux of gastric contents into the lower esophagus. Reflux esophagitis is a multifactorial disorder and has been shown to be related to frequent and protracted reflux of gastric juice. Thus, incompetence of the lower esophageal sphincter is an important predisposing factor. The acid and pepsin concentration as well as the bile content of the refluxed fluid are major factors in the production of inflammatory changes in the esophagus. In addition, disordered esophageal motility permits prolonged contact of the esophageal mucosa with caustic refluxed material (p. 801).

15. **(C)** Barrett's esophagus, a consequence of chronic gastrointestinal reflux, is characterized by metaplastic transformation of the stratified squamous epithelium of the normal esophageal mucosa to a columnar secretory type epithelium. Three types of metaplastic secretory epithelium have been described: (1) intestinal type with goblet cells and absorptive cells, (2) gastric antral type with mucus-secreting epithelial surface cells, and (3) gastric fundic type with both parietal cells and chief cells. The most important consequence of these metaplastic structures is an increased risk of adenocarcinoma of the esophagus, an otherwise rare entity.

Pseudomembrane formation typically occurs as a result of the severe mucosal injury of monilia esophagitis. Nuclear inclusion bodies occur in viral esophagitis produced by herpes or cytomegalovirus. Neither pseudomembranes nor intranuclear inclusions occur with esophageal reflux (p. 801).

16. **(E)** Stimuli for the secretion of gastric acid are numerous and varied. Chemical, mechanical, neurologic, and hormonal factors are known to be involved in the secretory process. Parasympathetic (vagal) stimulation of gastric parietal cells is the final common pathway for stimuli such as the sight, smell, and taste of food (the "cephalic phase" of stimulation) and mechanical stimulation by gastric distention ("gastric phase"). During the gastric stage, digested proteins and amino acids also chemically stimulate the release of gastrins by antral endocrine cells (G cells). This family of polypeptide hormones is the most potent stimulus to gastric acid secretion. The role of histamine in this process is still poorly understood, but it is clear that histamine acts as a potent acid secretagogue and may function as a mediator of gastrin and vagal stimulation. The final phase of the secretory process occurs when digested proteins enter the proximal small intestine (the "intestinal phase") and cause the release of a small intestinal polypeptide hormone, which in turn stimulates gastric acid secretion.

In the normal stomach, protection against the corrosive effects of the secreted acid is dependent upon the integrity of the tight intercellular junctions between gastric mucosal cells (the "gastric mucosal barrier"). Destruction of this barrier not only leads to gastric mucosal injury from back-diffusion of acid, but also causes further stimulation of gastric acid secretion. Thus, a truly vicious cycle is initiated (pp. 807–808).

17. **(D)** Although angiodysplasia of the colon is one of the most frequent causes of lower gastrointestinal bleeding in elderly patients, it has only recently received notice. Angiodysplasia is characterized by dilated, tortuous, submucosal veins and venules that may easily rupture to produce bleeding. These pathologic changes are always limited to the right colon and are most often located within the cecum. A' though it has been suggested that these lesions represent a congenital defect or even a neoplastic change, their pathogenesis is now believed to be related to bowel distention and increased intraluminal pressure from fecal impaction of the capacious cecum. Since these lesions are almost entirely intramucosal, they cannot be detected by conventional diagnostic methods and require selective mesenteric angiography for diagnosis *(p. 859)*.

18. (B) Melanosis coli is an innocuous condition that is virtually always asymptomatic but has an alarming gross appearance that may startle the unsuspecting colonoscopist. It is characterized by a diffuse, brown-black pigmentation of the colonic mucosa. The condition is associated with the use of cathartics of the anthracene type. It is always limited to the colon, curiously sparing the small intestine. Despite the name, melanosis coli, the brown-black pigment granules contained within lysosomes of macrophages in the mucosal lamina propria have not yet been definitively identified. Histochemical studies show that the pigment has characteristics of both melanin and lipofuscin. Melanosis coli has no association with either benign or malignant melanocytic tumors *(p. 858)*.

19. (C) Pseudomembranous colitis is an inflammatory disorder of the colon characterized by focal mucosal ulceration and the formation of fibrinomucinous exudate over denuded areas. This coagulum of fibrin and mucin containing inflammatory cells and necrotic mucosal epithelial cells comprises what is known as a pseudomembrane. The disorder is associated with the administration of broad-spectrum antibiotics, particularly clindamycin and lincomycin, which allow for the overgrowth of *Clostridium difficile*, a microorganism resistant to these antibiotics. Although the organism does not invade the bowel mucosa, it produces a toxin that is the cause of the mucosal injury. The diagnosis can be confirmed by isolation of *Clostridium difficile* or its toxin from the stool. The disease is cured promptly by the administration of vancomycin. Although pseudomembranous colitis caused by toxin-producing Clostridia is grossly indistinguishable from that produced by fungal infection, it does not resemble uremia-associated colitis. Although uremia may produce patchy ulcerations of the colonic epithelium, it is not associated with pseudomembrane formation *(pp. 836, 862, 997)*.

20. (A) Acute appendicitis occurs mainly in adolescents and young adults but may affect individuals of any age. It is characterized histologically by transmural neutrophilic infiltration and, in fulminant cases, mural necrosis. Lymphoid hyperplasia of the submucosa, however, is not an indication of acute appendicitis and may be considered a variation of the normal appendiceal morphology. Clinically, acute appendicitis is most commonly confused with acute mesenteric lymphadenitis, which is discovered at laparotomy. Although the etiology of the disorder remains obscure, luminal obstruction of the appendix by a fecalith, calculus, tumor, or worms can be demonstrated in the majority of cases *(pp. 874–876)*.

21. (True); 22. (False); 23. (True); 24. (False); 25. (True)
(**21**) The esophagus is lined throughout its length by stratified squamous epithelium, which does not keratinize under normal conditions. (**22**) Its outer surface lacks a serosa and is covered instead by loose connective tissue. (**23**) The muscular wall of this hollow tube is composed of striated muscle in the upper third and smooth muscle in the lower two thirds. (**24**) Although functional studies have shown that sphincter function exists in both the upper and lower aspects of the esophagus, no anatomic counterpart for these functional sphincters has been discerned by morphologic studies. (**25**) The esophageal lumen narrows slightly at the level of the bifurcation of the trachea and at two other levels—the cricoid cartilage and the diaphragmatic hiatus *(p. 797)*.

26. (True); 27. (True); 28. (False); 29. (True); 30. (False)
Esophageal varices are dilated, tortuous, submucosal veins that are produced when flow through the hepatic portal system is compromised, increasing portal venous pressure and diverting flow through the coronary veins of the stomach into the esophageal plexus. Portal hypertension is most commonly caused by hepatic cirrhosis, yet the incidence of this consequence varies markedly among the different forms of cirrhosis. (**26**) Portal hypertension and esophageal varices are most commonly found in association with alcoholic cirrhosis and occur in nearly two-thirds of the patients with this disorder. (**27**) Curiously, however, they rarely occur in association with biliary cirrhosis or cardiac cirrhosis. (**28**) Whatever the etiology, esophageal varices are asymptomatic until they rupture. Thus, epigastric pain in alcoholic patients would most likely indicate acute gastritis or reflux esophagitis rather than the presence of esophageal varices, although they may well coexist. (**29**) Once rupture has occurred, the consequences are dire, and death occurs with the first episode of bleeding in about half of the cases. (**30**) Even if the initial episode of bleeding can be controlled with medical measures or surgical ligation, rebleeding is likely to occur. Overall, only surgical procedures that reduce the pressure in the portal venous system are capable of altering the course of this highly lethal consequence of advanced cirrhosis *(pp. 802–803)*.

31. (False); 32. (True); 33. (False); 34. (True); 35. (True); 36. (False); 37. (True); 38. (False)
Peptic ulcers are perhaps the most common chronic gastrointestinal disorder in industrialized nations. (**31**) Although they may occur at any level of

the gastrointestinal tract exposed to gastric acid and pepsin, they occur most commonly in the first portion of the duodenum. The second most common site is the gastric antrum. (**32**) Peptic ulcers occur most commonly as solitary lesions. Occasionally, however, they may be multiple, especially in such disorders as the Zollinger-Ellison syndrome.

(**33**) Although approximately 1 in every 10 adult males in the United States develops a peptic ulcer before the age of 65, this statistic actually represents a drop in the incidence of peptic ulcer over the last half century. A steadily declining incidence of peptic ulcer disease has been observed in the general population in the United States and in other industrialized nations as well.

(**34**) Although the pathogenesis of chronic peptic ulcers remains largely unknown, it is clear that they are associated with gastric acid and pepsin secretion. In fact, without some level of acid/pepsin secretion, peptic ulcers do not develop and therefore are not seen in individuals with achlorhydria. (**35**) Epidemiologic evidence suggests that genetic factors are important in the predisposition to duodenal peptic ulcer but do not appear to be important in the genesis of gastric peptic ulcer. Duodenal ulcers occur approximately 3 times more commonly in first-degree relatives of affected patients than in the general population, and individuals of blood group O are more prone to develop these lesions than individuals of other blood types.

(**36**) Although some degree of gastric acid production has been shown to be requisite to the genesis of peptic ulcers, abnormally high levels of gastric acid have been demonstrated only in patients with duodenal peptic ulcers. Even in duodenal ulcer disease, this finding is not constant, and there is considerable overlap between measurements of mean basal acid output in duodenal ulcer patients and normal controls. Patients with gastric ulcers, in general, have low to normal levels of gastric acid.

(**37**) In 60 to 80% of cases of gastric ulceration, chronic antral gastritis is also present and frequently persists after the ulcer heals. This implies that chronic gastritis may be the primary condition and ulcer development is secondary. It has been suggested that both are etiologically related to the reflux of bile acids and lysolecithin into the gastric antrum, causing damage to the gastric mucosal barrier with back-diffusion of gastric acid.

(**38**) The characteristic gross appearance of a chronic peptic ulcer is that of a small, round to oval, sharply punched-out defect with straight walls and a smooth base due to the peptic digestion of any exudate. These features help to differentiate a peptic ulcer from an ulcerating carcinoma, which is characteristically irregular in shape with heaped-up, beaded borders and a shaggy base (*pp. 814–820*).

39. (**True**); 40. (**True**); 41. (**False**); 42. (**True**); 43. (**False**); 44. (**False**); 45. (**False**)

Diverticular disease is an idiopathic disorder characterized by the development of saccular outpouchings of the colonic mucosa, usually in the distal third of the colon, that are prone to fecal impaction. (**39**) In industrialized western countries, the disease is extremely common and appears to have increased in incidence since the turn of the century. In the United States, diverticular disease is currently found in approximately 50% of autopsies. (**40**) The incidence of the disease increases with increasing age. Although rare in those under 30 years of age, in the United States diverticular disease is found in approximately 50% of individuals over the age of 60.

(**41**) Because diverticula without superimposed inflammation may be symptomatic and conversely, inflamed diverticula may not be associated with symptoms of inflammatory disease, it is frequently impossible to differentiate between diverticulosis and diverticulitis. In fact, about half of the cases of diverticulitis do not produce fever or systemic leukocytosis. Thus, the terms diverticulosis and diverticulitis have been replaced by the more useful clinical term "diverticular disease."

(**42**) Inflammatory changes in diverticula are usually produced by perforation of these thin-walled structures, with leakage of the contents into the adjacent pericolonic fat. Although it may be quite florid, the inflammatory response is nonspecific. As might be expected, bacterial cultures usually grow a mixed bowel flora, with abundant *E. coli*.

(**43**) Perhaps the most significant histologic feature of colonic diverticula is their lack of muscularis. Microscopically, they appear as outpouchings of atrophic mucosa and compressed submucosa that project through the muscular wall of the colon into the pericolonic fat but are themselves devoid of a muscular layer. In fact, the delicacy of diverticular structures makes perforation an easily understood complication. The morphology of diverticula also suggests that they arise as a consequence of increased intraluminal pressure and subsequent herniation of the colonic mucosa through a muscular weakness in the colonic wall. (**44**) Although clinical studies have failed to confirm the need for increased intraluminal pressure in the pathogenesis of diverticular disease, they have shown that increased intraluminal pressure correlates well with symptomatic disease, irrespective of the presence or absence of inflammation. Thus, high-fiber diets that increase stool bulk and decrease peristaltic activity (hence intraluminal pressure) do not prevent the development of diverticular disease but are effective in reducing the symptomatology of this condition. (**45**) Happily, the majority of individuals with diverticular disease are asymptomatic and never come to medical attention. When inflammation does occur, however, it most often resolves spontaneously. Only a small percentage of patients require surgical intervention for obstruction, free perforation, or inflammatory complications (*pp. 856–857*).

46. (False); 47. (False); 48. (False); 49. (True); 50. (True); 51. (False); 52. (True)

Adenocarcinoma of the colon is by far the most common malignant tumor of the gastrointestinal tract.(46) Colon cancer is the second most common cause of death from cancer in the United States. Only lung cancer is associated with a higher mortality rate. (47) Nearly three-quarters of colonic carcinomas are located in the rectum, rectosigmoid, or sigmoid colon. The remainder occur with more or less equal frequency throughout the remainder of the colon. Approximately 10 to 15% occur in the right colon. (48) Cancers of the right colon tend to be *less* invasive than cancers of the left colon. Rather than being deeply infiltrating lesions like left-sided colonic carcinomas, tumors of the right colon tend to form fungating polypoid masses that project into the lumen. Eventually, of course, the tumor invades the underlying colonic wall and penetrates into the mesentery. (49) Despite the difference in the growth patterns of right-sided and left-sided tumors, the lesions tend to have a similar histologic appearance. Ninety-eight per cent of all carcinomas of the large intestine are adenocarcinomas, and the vast majority of these are moderately to well differentiated.

(50) Although the antigen is by no means unique to colonic carcinomas, carcinoembryonic antigen (CEA) is produced by most colonic cancers. With removal of the primary tumor mass, the serum levels of this antigen usually drop. Thereafter, the level of this antigen in the patient's serum can be used as a marker for recurrent or metastatic disease. (51) Although most colon carcinomas are capable of mucin production, those that produce copious amounts of mucin (known as mucinous or colloid carcinomas) tend to have a worse prognosis. It is believed that the elaboration of pools of extracellular mucin by the tumor aids in its ability to dissect through normal tissues and increases its potential for infiltration. (52) Not only does colon cancer occur with greater frequency in patients with ulcerative colitis (see Question 96), but it tends to be more highly invasive than other colon cancers, which do not arise in a background of inflammatory bowel disease (pp. 862, 869–873).

53. (False); 54. (False); 55. (True); 56. (True); 57. (True); 58. (True); 59. (True)

(53) Although they may occur in the lung as well as the breast, thymus, liver, gallbladder, ovary, or urethra, carcinoid tumors (argentaffinomas) arise most often in the gastrointestinal tract. (54) No matter what their site of origin, however, carcinoid tumors tend to have the same histologic appearance. They are composed of a uniform population of round cells showing little cytologic atypia. Thus, the ability of many of these tumors to invade and metastasize cannot be predicted from their histologic appearance. (55) Carcinoid tumor cells can be positively identified by their cytoplasmic content of secretory granules. These granules have a characteristic affinity for soluble silver salts. Thus, carcinoid tumors are also known as argentaffinomas. (56) These secretory granules may contain a variety of amine and peptide products, including ACTH, histamine, serotonin, 5-hydroxytryptophan, kallikrein, or prostaglandin. An ACTH-producing tumor could cause Cushing's syndrome as a paraneoplastic phenomenon.

(57) Although in general the biologic behavior of carcinoid tumors is somewhat unpredictable, carcinoids arising in the appendix (the most common site of gastrointestinal carcinoid tumors) are almost always indolent and rarely metastasize. Their behavior contrasts with that of extra-appendiceal carcinoid tumors, which tend to spread to local lymph nodes as well as the liver, lungs, and bone. (58) The carcinoid syndrome results from the systemic effects of the secretory products of carcinoid tumors, especially serotonin and histamine. Because these substances are readily metabolized in the liver, the carcinoid syndrome is rarely produced by small intestinal carcinoid tumors in the absence of liver metastases. The secretory products of hepatic metastases enter the systemic circulation directly and bypass hepatic degradation. (59) One of the most important and unfortunate features of gastrointestinal carcinoid tumors is their association with an increased incidence of other malignant tumors, both intestinal and extraintestinal. Concurrent malignant neoplasms are found in about 30% of patients with carcinoid tumors of the small intestine and in about 15% of those with appendiceal carcinoids. The majority of these concurrent cancers are found elsewhere in the gastrointestinal tract and are usually adenocarcinomas (pp. 842–845).

60. (B); 61. (B); 62. (A); 63. (A); 64. (C); 65. (D); 66. (B)

(60) Gastric carcinoma refers almost exclusively to adenocarcinomas that arise from the glandular epithelium of the gastric mucosa. Nearly all carcinomas of the esophagus, however, are squamous cell carcinomas. Exceptions to this are represented by esophageal adenocarcinomas that arise from the metaplastic epithelium of a Barrett's esophagus or, rarely, from esophageal mucus glands.

(61) In the United States, for reasons that are unknown at the present time, the incidence of gastric carcinoma has been declining for decades and still continues to drop. Esophageal carcinoma, however, does not appear to be changing significantly in incidence in the United States, where it represents about 10% of all cancers of the gastrointestinal tract. (62) Although the reasons are completely unknown, epidemiologic studies have shown that throughout the world the incidence of esophageal carcinoma is significantly higher among blacks than whites. No such racial predisposition has been demonstrated for gastric carcinoma. (63) It has been further shown by epidemiologic studies in the United States that

esophageal carcinoma occurs 6 to 7 times more frequently among smokers of cigarettes, cigars, or pipes than among nonsmokers. Cigarette smoking has not been demonstrated to influence the incidence of gastric carcinoma, however.

(64) Common to both esophageal and gastric carcinoma is the increased risk of malignancy. The respective incidence of esophageal carcinoma and gastric carcinoma is significantly higher among individuals with chronic esophagitis and chronic atrophic gastritis than in control groups.

(65) Unfortunately, both esophageal and gastric carcinoma tend to be diseases of insidious onset and rarely produce early symptoms that would bring the patient to clinical attention. Both diseases are characteristically asymptomatic until late in their course, when pain may develop as a symptom.

(66) Bilateral metastatic adenocarcinomas in the ovaries are known as Krukenberg tumors. Although the primary tumor may originate from any abdominal viscus, it is most frequently gastric adenocarcinomas that give rise to this metastatic pattern. Squamous carcinoma of the esophagus, by definition, never gives rise to Krukenberg tumors. Adenocarcinoma of the esophagus, for unknown reasons, does not produce this metastatic pattern (*pp. 804–806, 821–825*).

67. (A); 68. (A); 69. (B); 70. (A); 71. (D); 72. (A); 73. (B); 74. (D)

Acute gastritis is a gastric mucosal inflammatory process that is usually transient in nature; it commonly resolves completely following reversal of the etiologic condition or removal of the causative agent. Chronic gastritis, however, refers to a group of conditions with an extended clinical course and poorly understood etiologies. It is associated with atrophic, metaplastic, and dysplastic changes of the gastric mucosa. Chronic gastritis has a limited potential for reversibility and is often associated with autoimmune phenomena.

(67 and 68) Unlike chronic gastritis, acute gastritis may be produced by excessive alcohol consumption or heavy smoking. Alcohol, cigarette smoke, and aspirin, the three most common causes of acute gastritis, are all agents known to damage the gastric mucosal barrier. They disrupt the tight junctions between mucosal cells, potentiate their shedding, and allow back diffusion of gastric acids. Consequently, mucosal edema and inflammation and erosion of the gastric mucosal cells are produced.

(69) The production of autoantibodies directed against gastric mucosal cells is a feature associated exclusively with chronic forms of gastritis. In particular, patients with chronic fundal gastritis and pernicious anemia typically produce antibodies directed against gastric parietal cells. In addition, most of these patients produce antibodies directed against intrinsic factor. Patients with chronic antral gastritis have also been shown to produce autoantibodies against gastrin-producing cells in some cases.

Whether these antibodies represent a secondary response to exposed antigens on damaged gastric mucosal cells or whether they are indeed the causative agents in chronic forms of gastritis is still a moot point.

(70) Primary among the factors that are necessary to the maintenance of the gastric mucosal barrier is adequate mucosal blood flow. Shock and consequent hypoperfusion of the gastric mucosa therefore lead to breakdown of the barrier and acute gastritis. (71) Nitrosamine compounds are known to be carcinogenic in animals. Since nitrites (food preservatives) may be coupled to secondary amines in the stomach to form nitrosamines, nitrite ingestion has been implicated as a cause of gastric cancer. Nitrites are not associated with either acute or chronic gastritis, however.

(72) Only the acute form of gastritis, with its gastric epithelial cell damage, mucosal denudation, and exposure of delicate submucosal vessels, is associated with gastrointestinal bleeding. In chronic forms of gastritis, mucosal atrophy is the rule, but the mucosa characteristically remains intact.

(73) Only the antral form of chronic gastritis is commonly associated with concurrent gastric peptic ulcers. Thus, a common etiology for these two disorders has been suggested, and reflux of bile salts and possibly lysolecithin from the duodenum has been implicated as a cause.

(74) Although increased gastric acid production may occur as a secondary phenomenon in acute gastritis (see Question 16), neither acute nor chronic gastritis is felt to be etiologically related to hypersecretion of gastric acid. In contrast to gastritis, however, gastric peptic ulcers *are* believed to be a consequence of gastric hyperacidity (*pp. 809–813*).

75. (C); 76. (B); 77. (A); 78. (D); 79. (A); 80. (B); 81. (D)

Menetrier's disease and the Zollinger-Ellison syndrome are both considered forms of so-called hypertrophic "gastritis." Since neither is inflammatory in origin, these disorders are more accurately termed hypertrophic gastropathies. (75) Although they represent opposite ends of the histologic spectrum of disorders producing hyperplasia of the gastric epithelium, both Menetrier's disease and the Zollinger-Ellison syndrome are characterized grossly by striking cerebriform enlargement of rugal folds.

(76 and 80) The Zollinger-Ellison syndrome is produced by gastrin-producing tumors, usually of pancreatic origin. With continued excessive gastrin stimulation, hyperplasia of gastric glands occurs with increased numbers of both parietal and chief cells. Hypersecretion of gastric acid by parietal cells is induced, leading to the production of numerous intractable peptic ulcers, the hallmark of the syndrome. (77) In Menetrier's disease, the hypertrophic rugal folds are composed predominantly of hyperplastic surface mucous cells. These cells secrete ex-

cessive amounts of mucus and, in some patients, the loss of mucoprotein is severe enough to produce hypoproteinemia. Thus, Menetrier's disease sometimes constitutes a form of protein-losing gastroenteropathy.

(78) Although the heaped-up mucosal folds of Menetrier's disease and the Zollinger-Ellison syndrome may bear a superficial morphologic resemblance to the mucosal thickening seen in gastric lymphoma, neither disorder is actually associated with lymphoma. (79) Menetrier's disease, however, does impose a slightly increased risk of gastric carcinoma.

(81) The gastrin-producing pancreatic islet cell tumors of the Zollinger-Ellison syndrome may be part of a multiple endocrine neoplasia (MEN) syndrome. MEN syndromes can be divided into two major categories: those composed primarily of tumors of neural crest origin and those arising in endocrine organs that are not derived from the neural crest. The pancreatic adenomas of the Zollinger-Ellison syndrome belong to the latter group. They are associated with adenomas of the pituitary gland, the parathyroid, and the adrenal cortex. In contrast to this group of neoplasms, pheochromocytoma and medullary carcinoma of the thyroid are examples of tumors of neural crest origin and do not occur in association with pancreatic adenomas (pp. 812–813, 987–989, 1112–1113).

82. (B); 83. (D); 84. (C); 85. (B); 86. (A)

Although gastric polyps are in fact rare, they are among the most common benign neoplasms of the stomach. Histologically, gastric polyps are classified as either hyperplastic or adenomatous; the hyperplastic variety comprise 80 to 90% of all gastric polyps. (82) Adenomatous polyps, which are true neoplasms, tend to be large and average about 4.0 cm in diameter. Hyperplastic polyps are seldom over 2.0 cm in diameter. (83) Both hyperplastic and adenomatous polyps tend to occur singly, although multiple polyps may be present as part of the diffuse intestinal polyposis such as familial multiple polyposis, or Peutz-Jegher's syndrome. (84) Gastric polyps tend to be asymptomatic and are usually discovered incidentally. (85) The major significance of adenomatous gastric polyps is their tendency to undergo malignant transformation. Hyperplastic polyps represent regenerative non-neoplastic lesions and rarely, if ever, undergo malignant transformation. (86) Curiously, however, hyperplastic polyps are associated with coexistent gastric carcinoma elsewhere in the stomach, constituting perhaps the most significant feature of this otherwise innocuous lesion (p. 820).

87. (A); 88. (C); 89. (D); 90. (D); 91. (D); 92. (A); 93. (B); 94. (A); 95. (A); 96. (C); 97. (C)

Crohn's disease and ulcerative colitis are both idiopathic disorders with systemic manifestations that produce inflammatory disease of the bowel as their primary consequence. Although they have many overlapping features, leading to the hypothesis that the two diseases may actually represent opposite ends of the spectrum of host response to the same disease entity, in their classic forms the two processes can be distinguished on a number of bases.

(87) The distribution of the two diseases is usually quite distinctive. On the one hand, Crohn's disease involves the terminal ileum in the majority of cases (65%) and frequently affects the colon concurrently. The colon alone is involved in 20 to 30% of cases, but the lesions of Crohn's disease may be found at any level of the gastrointestinal tract, including the stomach. On the other hand, ulcerative colitis is a process largely limited to the large intestine, although the terminal ileum is involved in 10% of cases.

(88) In both conditions, extraintestinal involvement may occur. The systemic complications are similar in both diseases and include: migratory polyarthritis, sacroiliitis, ankylosing spondylitis, uveitis, hepatic involvement, and skin lesions. (89) One of the primary pathologic features that distinguishes Crohn's disease from ulcerative colitis is the presence of granulomata. These appear in affected bowel segments in approximately 60% of the cases. The presence of granulomata is by no means pathognomonic for Crohn's disease, however. When granulomata are observed, specific causes of granulomatous enterocolitis such as tuberculosis or fungal infection must be considered, and special stains for these organisms should be performed. In Crohn's disease, special stains for bacteria, fungi, or acid-fast bacilli fail to reveal microorganisms.

(90) The search for a specific etiologic microorganism in ulcerative colitis and Crohn's disease has proven unfruitful. Although various viruses have been suspected to be causative agents, the evidence for a viral etiology of inflammatory bowel disease is inconclusive. Although viruses have been cultured from diseased portions of bowel in a small number of cases, electron and immunohistochemical microscopic studies have failed in most cases to confirm the presence of viral particles in diseased tissue. Moreover, the issue is further clouded by the possibility that viral particles, when present, represent only secondary infection of diseased bowel.

(91) Crohn's disease and ulcerative colitis share many epidemiologic similarities, including age, race, and sex distribution, but no specific HLA profiles have been identified in association with these diseases. Although previous reports link HLA-B27 to Crohn's disease with ankylosing spondylitis, it is now clear that the antigen is associated only with the latter disorder with or without Crohn's disease.

(92) In general, the gross appearance of the affected bowel in the two diseases differs in several specific aspects. In Crohn's disease the inflammation is characteristically transmural and leads to marked fibrosis (scarring) of the submucosa and muscularis propria.

Thus, the wall of the affected bowel becomes rigid, thickened, and narrowed. (**93**) In ulcerative colitis, the inflammatory process is usually limited to the mucosa, and the bowel wall is not significantly thickened. Occasionally, however, a severe acute attack of fulminant ulcerative colitis may produce sudden cessation of bowel function with dilatation of the colon and acute transmural inflammation, with fraying and thinning of the muscularis propria (toxic megacolon). The danger of perforation in this situation is great, and the consequences may be lethal. Curiously, this important complication of ulcerative colitis is virtually never seen in Crohn's disease.

(**94**) Another major distinguishing feature between ulcerative colitis and Crohn's disease is the distribution of lesions in the involved bowel. The lesions of Crohn's disease are typically discontinuous; affected areas are interrupted by uninvolved patches of bowel (known as "skip lesions"). This pattern contrasts with that of ulcerative colitis in which the lesions are usually confluent and continuous. (**95**) Furthermore, the transmural nature of the inflammatory process in Crohn's disease leads to the formation of deep mural fissures and fistulous tracts, which are among the most important complications of this disease. Ulcerative colitis does not produce these deeply penetrating lesions; ulcerative colitis is characterized instead by the shallow superficial mucosal ulcerations from which the disease derives its name.

(**96**) One of the most important yet most unfortunate similarities between ulcerative colitis and Crohn's disease is the increased frequency of colonic carcinoma with which they are both associated. Although the overall risk of gastrointestinal carcinoma is smaller in Crohn's disease than in ulcerative colitis, in both disorders the risk increases with increasing duration of the disease. (**97**) In addition, both Crohn's disease and ulcerative colitis impose an increased risk of primary gastrointestinal lymphoma (*pp. 836–841, 859–862*).

98. (A); 99. (A); 100. (A); 101. (C); 102. (B); 103. (C); 104. (A)
Ischemic bowel disease is a broad term used to describe hypoxic injury to the gastrointestinal tract caused by any disorder that leads to enteric hypoperfusion. In general, the extent of the injury produced in the bowel is directly related to the severity of the reduction in blood flow. On the one hand, transmural infarction represents maximal injury to the bowel, producing ischemic necrosis of all layers of the bowel wall. Mural infarction, on the other hand, is the result of minimal ischemic damage, involving only that layer of the wall which is most remote from the arterial blood supply. Thus, in mucosal infarction, ischemic injury and necrosis are limited to the mucosa and submucosa and spare the muscularis and the serosa. (**98**) Mucosal infarction may occur at any level of the bowel from stomach to anus without particular predilection for any specific

region. Transmural infarction, however, most commonly affects the small bowel. Unlike the colon, which throughout most of its length receives collateral circulation from the posterior abdominal wall to which it is attached, the small bowel is entirely dependent on the mesenteric vascular supply.

(**99 and 100**) Although transmural infarction is most often produced by arterial occlusion with total or near total reduction in blood flow, it occurs as a result of venous thrombosis in a minority of cases. In contrast to total arterial or venous occlusion, which completely halt the flow of blood, conditions that reduce but do not arrest the flow of blood may produce mucosal injury but rarely lead to transmural infarction. (**101**) The combination of atherosclerosis and hypotension may, according to the severity of these elements, produce any degree of ischemic injury, from mucosal to transmural infarction. (**102**) In the absence of significant atherosclerosis, hypotension alone virtually never produces transmural infarction. Conversely, low flow states (shock) with reflex splanchnic vasoconstriction are the major causes of mucosal infarction.

(**103**) Ischemic bowel disease, no matter what the level of injury, commonly appears hemorrhagic. In mucosal infarction, the hemorrhage is limited to the superficial layers of the gut, but in transmural infarction hemorrhage may be seen throughout the deeper levels as well. (**104**) Because the hemorrhagic necrosis of mucosal infarction is of a limited and superficial nature, it rarely has grave consequences. Transmural infarction, in contrast, is a highly lethal disorder that is associated with a mortality rate of 50 to 75%. It requires prompt diagnosis and surgical intervention (*pp. 831–833*).

105. (D); 106 (A); 107. (C); 108. (B); 109. (B)
Tropical sprue and Whipple's disease are two uncommon causes of malabsorption that are suspected to be of infectious etiology, but a causative microbiologic agent has not yet been identified for either disease. (**105**) Neither tropical sprue nor Whipple's disease has a strong female predominance. On the contrary, Whipple's disease occurs 10 times more commonly in males than in females, and tropical sprue occurs with equal frequency in the two sexes. (**106**) Only tropical sprue is associated with travel to an endemic area (the Caribbean, for example). In fact, because the pathologic changes in the small bowel are so variable and nonspecific in this disease, a history of travel to an endemic area is essential to its diagnosis.

(**107**) Despite the fact that no etiologic microorganism has been identified for either disease, both tropical sprue and Whipple's disease can be cured by antibiotic therapy. The dramatic response of these diseases to antibiotics strongly suggests that they are indeed of bacterial origin. (**108**) Although Whipple's disease was once thought to be a process limited to the small bowel, it is now clear that the disorder is systemic in distribution. The skin, central nervous system, joints, heart, blood vessels, kidney, lungs, serosal membranes, lymph nodes, spleen, and liver may all be involved. Tropical sprue, in contrast, produces disease only in the small intestine. (**109**) One of the primary pathologic features of Whipple's disease is the presence of PAS-positive glycoprotein-laden macrophages in the small bowel mucosa that contain unidentified, rod-shaped bacilli. Although it is suspected that these rod-shaped bacteria are etiologic, this remains to be confirmed (*pp. 848–851*).

110. (C); 111. (B); 112. (C); 113. (C); 114. (D)

Congenital anomalies may occur at any level of the gastrointestinal tract and lead to bowel obstruction and other serious gastrointestinal problems in the neonate. Since many of these developmental defects are life-threatening and must be recognized early, knowledge of the most prevalent lesions and their most common sites of occurrence is critical. (**110**) Congenital atresia (failure of a bowel segment to develop, leaving behind a solid cord-like remnant) occurs most often in the small intestine (*p. 830*).

(**111**) Intestinal stenosis refers to luminal narrowing from any cause. The most frequent developmental abnormality producing intestinal stenosis is hypertrophy of the gastric pylorus. Hypertrophic pyloric stenosis is unique among the congenital stenoses, since most of the others are caused by hypoplastic, rather than hyperplastic, segments of bowel wall or luminal strictures (*p. 808*).

(**112**) Congenital duplication occurs as a consequence of a defect in transformation from the solid to the hollow luminal phase of bowel development early in gestation. Although rare, this anomaly occurs most frequently in the small intestine (*p. 830*).

(**113**) Congenital diverticula, which represent herniations or outpouchings of the intestinal wall, are uncommon lesions and are often asymptomatic. The most common congenital diverticulum, known as Meckel's diverticulum, is located in the small intestine and represents a remnant of the vitelline duct (see Question 126). Other congenital diverticula represent primary defects in the bowel wall and are unrelated to other embryologic structures (*p. 830*).

(**114**) Ganglion cells, which are critical to the transmission of the parasympathetic stimulus to peristalsis, migrate into the gut from the neural crest. Most commonly, they fail to reach the most distal bowel segment, the rectosigmoid region of the large bowel. The aganglionic segment cannot propagate a peristaltic wave and acts as a functional bowel obstruction (see Question 8) (*p. 855*).

115. (C); 116. (B); 117. (B); 118. (D); 119. (E); 120. (E)

(**115**) Gastrin, a peptide hormone that stimulates hydrochloric acid production by gastric parietal cells, is primarily produced in the gastric antrum, which itself is devoid of parietal cells. (**116**) Pepsin is pro-

duced by the zymogenic chief cells of the gastric glands in the body and fundus of the stomach that produce pepsin. (**117**) It is also in the gastric glands of the body and fundus of the stomach that the gastric parietal cells are located. In addition to the production of hydrochloric acid, parietal cells elaborate intrinsic factor—a glycoprotein that plays an essential role in the absorption of vitamin B_{12} (see Chapter 3, Question 17). (**118**) Gastric endocrine cells (enterochromaffin cells) are scattered throughout the glands of all the gastric regions and indeed throughout the entire gut, making the gastrointestinal tract the largest endocrine organ in the body. (**119**) The goblet cell, however, is a cell type characteristically found in the small and large intestine but not in the normal stomach. Mucus-secreting surface cells and neck cells of the gastric glands contain finely dispersed mucigen granules rather than a single large mucin-containing apical vacuole that characterizes the intestinal goblet cell. (**120**) Similarly, in the normal gastrointestinal tract, the Paneth cell is found only in the small intestine. Therefore, the appearance of Paneth cells or goblet cells in the gastric mucosa indicates a pathologic metaplastic change and usually occurs in association with chronic gastritis (*pp. 806–807, 812*).

121. (D); 122. (C); 123. (A); 124. (D); 125. (C); 126. (C); 127. (D)

(**121**) Two microscopic features that are unique to the normal small intestine allow for its ready histologic identification. On a cytologic level, the easily recognizable, intensely eosinophilic Paneth cells, a cell type that occurs almost exclusively in the small bowel, can be identified in the mucosal crypts of all small bowel segments. The second singular feature of the small bowel is the architecturally unique arrangement of the surface mucosal epithelium into villous projections (known simply as villi). (**122**) Peyer's patches are prominent lymphoid nodules (germinal centers) that characterize the ileal segment of small bowel, whereas (**123**) Brunner's glands, elaborately branched submucosal mucus glands, are found only in the duodenal segment. (**124**) Endocrine cells (argentaffin or enterochromaffin cells), many of which secrete serotonin, are found in the mucosal crypts throughout the length of the small intestine. Although histologically identical, endocrine cells represent a family of unique cell types, each capable of elaborating a particular gut hormone. Besides serotonin, these cells are known to produce gastrin, somatostatin, substance P, vasoactive intestinal peptides, bombesin, and possibly glucagon. However, serotonin-producing endocrine cells do not appear to be anatomically segregated from endocrine cells producing any of these other intestinal hormones and are found scattered among other argentaffin cells in all small bowel segments. (**125**) Like the intestinal endocrine cells, mucosal absorption cells in the small bowel are histologically identical but, at least in some aspects, functionally unique. The best studied example of such functional uniqueness is that of vitamin B_{12}–intrinsic factor absorption by the surface absorptive cells of the ileum. These cells produce a specific receptor protein for intrinsic factor–vitamin B_{12} complex, which they display on the luminal surface of their cell membrane. The receptor protein is not produced by absorptive cells elsewhere in the small intestine; thus, vitamin B_{12} deficiency is a common consequence of ileal resection. (126) Meckel's diverticulum is a remnant of the omphalomesenteric duct, an embryologic structure that connects the primitive gut with the yolk sac. Although it may vary slightly in position, it is always located in the ileal segment of small bowel, usually within 12 inches of the ileocecal valve. (127) Pancreatic rests, on the other hand, may occur anywhere in the small bowel. They occur as small foci of ectopic, yet normal, pancreatic tissue that are considered to be congenital anomalies but, unlike Meckel's diverticula, have no normal embryologic counterpart. Their occurrence may have clinical significance, however, as they may give rise to acute pancreatitis or even pancreatic adenocarcinoma (pp. 828, 830).

128. (B); 129. (A); 130. (D); 131. (C); 132. (D); 133. (B); 134. (D)

The pathologic characteristics of bacterial enterocolitides vary according to three basic properties of the infecting agent: (1) invasive potential, (2) toxin production, and (3) antigenic potential (ability to elicit immune responses in the host). The infective enterocolitides produced by Salmonella, Shigella, and Vibrio cholerae organisms are major causes of infectious gastrointestinal disease that represent classic examples of these three pathogenetic features. (128) The Shigella bacillus is the cause of the clinical syndrome known as bacillary dysentery. This organism directly penetrates the bowel mucosa through the epithelial cells and replicates within the lamina propria. Here the organism liberates an endotoxin that is cytodestructive and leads to shallow mucosal ulcerations, the characteristic feature of Shigella enterocolitis. (129) Although Salmonella organisms are capable of mucosal penetration and liberation of endotoxins, mucosal ulceration is not a prominent feature. Instead, Salmonella enterocolitis is characterized by an intense immune response producing massive hypertrophy of submucosal lymphoid follicles. In the prototypic Salmonella gastroenteritis, typhoid fever, Salmonella typhi organisms tend to localize within the Peyer's patches of the ileum, which become greatly hypertrophied and are seen grossly as plaque-like mucosal elevations often 6.0 to 8.0 cm in diameter. The mucosa overlying these hypertrophied follicles undergoes secondary necrosis, presumably due to pressure-induced ischemia but not as a direct consequence of bacterial toxicity. (130) Granulomatous inflammation is not produced by any of these three organisms. The presence of granulomata would suggest infection with mycobacteria (tuberculosis), fungi,

or, rarely, strains of bacteria, such as Brucella, that induce granulomatous inflammation.

(131) Enterocolitis produced by Vibrio cholerae organisms causes few anatomic changes in the affected bowel. Because the organism does not invade the bowel mucosa, no mucosal ulcerations are produced. The profuse watery diarrhea that is the hallmark of this infection is caused by an enterotoxin elaborated by the bacillus. The enterotoxin activates membrane-bound adenyl cyclase, causing increased intracellular levels of cAMP. Thus, salt and water absorption are inhibited, and active secretion of water, chloride, and bicarbonate by mucosal crypt cells is stimulated. (132) As indicated above, all three of these organisms are capable of toxin production. In Shigella enterocolitis and cholera, toxin production by the causative organism is the principal pathogenetic factor.

(133) Among these three forms of enterocolitis, only shigellosis preferentially involves the large bowel. The tissue damage in Shigella enterocolitis is almost entirely limited to the mucosa of the colon, although the ileum is sometimes involved. Salmonella enterocolitis classically involves both small and large intestine, whereas cholera is primarily a disease of the small bowel.

(134) Although ulcero-inflammatory proctitis of infectious etiology may be seen among homosexual males, it is not associated with any of the above forms of bacterial enterocolitis. The most common causative agents are Treponema pallidum, gonococci, chlamydia, and herpes simplex (pp. 319–323, 835).

135. (A); 136. (C); 137. (C); 138. (B); 139. (D); 140 (C); 141. (D)

Any benign proliferation of colonic mucosal elements that has an exophytic growth pattern and protrudes above the level of the surrounding mucosa is called a colonic polyp. The term, however, refers only to the gross morphology of the lesion. Microscopically, colonic polyps can be divided into two basic categories: hyperplastic lesions and true neoplasms (adenomas). Among the adenomas, several different morphologic types may be distinguished that correspond to differing tendencies to undergo neoplastic transformation.

(135) The hyperplastic polyp is the most common type of colonic polyp, comprising 90% of all colonic epithelial polyps at autopsy. Clinically, they are usually only discovered incidentally, since they are virtually always asymptomatic. Hyperplastic polyps are not considered to be true neoplasms but rather reactive proliferations of mature, well-differentiated, non-neoplastic epithelial cells separated by connective tissue resembling the lamina propria.

(136) Although the definitive identification of any colonic polyp depends upon its histologic appearance, the gross size and configuration of the polyp often provide clues to the recognition of specific types. Overall, villous adenomas are the largest in size.

They are slow-growing velvety lesions that, unlike other types of adenomatous polyps, are rarely pedunculated. In general, hyperplastic polyps are the smallest lesions. Tubular adenomas and hamartomatous polyps tend to be intermediate in size between hyperplastic polyps and villous adenomas.

(137) In true adenomatous polyps (tubular adenomas, villous adenomas, and tubulovillous adenomas, a histologic composite of these two types), there is a positive correlation between the size of the lesion and the probability of neoplastic transformation. Thus, villous adenomas, the largest of the adenomatous polyps, have the highest likelihood of containing carcinoma. Nonadenomatous polyps (hyperplastic polyps and hamartomatous polyps) virtually never undergo neoplastic transformation.

(138) Familial polyposis is a hereditary autosomal dominant disorder characterized by the formation of extremely large numbers of adenomatous polyps in the colon and occasionally the small bowel and stomach as well. Typically, the entire colonic mucosa is covered by closely packed polyps, giving the surface a shaggy appearance. The vast majority of the polyps are small tubular adenomas, although an occasional villous adenoma may occur. Eventual malignant transformation of one or more of these polyps is virtually inevitable in this disease; therefore, it is commonly treated with total colectomy at an early age.

(139) The Peutz-Jeghers syndrome is also an auto-somal dominant disorder characterized by diffuse intestinal polyposis. In contrast to familial polyposis, however, the polyps of Peutz-Jeghers syndrome occur mainly in the small intestine and are of the hamartomatous variety. Since hamartomatous polyps do not undergo malignant transformation, the Peutz-Jeghers syndrome imposes no increased risk of gastrointestinal carcinoma.

(140) Villous adenomas in general tend to be symptomatic more often than other adenomatous polyps and often cause rectal bleeding. Occasionally, villous adenomas may be associated with copious mucin production, causing a protein-losing enteropathy, a complication not usually associated with other types of colonic polyps.

(141) Although the hamartomatous polyps of the Peutz-Jeghers syndrome resemble tubular adenomas grossly, they are easily differentiated from the latter by histologic examination. Instead of the closely aggregated neoplastic glands of tubular adenomas, hamartomatous polyps are composed of dilated, mucin-filled cysts that are lined primarily by normal-appearing goblet cells. The cysts are often separated by strands of smooth muscle. As the name implies, hamartomatous polyps are composed of proliferations of the three normal elements of the colonic mucosa: mucosal epithelial cells, loose connective tissue (lamina propria), and smooth muscle (muscularis mucosae) (*pp. 867–868*).

9

THE LIVER, BILIARY TREE, AND PANCREAS

DIRECTIONS: For Questions 1 to 12, choose the ONE BEST answer to each question.

1. Conditions that predispose to gallstone formation include all of the following EXCEPT:

   A. Type IV hyperlipidemia
   B. Crohn's disease
   C. Clofibrate therapy
   D. Diabetes mellitus
   E. Ulcerative colitis

2. All of the following characteristically cause fatty change in the liver EXCEPT;

   A. Reye's syndrome
   B. Diabetes mellitus
   C. Total parenteral nutrition
   D. Tetracycline toxicity
   E. Acute viral hepatitis

3. Which of the following histologic features of hepatocollular injury is prognostically LEAST favorable?

   A. Councilman body formation
   B. Bile infarct formation
   C. Collagen formation
   D. Ballooning of hepatocytes
   E. Lobular inflammatory cell infiltrates

4. The hepatorenal syndrome refers to which of the following:

   A. Functional failure of a morphologically normal kidney associated with severe liver disease
   B. Simultaneous toxic damage to the liver and kidneys with functional failure of both
   C. Immune complex glomerulopathy from chronic antigenemia associated with chronic viral hepatitis
   D. Acute tubular necrosis from hypotension following a gastrointestinal bleed in the cirrhotic patient
   E. All of these

5. Which one of the following statements about central hemorrhagic necrosis of the liver is TRUE?

   A. Pressure necrosis from distended central veins and sinusoids is the major causal factor
   B. Congestive heart failure is the most common cause
   C. Its gross appearance is identical to that of nutmeg toxicity ("nutmeg liver")
   D. In chronic cases, micronodular cirrhosis frequently develops
   E. Severe involvement with bridging necrosis is known as an "infarct of Zahn"

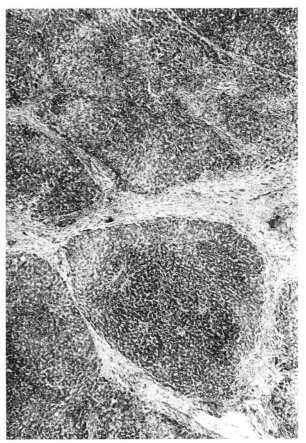

Figure 9–1

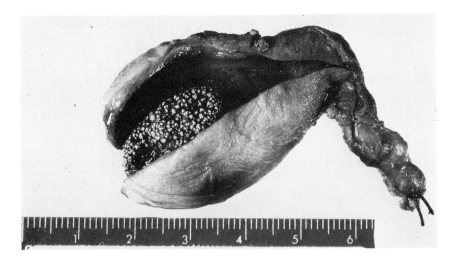

Figure 9–2

6. All of the following statements about fulminant viral hepatitis are true EXCEPT:

    A. It is less common than fulminant hepatitis caused by drugs

    B. Its severity is proportional to the immune response to the virus

    C. Death usually occurs within 24 hours of the onset of symptoms

    D. Histologically, it is commonly indistinguishable from drug-induced fulminant hepatitis

    E. Survivors usually have lifelong immunity to recurrent infection

7. The liver condition pictured in Figure 9–1 predisposes to all of the following disorders EXCEPT:

    A. Hemorrhoids

    B. Mixed gallstones

    C. Hyperaldosteronism

    D. Splenomegaly

    E. Hepatocellular carcinoma

8. Causes of cirrhosis in infancy include all of the following EXCEPT:

    A. Wilson's disease

    B. Alpha-1-antitrypsin deficiency

    C. Total parenteral nutrition

    D. Extrahepatic biliary atresia

    E. Galactosemia

9. All of the following statements about Wilson's disease are true EXCEPT:

    A. It is caused by increased copper absorption

    B. Kayser-Fleischer rings in the eyes are diagnostic

    C. Excess copper in the liver is rarely visible on liver biopsy

    D. Cirrhosis eventually develops in virtually all patients

    E. Serum ceruloplasmin levels are characteristically low

10. All of the following features are associated with hepatocellular carcinoma EXCEPT:

    A. Bile production

    B. Alpha-fetoprotein production

    C. Mucin production

    D. Tumor embolization to the lung

    E. Intraperitoneal hemorrhage

11. Conditions that predispose to the disorder pictured in Figure 9–2 include all of the following EXCEPT:

    A. Obesity

    B. Crohn's ileitis

    C. Diabetes mellitus

    D. Clofibrate therapy

    E. Chronic hemolytic anemia

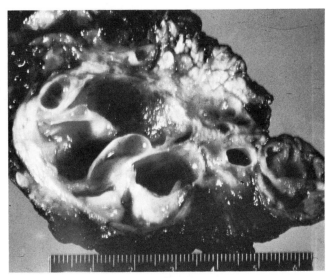

12. The lesion pictured in Figure 9–3 was removed from the head of the pancreas and was lined by epithelium forming papillary projections. This lesion is associated with:

A. Angiomas of the retina and cerebellum
B. Pancreatitis
C. Mucin-producing adenocarcinoma
D. Pancreatic duct obstruction
E. None of these

Figure 9–3

DIRECTIONS: For Questions 13 to 22, ONE or MORE of the completions given correctly finishes the incomplete statement. Choose:

A—if only *1, 2, and 3* are correct
B—if only *1 and 3* are correct
C—if only *2 and 4* are correct
D—if only *4* is correct
E—if all are correct

13. In which of the following conditions is the indirect fraction of bilirubin increased more than the direct fraction?

1. Primary biliary cirrhosis
2. Recurrent jaundice of pregnancy
3. Rotor syndrome
4. Thalassemia

A. 1,2,3   B. 1,3   C. 2,4   D. 4 Only   E. All

14. Metabolic effects of alcohol that contribute to fatty change in the liver include:

1. Increased lipid absorption from the small bowel
2. Increased lipid mobilization from adipose tissue
3. Decreased triglyceride formation in hepatocytes
4. Decreased fatty acid oxidation

A. 1,2,3   B. 1,3   C. 2,4   D. 4 Only   E. All

15. In which of the following conditions is Mallory's hyaline found within hepatocytes?

1. Carbon tetrachloride toxicity
2. Wilson's disease
3. Viral hepatitis
4. Alcoholic liver disease

A. 1,2,3   B. 1,3   C. 2,4   D. 4 Only   E. All

16. Hepatic encephalopathy:

1. Characteristically causes asterixis
2. Frequently responds to antibiotic treatment
3. Is frequently associated with generalized cerebral edema
4. Does not occur when serum ammonia levels are normal

A. 1,2,3   B. 1,3   C. 2,4   D. 4 Only   E. All

17. Hepatic disorders that are incompatible with survival to adulthood include:

1. Crigler-Najjar syndrome type 1
2. Gilbert's disease
3. Extrahepatic biliary atresia
4. Wilson's disease

A. 1,2,3   B. 1,3   C. 2,4   D. 4 Only   E. All

18. Hepatitis A virus infection:

1. Produces a viral carrier state in about 1% of cases
2. Produces chronic hepatitis in about 5% of cases
3. Is most often acquired from contaminated shellfish
4. Produces fatal fulminant hepatitis in about 0.1% of cases

A. 1,2,3   B. 1,3   C. 2,4   D. 4 Only   E. All

19. Causes of chronic active hepatitis include:

1. Wilson's disease
2. Methyldopa
3. Alpha-1-antitrypsin deficiency
4. Alcohol

    A. 1,2,3 B. 1,3 C. 2,4 D. 4 Only E. All

20. Acetaminophen hepatotoxicity is related to:

1. Dose of the drug
2. Glutathione content of the liver cell
3. Previous alcohol ingestion
4. T cell sensitization to the drug

    A. 1,2,3 B. 1,3 C. 2,4 D. 4 Only E. All

21. Primary idiopathic hemochromatosis:

1. Inevitably produces cirrhosis
2. Is associated with HLA-A3
3. Predisposes to hepatocellular carcinoma
4. Commonly occurs in diabetic patients

    A. 1,2,3 B. 1,3 C. 2,4 D. 4 Only E. All

22. Carcinoma of the pancreas:

1. Arises from pancreatic acinar cells
2. Is decreasing in incidence in the United States
3. Occurs most often in the tail of the pancreas
4. Is associated with spontaneous venous thrombosis

    A. 1,2,3 B. 1,3 C. 2,4 D. 4 Only E. All

DIRECTIONS: For Questions 23 to 41, you are to decide whether EACH choice is TRUE or FALSE.

For each of the following statements about hepatitis B virus (HBV) infection, choose whether it is TRUE or FALSE.

23. The virus causes cytotoxic damage to the liver cells

24. Antibody production to the HBV surface antigen is defective in HBV carriers

25. Antibody production to the HBV core antigen confers lifelong immunity

26. The presence of HBV "e" antigen in serum indicates infectivity

27. HBV is the only hepatotrophic virus associated with an asymptomatic carrier state

28. The histologic finding of "ground glass" cytoplasm in liver cells is diagnostic of hepatitis B

29. HBV infection is the most common cause of chronic active hepatitis

For each of the following statements about extrahepatic biliary obstruction, choose whether it is TRUE or FALSE.

30. Increased synthesis of cholesterol by liver cells contributes to the associated hypercholesterolemia

31. The increased serum levels of alkaline phosphatase help to differentiate it from primary biliary cirrhosis

32. The increased serum levels of conjugated bilirubin cause pruritus

33. The associated bleeding diathesis is a result of platelet dysfunction

34. The associated darkening of the urine differentiates it from hemolytic causes of jaundice

35. It is most frequently produced by impaction of a gallstone in the cystic duct

36. The histologic finding of bile lakes is pathognomonic

For each of the following statements about acute cholecystitis, choose whether it is TRUE or FALSE.

37. Virtually all patients with gallstones eventually develop acute cholecystitis

38. Bacterial infection is the initiating factor in acute cholecystitis in the majority of cases

39. Chronic cholecystitis is usually preceded by repeat episodes of acute cholecystitis

40. Right upper quadrant pain is the most common presentation of acute cholecystitis

41. Surgical removal of the gallbladder is the treatment of choice

DIRECTIONS: For Questions 42 to 67, the set of lettered headings is followed by a list of numbered words or phrases. For each numbered word or phrase choose:

A—if the item is associated with (A) only
B—if the item is associated with (B) only
C—if the item is associated with *both* (A) and (B)
D—if the item is associated with *neither* (A) nor (B)

For each of the following characteristics, choose whether it describes hepatic vein thrombosis, portal vein thrombosis, both, or neither.

A. Hepatic vein thrombosis
B. Portal vein thrombosis
C. Both
D. Neither

42. Associated with a high mortality rate
43. Known as the Budd-Chiari syndrome
44. Produces an enlarged and tender liver
45. Frequently occurs as a result of tumor invasion
46. Strongly related to oral contraceptive use
47. Frequently caused by peritoneal sepsis
48. Occasionally caused by pancreatitis

For each of the statements listed below, choose whether it describes cholangitis, pericholangitis, both, or neither.

A. Cholangitis
B. Pericholangitis
C. Both
D. Neither

49. Characterized by a neutrophilic inflammatory infiltrate
50. Associated with cholelithiasis (gallstones)
51. Associated with inflammatory bowel disease
52. Produces an elevated serum alkaline phosphatase
53. Usually accompanied by bile stasis
54. Responds to antibiotic therapy
55. Predisposes to cholangiocarcinoma

For each of the characteristics listed below, choose whether it describes primary biliary cirrhosis, sarcoidosis, both, or neither.

A. Primary biliary cirrhosis
B. Sarcoidosis
C. Both
D. Neither

56. Productive of granulomas in the liver
57. Associated with Sjögren's syndrome
58. Associated with a hyperglobulinemia
59. Associated with cutaneous anergy
60. Associated with antimitochondrial antibody

For each of the characteristics listed below, choose whether it describes acute cholecystitis, acute pancreatitis, both, or neither.

A. Acute cholecystitis
B. Acute pancreatitis
C. Both
D. Neither

61. Strongly resembles perforated peptic ulcer on clinical presentation
62. Associated with gallstones
63. Associated with hyperlipidemia
64. Associated with hypercalcemia
65. Associated with alcoholism
66. Causes markedly elevated serum amylase levels
67. Causes adult respiratory distress syndrome

DIRECTIONS: Questions 68 to 81 are matching questions. For each numbered item, choose the most likely associated lettered item from those provided. Each numbered item has ONLY ONE answer. Within each group, each lettered item may be the answer to one, more than one, or none of the numbered items.

For each of the characteristics listed below, choose whether it describes liver cell adenoma, hepatocellular carcinoma, angiosarcoma of the liver, gallbladder carcinoma, or none of these.

A. Liver cell adenoma
B. Hepatocellular carcinoma
C. Angiosarcoma of the liver
D. Gallbladder carcinoma
E. None of these

68. Associated with cirrhosis
69. Associated with cholelithiasis
70. Usually produces elevated serum levels of alpha-fetoprotein
71. Associated with polyvinyl chloride exposure
72. Associated with oral contraceptive use
73. Occasionally causes the Budd-Chiari syndrome
74. Usually produces elevated serum levels of human chorionic gonadotropin

For each of the following causes of hepatic injury, choose the histologic feature with which it is commonly associated:

A. Fatty change
B. Cholestasis
C. Councilman bodies
D. Granulomas
E. None of these

75. Hepatic duct obstruction
76. Hypersensitivity response to sulfa drugs
77. Toxicity from anovulatory steroids ("the pill")
78. High-dose corticosteroid toxicity
79. Yellow fever
80. Acute viral hepatitis
81. Cardiogenic shock

9

THE LIVER, BILIARY TREE, AND PANCREAS

ANSWERS

1. (E) Most gallstones (approximately 90%) are composed largely of cholesterol. Cholesterol is a water-insoluble substance; its solubility in bile in the form of micelles is dependent upon the presence of bile salts and phospholipids. In normal bile the ratio of concentration of bile salts and phospholipids to cholesterol usually exceeds 13:1. When this equilibrium is disturbed by either an increase in the concentration of cholesterol or a decrease in bile salts or lecithin, cholesterol may precipitate out and form stones. Type IV hyperlipidemia, clofibrate therapy, and diabetes mellitus all increase the serum and biliary concentrations of cholesterol and predispose to gallstone formation. Crohn's disease most commonly affects the terminal ileum—the site of bile salt resorption—leading to loss of bile salts from the enterohepatic circulation. The loss of bile salts disturbs the bile salt/lecithin:cholesterol ratio, predisposing to stone formation. In contrast to Crohn's disease, ulcerative colitis produces enteric disease that is limited to the large bowel and usually does not interfere with the enterohepatic circulation of bile salts *(pp. 944–945)*.

2. (E) The accumulation of fat within liver cells is one of the most common patterns of hepatic injury. Although the pathogenesis is not fully understood in some cases such as Reye's syndrome, most conditions that cause fatty liver are believed to involve one or more of the following metabolic/biochemical abnormalities in hepatocyte lipid metabolism: (1) excessive entry of free fatty acids into the liver; (2) interference with conversion of fatty acids to phospholipids; (3) increased esterification of fatty acids to triglycerides; (4) decreased apoprotein synthesis; (5) impaired coupling of lipid with apoproteins; or (6) impaired lipoprotein secretion from the liver.

Diabetes mellitus is one of the most common systemic diseases associated with fatty change in the liver. Diabetes causes excessive breakdown of fat stores and an increased presentation of fatty acids to the liver. The lipid content of total parenteral nutritional solutions also represents an increased free fatty acid load for the liver. Tetracycline commonly causes fatty change in the liver and is thought to do so by reducing apoprotein synthesis. Acute viral hepatitis, however, is not a disease associated with fatty change in the hepatocytes. In this disorder, the lymphocyte-mediated immune attack on the virally infected cell causes focal hepatocyte necrosis and is not preceded by any biochemical abnormality that would lead to accumulation of lipid in the liver cells *(pp. 18–20, 906, 941)*.

3. (C) The liver is an organ with impressive regenerative capacity and may recover fully from disorders that cause liver cell death. However, the severity, duration, and type of injury are counterbalancing factors in the recovery process. Chronic or profound injuries frequently lead to scar (collagen) formation in the damaged liver. Although fibrosis is reversible to a variable extent during the early stages of chronic injury if the source of the injury is removed, removal of the injurious agent is frequently difficult (alcoholism) or impossible (chronic active viral hepatitis or primary biliary cirrhosis). Thus, collagen formation often heralds the development of cirrhosis and is prognostically the least favorable histologic feature of hepatic injury.

Councilman body formation and ballooning degeneration of hepatocytes are the histologic manifestations of coagulative necrosis or cell membrane damage with cell swelling, respectively. They are examples of single-cell hepatocyte necrosis, whereas infarct formation corresponds to death of small groups of hepatocytes from chemical (bile) injury. The liver, through regeneration, may recover fully from any of these events.

Lobular inflammatory infiltrates may be the cause of or the result of hepatocyte necrosis and are a variable feature of hepatocyte injury. They may resolve completely ·or contribute to the formation of fibrosis and thus have less prognostic significance than fibrosis itself *(pp. 70, 908, 929)*.

4. (A) The hepatorenal syndrome is defined as functional renal failure in the absence of morphologically overt renal damage. It occurs in patients with severe liver disease, most often advanced cirrhosis. Although the pathogenesis of the hepatorenal syndrome has not been fully elucidated, there is evidence that it may be related to generalized renal vasoconstriction, which is more marked in the cortex than in the medulla. The cause of the vasoconstriction is unknown. Although hepatic and renal failure may occur simultaneously in toxic or immune complex disorders, these specific cases are defined by their underlying etiology and are not included in the concept of the hepatorenal syndrome. Likewise, acute tubular necrosis from hypotension following a gastrointestinal bleed in a patient with cirrhosis would be excluded according to the above definition (*p. 893*).

5. (B) Central hemorrhagic necrosis of the liver results from severe chronic passive congestion of the centrilobular area and is most commonly caused by congestive heart failure. Necrosis of hepatocytes in the centrilobular zone is primarily the result of hypoxia secondary to arteriolar hypoperfusion, although pressure necrosis may play a minor role. Gross appearance of the severely congested liver with its deep red centrilobular zone surrounded by pale tan peripheral zone hepatocytes resembles the cut surface of a nutmeg and thus has become known as "nutmeg" liver. In chronic cases, delicate scarring may result, but true cirrhosis rarely develops. Infarcts of Zahn refer to a sharply demarcated area of red-blue discoloration of the hepatic parenchyma caused by occlusion of an intrahepatic branch of the portal vein and are not related to central hemorrhagic necrosis (*p. 897*).

6. (C) Fulminant hepatitis refers to an uncommon but often lethal complication of hepatocellular disease characterized by submassive to massive necrosis of liver cells and precipitous hepatic failure. Most cases (about 40%) are caused by hepatotoxic drugs, but 25% of cases are related to viral hepatitis, the second most common cause. In contrast to the drug-induced form of fulminant hepatitis in which the liver cell is damaged by a toxic compound produced during the metabolic breakdown of the offending drug, fulminant viral hepatitis is an immunologically induced phenomenon. None of the hepatitis viruses are cytotoxic. Liver injury in viral hepatitis is produced by the immune response to the virally infected, antigenically altered hepatocytes, and the severity of the injury is proportional to the strength of the immune response.

Histologically, all forms of fulminant hepatitis tend to look alike. Massive "dropout" necrosis (liquefactive necrosis) of the liver cells occurs, leaving only a collapsed reticulin framework and intact portal structures. The severity and distribution of the necrosis tends to be variable. Although the mortality rate in fulminant viral hepatitis is high, those who do survive almost never become carriers but acquire lifelong immunity to recurrent infection.

Despite the fact that this disorder is termed "fulminant," death rarely occurs within the first few days of onset of the necrotizing process. The course is usually measured in weeks, and by definition, death within 8 weeks of the onset of acute symptoms is termed "fulminant hepatic failure" (*pp. 909–910*).

7. (B) Micronodular cirrhosis, most commonly caused by alcohol abuse, is pictured in the micrograph. The fibrous scarring and regenerative nodules of the scler-

otic liver greatly increase resistance to flow through the portal venous system, and the hydrostatic pressure in the portal vein increases. With the rising portal pressure, flow is diverted into the systemic venous system through common portosystemic collateral channels. The principal sites of these portosystemic shunts are the veins around the rectum (hemorrhoids), gastroesophageal junction (esophageal varices), retroperitoneum, and the falciform ligament of the liver (periumbilical or abdominal wall varices). Blood flow is also preferentially diverted into the splenic vein, which is a major tributary of the portal vein, and congestive splenomegaly results. Secondary hyperaldosteronism and sodium retention also occur in association with cirrhosis. It is thought to be due to sequestration of blood within the splanchnic bed, leading to a decrease in circulating blood volume, a decrease in renal blood flow, and renin release from the juxtaglomerular cells. In addition to increased aldosterone secretion, impaired hepatic metabolism and excretion of the hormone contribute to the hyperaldosteronism.

Cirrhosis is an important predisposing factor to the development of hepatocellular carcinoma. In the United States, about 80% to 90% of liver cell carcinomas arise in cirrhotic livers. The risk of developing hepatocellular carcinoma varies with different etiologic types of cirrhosis, but all forms impose some risk. Worldwide, cirrhosis following chronic active hepatitis from hepatitis B virus (HBV) infection imposes the greatest risk of subsequent development of hepatocellular carcinoma. In the United States, where persistent HBV infection is relatively infrequent, other forms of cirrhosis such as pigment cirrhosis are relatively more frequently associated with hepatocellular carcinoma.

Although mixed gallstones may be associated with cirrhosis, they are a cause rather than a result of cirrhosis. Chronic impaction of gallstones and large duct obstruction may produce secondary biliary cirrhosis, but this is now unusual since surgical therapy for cholelithiasis is widely available. Production of gallstones is the result of elaboration by the liver of bile with abnormal proportions of cholesterol and bile salts, a feature not typically associated with cirrhosis. For obscure reasons, however, alcoholic cirrhosis predisposes to the formation of pigment gallstones, an infrequent complication (*pp. 916–923, 945*).

8. (A) A wide variety of hereditary metabolic defects, congenital anomalies, and iatrogenic disorders produce severe liver injury early in life and cirrhosis in infancy or early childhood. Although the hepatic manifestations of alpha-1-antitrypsin deficiency are extremely varied, in severe cases neonatal hepatitis and childhood cirrhosis are produced. Prolonged total parenteral nutrition administered in infancy is now known to produce significant hepatocellular damage, and cases of cirrhosis have been reported. Extrahepatic biliary atresia is a congenital condition characterized by defective development of the extrahepatic biliary tree, which may be incomplete and/or lack luminal patency. This is a rare and catastrophic condition that is incompatible with life unless surgically corrected before the inevitable production of secondary biliary cirrhosis early in life. Galactosemia and tyrosinemia are two of the more common errors of metabolism that produce cirrhosis in infancy if survival is sustained long enough.

Wilson's disease, in contrast, is an autosomal recessive disorder of copper metabolism that rarely becomes symptomatic before 5 to 10 years of age and in half of the patients remains asymptomatic until adolescence. Ultimately, cirrhosis is produced, and Wilson's disease is among the most common causes of cirrhosis in the older child but is compatible with survival into adulthood *(pp. 492, 931–933, 940)*.

9. (A) Wilson's disease (hepatolenticular degeneration) is a hereditary defect of copper metabolism with an impairment of *excretion* of copper by the liver. Copper accumulates in the parenchyma of various organs, most importantly the liver and brain. Deposition of copper granules in Descemet's membrane close to the limbus of the cornea produces one of the most characteristic and diagnostic features of Wilson's disease, the Kayser-Fleischer rings. Although toxic accumulations of copper in the liver may first produce active hepatitis, the disease inevitably produces cirrhosis. Ironically, however, copper may be difficult to identify on liver biopsy in Wilson's disease. Copper is rarely visible in routine histologic preparations and may or may not be demonstrable with special histochemical techniques. A more easily identified abnormality consistently present in all patients with Wilson's disease, however, is a reduction of the serum ceruloplasmin level. Ceruloplasmin is an alpha$_2$ globulin produced by the liver to which copper is bound and released from the liver cells. Normally, it accounts for 90% to 95% of the total plasma copper. In Wilson's disease, the ceruloplasmin is consistently reduced, but the "free" copper loosely bound to albumin increases so that the total serum copper approaches normal levels *(pp. 932–933)*.

10. (C) Hepatocellular carcinoma is a malignancy with many distinctive features that help to differentiate it from other forms of carcinoma. A feature that distinguishes liver cells from any other cell type is their ability to produce bile; likewise, bile production by their malignant counterpart, the hepatocellular carcinoma, is a diagnostic feature. The production of alpha-fetoprotein by hepatocellular carcinoma is also highly characteristic but not diagnostic since other tumor types, such as germ cell tumors, may also manufacture this protein. The production of alpha-fetoprotein by hepatocellular carcinoma recapitulates the characteristic production of this protein by the embryonic liver. Hepatocellular carcinoma is a tumor with a striking propensity for venous invasion. It commonly invades the hepatic vein and may extend into the inferior vena cava. Fragments of intravascular tumor may then break off and embolize to the lung, a phenomenon associated with only a few other tumors, including renal cell carcinoma, choriocarcinoma, and gastric or breast carcinoma metastatic to the liver. Another distinctive pattern of growth that hepatocellular carcinomas exhibit is direct extension through the liver capsule with penetration of surrounding structures. Capsular penetration may give rise to severe intraperitoneal bleeding, which is occasionally the presenting feature of the disease.

It is important to recognize, however, that hepatocellular carcinoma is not an adenocarcinoma and does not secrete mucin. Rather, primary mucin-secreting adenocarcinomas arising in the liver originate from the bile duct epithelium and are known as cholangiocarcinomas. Occasionally, hepatocellular carcinoma and cholangiocarcinoma may exist simultaneously in a so-called "mixed" pattern, but the two elements may be differentiated on the basis of bile production and mucin production respectively. Of course, adenocarcinomas involve the liver far more frequently than any other tumor type, but the vast majority of these are metastatic *(pp. 936–938)*.

11. (E) The gallbladder pictured contains a large crystalline, yellow-flecked, mixed gallstone. Mixed stones are by far the most common type of gallstones and account for about 90% of biliary calculi. They are termed "mixed" gallstones because they contain varying proportions of all three stone-forming elements of bile: cholesterol, bilirubin, and calcium carbonate. Their primary constituent is cholesterol, a water-insoluble molecule, which crystallizes out of a supersaturated bile. Thus, conditions that affect lipid metabolism and increase the cholesterol content of the bile, such as obesity, diabetes mellitus, and clofibrate therapy, predispose to the formation of cholesterol-containing stones.

In normal bile, cholesterol is kept in solution by bile salts and lecithin. These polar molecules form a hydrophilic shell around cholesterol, and the resultant water-soluble complex is known as a "micelle." Conditions that lead to loss of bile salts from the enterohepatic circulation and reduce their availability for micelle formation also predispose to cholesterol-containing calculus formation. Therefore, diseases such as Crohn's disease that primarily affect the ileum, the principal site of bile salt resorption, predispose to mixed stone formation.

Chronic hemolytic anemia is an example of a disorder that increases only the bilirubin content of the bile and predisposes to the formation of *pigment* (calcium bilirubinate) stones but not cholesterol-based calculi. Pigment stones are small, occur multiply, and are jet black *(pp. 945–946)*.

12. (C) The lesion pictured is a multiloculated neoplastic pancreatic cyst known as a cystadenoma.

These lesions are uncommon but are important to recognize because of their premalignant potential. The epithelial lining of these tumors may be either serous or mucinous, the mucinous variety having the greatest premalignant potential. Extensive histologic examination of these tumors is required to rule out the presence of a mucin-producing adenocarcinoma in some portion of the wall. These lesions must be differentiated clinically from congenital cysts, retention cysts, or pseudocysts of the pancreas. It is the congenital cyst of the pancreas, believed to develop from anomalous pancreatic ducts, that is associated with a rare entity called von Hippel–Lindau disease. In this syndrome, angiomas are found in the retina and cerebellum or brainstem in association with cysts of the pancreas as well as cysts of the liver and kidney. Pancreatitis is associated with the formation of pseudocysts that are the result of inflammation and necrosis with subsequent fibrosis and fluid accumulation, forming a cystic lesion that lacks a true epithelial lining (therefore called a pseudocyst). Retention cysts refer to dilated pancreatic ducts that develop from ductal obstruction and are lined by ductal epithelium. Congenital cysts, pseudocysts, and retention cysts all tend to be unilocular lesions. The presence of a multilocular cyst, such as the one pictured, suggests a neoplastic lesion, a cystadenoma, or a cystadenocarcinoma (*p. 968*).

13. (D) Bilirubin is a catabolic product of heme metabolism that is delivered to the liver bound to albumin, taken up by the hepatocytes, conjugated with glucuronide, and excreted in bile. Disorders that cause defects in the excretion of bile from the hepatocyte or block its flow through the biliary tree cause an increase in serum levels of conjugated bilirubin (direct fraction). Unconjugated bilirubin (indirect fraction) is elevated in disorders that increase the amount of bilirubin delivered to the liver, impair hepatic uptake of unconjugated bilirubin, or impair the conjugation process within the liver cells. In thalassemia, for example, bilirubin production is greatly increased as a result of hemolysis, the conjugation capacity of the liver is overwhelmed, and the *indirect* fraction of bilirubin in the serum rises.

Primary biliary cirrhosis, recurrent jaundice of pregnancy, and the Rotor syndrome all cause increases in the *direct* fraction of bilirubin. They are examples of underexcretion rather than overproduction of bilirubin. The capacity of the liver cell to conjugate bilirubin is unimpaired in these conditions. In primary biliary cirrhosis, intrahepatic bile ducts are injured, and flow through the injured duct is consequently impaired. In the Rotor syndrome and recurrent jaundice of pregnancy, secretion of bile into the bile canaliculus is impaired. Consequently, bilirubin conjugated in the hepatocytes cannot be eliminated and backs up into the serum. The secretory defect of the liver cells is hereditary in the Rotor syndrome and in recurrent jaundice of pregnancy is

believed to be induced by an exaggerated response to estrogens (*p. 892*).

14. (C) Alcohol is the most common cause of fatty change in the liver. The abnormal accumulation of neutral fat in the hepatocytes is the result of a combination of pathogenetic mechanisms. Alcohol causes increased mobilization of lipid from adipose tissue stores, leading to excessive entry of free fatty acids into the liver. Concomitantly, alcohol *increases* the esterification of fatty acids to triglycerides while reducing fatty acid oxidation. In addition, the formation of lipoproteins and their release from the hepatic cells are also impaired by alcohol. Alcohol has no known effect on lipid absorption from the small bowel, however (*pp. 18–19*).

15. (C) Mallory's hyaline is a finely granular eosinophilic material that is found in the liver cell cytoplasm in certain forms of hepatocellular injury. It is considered to be highly characteristic of alcoholic injury but also occurs in less common disorders such as Wilson's disease and primary biliary cirrhosis. Mallory's hyaline is made up of retained proteins that appear in the electron microscope as aggregates of intermediate filaments. Their pathogenesis is now believed to result from defective assembly of microtubules required for intracytoplasmic transport of protein, leading to decreased protein secretion and increased protein retention. This pattern of injury occurs in relatively few hepatocellular disorders, however, and is not seen in carbon tetrachloride toxicity or viral hepatitis (*pp. 12, 904–909, 918–919, 932–933*).

16. (A) Hepatic encephalopathy, a complication of liver failure, is a metabolic disorder of the central nervous system characterized by alteration in consciousness, neurologic signs, and electroencephalographic changes. Characteristically it produces a flapping tremor of the upper extremities known as asterixis. Although the pathogenesis of these manifestations is unknown, it is believed to be related to the production of a toxin in the intestine derived from protein metabolism by intestinal bacteria. With cirrhosis and portal hypertension, toxic substances absorbed from the bowel would be shunted into the inferior vena cava from the portal system through intra- or extrahepatic anastomoses, bypassing liver cells and escaping detoxification. Support for this concept is derived from the observation that antibiotics administered to reduce the intestinal flora are effective in treatment of hepatic encephalopathy. Although ammonia has been implicated as the toxic agent, hepatic encephalopathy may occur in the absence of hyperammonemia. Pathologic findings in the brain are inconsistent in hepatic encephalopathy but usually include generalized cerebral edema as well as alterations in neurones and laminar necrosis (*pp. 893–894*).

17. (B) The Crigler-Najjar syndrome type 1 is characterized by the near complete impairment of glucuronyl transferase. Death inevitably occurs in infancy from extensive brain damage caused by severe unconjugated hyperbilirubinemia, Extrahepatic biliary atresia inevitably leads to secondary biliary cirrhosis in infancy and causes death from hepatic failure unless surgical correction is possible. Gilbert's disease, in contrast, is a benign hereditary disorder producing mild defects in hepatocyte uptake of unconjugated bilirubin, mild deficiencies in glucuronyl transferase, and in 50% of the cases a mildly increased hemolysis. There are no pathologic alterations in the liver and the disease is usually asymptomatic, at most producing a mild jaundice. Wilson's disease, although a much more serious condition, usually remains asymptomatic until adolescence. Wilson's disease is caused by an impairment in hepatic excretion of copper, leading to the accumulation of toxic levels of this metal in the liver, brain, and other organs. The process of accumulation is slow, however, and the liver damage (hepatitis or cirrhosis) and degenerative changes in the brain develop during adulthood (see Question 9) (*pp. 895–896, 932, 940*).

18. (D) In the vast majority of cases, hepatitis A virus infection is a benign, transient disease from which lifelong immunity is acquired. The hepatitis A virus produces neither a carrier state nor a chronic disease process. The infection is usually contracted by the fecal-oral route from infected humans, the natural reservoir of the virus, during the stage of fecal viral shedding. Less often, the infection is contracted from contaminated food, water, milk, or shellfish. Only rarely does infection with hepatitis A virus produce fulminant hepatitis; thus, the mortality rate for this disease is less than 0.1%. Overall, hepatitis A virus is responsible for less than 1% of all fulminant hepatitis (*p. 900*).

19. (E) Chronic active hepatitis is a serious disorder of varied etiology that is characterized by chronic destructive inflammation and fibrosis in the liver. It is a progressive disorder that often ends in cirrhosis and death. Although well known to occur in about 3% of cases of acute hepatitis B and even more frequently following non-A–non-B hepatitis, chronic active hepatitis may also occur in association with Wilson's disease, drug toxicity, or hypersensitivity, alpha-1-antitrypsin deficiency, and alcohol consumption. The most common drugs known to cause chronic active hepatitis are methyldopa, oxyphenacetin, isoniazid, and acetaminophen (*pp. 913–914, 919–920, 930–933*).

20. (A) Acetaminophen hepatotoxicity is an example of liver injury produced by the bile transformation of the drug by the liver into a toxic product. This pattern of drug injury is termed "direct" hepatotoxicity to distinguish it from "indirect" drug-related hepato-toxicity in which the drug acts as a hapten to convert an intracellular protein into an immunogenic molecule. T cell sensitization to the immunogen in turn effects an immune attack on the hapless liver cell.

In acetaminophen hepatotoxicity, the extent of hepatic injury is related to (1) the dose of the drug, (2) the glutathione content of the hepatocyte, and (3) previous ingestion of substances such as alcohol that induce the P-450 enzymes of the mixed function oxidase system. Glutathione, a molecular constituent of the hepatocyte cytoplasm, is the keystone of one of the major drug detoxification systems in the liver. Conjugation of drug metabolites to glutathione renders them nontoxic, water-soluble, and amenable to excretion in the urine. When the glutathione content of liver cell is exhausted, toxic drug metabolites accumulate in the cytoplasm. Since the great majority of drugs are metabolized by the mixed function oxidase system of the hepatocyte, induction of this enzymatic system by one drug (e.g., alcohol or barbiturate) will accelerate metabolic transformation of other drugs by the same activated enzymes. In the case of acetaminophen, the greater the rate of metabolic biochemical transformation, the greater the production of the toxic metabolite. T cell sensitization to acetaminophen with indirect hepatocellular injury is not believed to contribute to the hepatotoxicity of this drug (*pp. 912–913*).

21. (A) Primary idiopathic hemochromatosis is a hereditary disorder of iron metabolism transmitted as an autosomal recessive trait and associated with HLA-A3. Severe systemic iron overload is the result of this as yet undefined metabolic defect, and profound parenchymal damage from iron toxicity is produced in liver, pancreas, myocardium, pituitary, adrenal, thyroid and parathyroid, joints, and skin. Micronodular "pigment" cirrhosis results from damage to the liver, characteristically the most severely affected organ. Pigment cirrhosis poses a considerable risk to the subsequent development of hepatocellular carcinoma that occurs in about 30% of cases.

In the pancreas, iron is deposited both in the exocrine and the endocrine cells. The pancreas undergoes atrophy and fibrosis. Loss of pancreatic islets produces a secondary type of diabetes late in the course of the disease. Primary idiopathic diabetes mellitus, however, is unrelated to primary hemochromatosis. In short, diabetes commonly occurs in primary hemochromatosis, but hemochromatosis does not commonly occur in diabetic patients (*pp. 924–928*).

22. (D) The term "carcinoma of the pancreas" refers to neoplastic transformation of the pancreatic *ductal* elements. Pancreatic acini may give rise to malignant tumors but do so rarely and make up less than 1% of all pancreatic malignancies. The pathogenesis of pancreatic carcinoma is still obscure, and the incidence of this malignancy continues to be on the rise for unknown reasons. The adjusted death rate has *increased 3-fold* over the last 40 years. The malignancy arises most often in the *head* of the pancreas, where 60% to 70% of these tumors are located. Only 5% to 10% arise in the tail of the pancreas, but these are of great clinical significance since they may grow silently for long periods of time and are often metastatic by the time the patient comes to clinical attention. One of the most characteristic paraneoplastic syndromes associated with pancreatic carcinoma is that of spontaneous venous thrombosis, also referred to as migratory thrombophlebitis and associated clinically with Trousseau's sign. The pathogenesis of this condition is thought to be related to a thromboplastic factor produced by the malignancy, leading to a hypercoagulable state *(pp. 968–972)*.

23. (False); 24. (True); 25. (False); 26. (True); 27. (False); 28. (True); 29. (False)

(**23**) Hepatitis B virus is one of a small group of hepatotropic viruses that themselves are not cytotoxic for liver cells. Damage to the liver is produced by the host immune responses mounted against the virally infected liver cells. (**24**) Individuals who fail to respond immunologically to HBV harbor the virus indefinitely but fail to sustain liver disease. Such individuals are known as "healthy" carriers. (**25**) Although in normal individuals antibody to the HBV core antigen is produced earliest in the course of the disease, it serves only as a marker of current or recent past infection and does not confer immunity. Only antibody to the hepatitis B surface antigen is capable of erradicating the HBV infection and conferring lifelong immunity. (**26**) HBV "e" antigen is associated with the DNA-containing viral core but is immunologically distinct from both HBV core antigen and surface antigen. The "e" antigen is detectable in the serum early in the course of acute infection when the disease is most transmissible and disappears before the onset of recovery. Thus, it is a marker of infectivity.

(**27**) Although HBV is associated with an asymptomatic carrier state as outlined above, it is not the only hepatotropic virus to produce such a condition. The less well defined non-A–non-B virus (NANBV) or viruses have been shown by epidemiologic evidence to occasionally produce a chronic carrier state. There is, however, no known chronic carrier state for hepatitis A virus.

(**28**) Overall, the histologic findings in acute viral hepatitis are the same whether produced by hepatitis A virus, HBV, or NANBV. Since the histologic findings are so nonspecific in these three disease states, the best way to distinguish them is through serologic studies. Occasionally, however, hepatocytes infected with HBV may show an amorphous eosinophilic area within their cytoplasm known as "ground-glass" cytoplasm. This finding represents

focal collections of virions and is pathognomonic for HBV infection. Unfortunately, it is only infrequently present in acute hepatitis B.

(**29**) Chronic active hepatitis, a progressive fibrosing inflammatory disorder, follows about 3% of attacks of acute hepatitis B and about 30% of posttransfusion non-A–non-B hepatitis. The most common cause of chronic active hepatitis, however, is drug toxicity or hypersensitivity. Hepatitis A has not been known to produce chronic active hepatitis *(pp. 900–907)*.

30. (True); 31. (False); 32. (False); 33. (False); 34. (True); 35. (False); 36. (True)

Extrahepatic biliary obstruction causes hepatic cholestasis, secondary hepatocellular dysfunction, and malabsorption from the absence of bile acids in the gut. (**30**) Extrahepatic cholestasis is characterized by hyperlipidemia with increased plasma levels of cholesterol and phospholipids. Although not fully understood, the cause of the hyperlipidemia in cholestasis is thought to be mainly the result of increased synthesis of cholesterol by hepatocytes. (**31**) Increased serum levels of alkaline phosphatase originating from damaged ductal epithelial cells occur in extrahepatic duct obstruction but do not help to differentiate this disorder from other causes of cholestasis. Indeed, in primary biliary cirrhosis, significant elevations of alkaline phosphatase result from the widespread destruction of bile ducts, the hallmark of this disease. (**32**) One of the most characteristic clinical features of extrahepatic cholestasis is the development of pruritus, believed to be caused by the accumulation of bile acids in the serum. The elevated serum levels of conjugated bilirubin occurring in extrahepatic cholestasis cause jaundice, not pruritus.

(**33**) The absence of bile salts from the intestine seriously affects the absorption of fat and fat-soluble vitamins, including vitamin K. The synthesis of prothrombin and other vitamin K–dependent coagulation factors may become seriously impaired in extrahepatic cholestasis and may cause a bleeding diathesis. Platelet function is not known to be altered, however.

(**34**) In hemolytic causes of jaundice, excessive production of bilirubin results in an unconjugated hyperbilirubinemia. Unconjugated bilirubin is water insoluble and is bound to albumin in the serum; thus it is not filtered across the glomerulus into the urine. In extrahepatic biliary obstruction, however, jaundice is produced by conjugated hyperbilirubinemia. Since conjugated bilirubin is water soluble, it appears in the glomerular filtrate and produces a characteristically dark-colored urine (choluric jaundice).

(**35**) By far the most common cause of obstruction of the extrahepatic biliary tree is gallstones. In order to cause cholestasis in the liver, however, the stone must lodge in either the hepatic duct or the common bile duct. If lodged in the cystic duct, it may give rise to acute cholecystitis, but since hepatic biliary drainage is unimpaired, extrahepatic cholestasis will not occur.

(36) The histologic features of both intrahepatic and extrahepatic cholestasis include inspissated bile plugs in canaliculi, bile pigment in hepatocytes and Kupffer cells, feathery degeneration of hepatocytes, and, eventually, bile duct damage and portal fibrosis. Only in extrahepatic biliary obstruction, however, does the formation of bile lakes (bile infarcts) occur. They are believed to result from the extravasation of bile from cholangioles, resulting in necrosis of surrounding liver cells, and are pathognomonic for extrahepatic cholestasis (pp. 929–930).

37. (False); 38. (False); 39. (False); 40. (True); 41. (True)

(37) Although the great majority (about 90%) of cases of acute cholecystitis are associated with gallstones, the converse is not true. In fact, most cases of cholelithiasis (perhaps 80%) are asymptomatic.

(38) Bacterial infection may be a contributing factor to the pathogenesis of acute cholecystitis in 5% to 10% of cases; however, the major etiologic factor in most cases is direct chemical irritation of the gallbladder wall by concentrated bile.

(39) Although repeat attacks of acute cholecystitis may result in chronic changes with fibrosis of the gallbladder wall, this rarely occurs. Chronic cholecystitis is classically an insidious disorder producing vague complaints and is not associated with acute bouts of severe inflammation.

(40) In contrast to the intolerance to fatty foods, belching, and epigastric distress that characterize chronic cholecystitis, acute cholecystitis usually manifests itself as an acute abdominal emergency. It commonly produces right upper quadrant pain, often referred to the right shoulder.

(41) The treatment of choice in acute cholecystitis is surgical removal of the gallbladder to prevent catastrophic complications such as perforation of the gallbladder with pericholecystic abscess formation, generalized peritonitis, ascending cholangitis, liver abscess formation, subdiaphragmatic abscesses, or septicemia (pp. 947–949).

42. (A); 43. (A); 44. (A); 45. (C); 46. (D); 47. (B); 48. (B)

(42, 43, 44) The Budd-Chiari syndrome is a rare but catastrophic event caused by thrombosis of the hepatic veins. Because the liver has a dual blood supply from the hepatic artery and the portal vein but a single venous outflow from the hepatic veins, occlusion of the latter has the most serious consequences of any form of major vascular occlusion to the liver. Occlusion of the hepatic veins is associated with a high mortality rate, many patients dying within days of its onset, most dying within months. The liver is enlarged and tender, and intractable ascites is produced. This condition contrasts with portal vein

thrombosis, which is much better tolerated. In portal vein thrombosis, the liver is neither enlarged nor tender, and the outlook for survival is good when the problem is corrected surgically with a splenorenal shunt.

(45) One of the most common causes of thrombosis of either the portal or hepatic vein is vascular invasion by tumor. Hepatic vein thrombosis is frequently caused by tumors with a propensity for invasion of the vena cava such as hepatocellular, renal cell, or adrenal carcinoma, whereas portal vein thrombosis is caused most often by tumors arising within the abdominal cavity.

(46) Although oral contraceptives have been implicated in the past as a cause of hepatic vein thrombosis, the association is now believed to be circumstantial. There is no evidence that oral contraceptives are related to portal vein thrombosis.

(47) Intrahepatic rather than peritoneal infections are a common cause of hepatic vein thrombosis. Portal vein thrombosis, in contrast, is associated with intraperitoneal sepsis and secondary portal phlebitis. (48) Furthermore, since the portal vein is anatomically continuous with the splenic vein, disorders that initiate thrombosis in the splenic vein, such as pancreatitis or pancreatic carcinoma, may produce portal vein thrombosis through retrograde propagation of the thrombus. Pancreatitis, however, does not cause thrombosis of the hepatic veins (pp. 897–899).

49. (A); 50. (A); 51. (B); 52. (C); 53. (A); 54. (A); 55. (D)

(49) Cholangitis refers to suppurative inflammation of the intrahepatic or extrahepatic bile ducts and is characterized histologically by neutrophilic inflammatory infiltrates within the walls or lumens of affected ducts. (50) Cholangitis is almost always produced by extrahepatic duct obstruction, which is most commonly caused by impaction of a gallstone in the common bile duct.

(51) Pericholangitis, as the name implies, refers to inflammatory infiltrates in portal triads around, but not involving, bile ducts. In contrast to cholangitis, the inflammatory infiltrates in pericholangitis consist predominantly of lymphocytes and macrophages. Although pericholangitis is a rather common and nonspecific histologic finding, its strongest association is with inflammatory bowel disease.

(52) Both cholangitis and pericholangitis produce elevated serum alkaline phosphatase levels. Compared with cholangitis, however, the degree of alkaline phosphatase elevation occurring with pericholangitis is usually modest.

(53) Since cholangitis is almost always caused by extrahepatic duct obstruction, it is almost invariably accompanied by bile stasis. In pericholangitis, bile stasis may occur but is a much less predictable feature.

(54) Antibiotic therapy is usually effective in cho-

langitis, a process caused by direct bacterial infection of the bile duct. In contrast, pericholangitis is believed to be caused by drainage of bacterial products or other toxic substances through the portal system or peribiliary lymphatics and does not commonly respond to antibiotic therapy. (55) Neither cholangitis nor pericholangitis is associated with subsequent neoplastic transformation of bile ducts (pp. 910–912).

56. (C); 57. (A); 58. (C); 59. (C); 60. (A)

(56) Primary biliary cirrhosis and sarcoidosis are both idiopathic diseases that are associated with abnormal immunologic findings and may produce granulomas in the liver. (57) Primary biliary cirrhosis is thought to be an autoimmune disease whose primary target is the intrahepatic biliary tree. The disease is associated with other autoimmune diseases such as rheumatoid arthritis, Hashimoto's thyroiditis, and Sjögren's syndrome. Sarcoidosis is characterized by hyperreactive cellular and humoral immunity but is not believed to be autoimmune in nature. (58) Both diseases are associated with a hyperglobulinemia. In sarcoidosis, abnormally high levels of antibodies to commonly encountered antigens typically occur. In primary biliary cirrhosis, the hyperglobulinemia is usually of the IgM class and is believed to result from a failure of the immune response to convert IgM to IgG in antibody synthesis. (59) Abnormal cellular immunity is also observed in both diseases, and impaired T cell reactivity with cutaneous anergy is characteristic. (60) Primary biliary cirrhosis can usually be distinguished, however, on the basis of the histologic picture of a nonsuppurative injury to bile ducts and by the presence of an antimitochondrial antibody in the serum of 90% to 100% of patients with this disorder (pp. 390–392, 928–930).

61. (C); 62. (C); 63. (C); 64. (B); 65. (B); 66. (B); 67. (B)

(61) Acute cholecystitis and acute pancreatitis are diseases that may closely resemble one another at presentation, since the onset of both diseases is usually marked by the sudden development of acute abdominal pain, a situation known as an "acute abdomen." Thus, they must be differentiated not only from one another but from other common causes of acute abdomen such as perforated peptic ulcer or bowel infarction. (62) The two diseases share some etiologic conditions as well. Gallstones are implicated in the pathogenesis of almost all (90%) cholecystitis and over half (40% to 60%) of acute pancreatitis. However, only a small percentage of patients with gallstones develop either of these conditions. Direct damage to the organ caused by bile salts and lecithin is believed to be the underlying etiologic factor in both disorders.

(63) Both acute cholecystitis and pancreatitis are also more common among individuals with hyperlipidemia. Type IV hyperlipidemia predisposes to biliary calculus formation, which, as mentioned, is strongly related to the pathogenesis of acute cholecystitis. Types I and V hyperlipidemia are more closely associated with acute pancreatitis. In contrast to acute cholecystitis, acute pancreatitis associated with hyperlipidemia is believed to develop from activation of pancreatic lipase with local production of free fatty acids that are toxic to acinar cells and blood vessels. (64) Similarly, direct activation by calcium of another pancreatic enzyme, trypsinogen, is believed to be the underlying cause of acute pancreatitis associated with hypercalcemia. Trypsin, in turn, is able to activate the majority of proenzymes in the pancreas, such as proelastase and prophospholipase, initiating a catastrophic process of autodigestion in the pancreas. Very rarely, calcium may be the major constituent of gallstones (calcium carbonate gallstones), which could conceivably cause duct obstruction and acute cholecystitis; however, the formation of these calculi is poorly understood and does not appear to be related to hypercalcemia.

(65) One of the conditions most strongly associated with acute pancreatitis is chronic alcoholism. Although the exact role of alcohol in the pathogenesis of this disorder is unclear, it is known that alcohol is a potent stimulator of pancreatic secretion. At the same time, alcohol may increase pancreatic sphincteric tone, leading to partial pancreatic ductal obstruction. Alcoholism does not appear to be related to the pathogenesis of acute cholecystitis, however.

(66) Amylase is one of many pancreatic enzymes released into the serum during an attack of acute pancreatitis. Elevation of serum amylase usually occurs within the first 24 hours of an acute attack and serves as an early marker for the disease. Although amylase is somewhat less specific for pancreatic disease than other pancreatic enzymes, assay methods for amylase are simple and widely used. Serum amylase remains elevated during the active phase of the disease and falls to basal levels 2 to 5 days after the acute attack. Amylase is not an enzyme produced by the gallbladder or associated with cholecystitis.

(67) The adult respiratory distress syndrome (diffuse alveolar damage in the lungs) is an ominous complication of acute pancreatitis. The pathogenesis is thought to be related to enzymatic destruction of pulmonary surfactants by circulating pancreatic phospholipase released into the serum during an acute attack of pancreatitis (pp. 947–948, 963–966).

68. (B); 69. (D); 70. (B); 71. (C); 72. (A); 73. (B); 74. (E)

(68) Although chronic infection with hepatitis B virus is the most common condition associated with

hepatocellular carcinoma on a worldwide basis, cirrhosis is the most common predisposing condition in countries such as the United States, where the hepatitis B virus is not endemic. The risk of developing hepatocellular carcinoma varies among the specific forms of cirrhosis. Hepatoma occurs with high frequency in pigment cirrhosis and postnecrotic cirrhosis resulting from chronic active B viral hepatitis. Although alcoholic cirrhosis is the most common form of cirrhosis in the United States, hepatocellular carcinoma is relatively rare in this disease, perhaps because the natural course of the disease is usually relatively short.

(69) Gallstones are present in the great majority of cases (65–95%) of carcinoma of the gallbladder. It is postulated that chronic inflammation of the gallbladder associated with gallstones may be an important factor in the pathogenesis of gallbladder carcinoma. Furthermore, metabolic derivatives of cholic acid, a bile component, are known to be potent carcinogens and may also contribute to the origin of this malignancy.

(70) High serum levels of alpha-fetoprotein are present in up to 75% of patients with hepatocellular carcinoma. Although mildly elevated serum levels of alpha-fetoprotein may occur in nonmalignant liver disease, very high levels (greater than 1000 ng/ml) strongly suggest the presence of either of the two malignant tumors known to produce large quantities of this protein: hepatocellular carcinoma and yolk sac tumors of germ cell origin.

(71) Angiosarcoma of the liver is a very rare malignancy, but it occurs with increased frequency in individuals exposed to polyvinyl chloride (e.g., plastics workers). This tumor is also associated with chronic arsenic poisoning and exposure to Thorotrast.

(72) Liver cell adenoma used to be a very rare tumor. Although still uncommon, it now appears more frequently in women between 20 and 40 years of age who have used oral contraceptives.

(73) Hepatocellular carcinoma has a propensity for hepatic vein invasion and may even extend into the inferior vena cava and right side of the heart. With extensive hepatic vein invasion, venous outflow from the liver is blocked and the Budd-Chiari syndrome is produced.

(74) With rare exceptions, the only malignancies that produce elevated levels of human chorionic gonadotropin are those that originate from germ cells and have trophoblastic differentiation. The primary hepatic and biliary neoplasms discussed do not produce this hormone *(pp. 935–939, 952–954)*.

75. (B); 76. (E); 77. (B); 78. (A); 79. (C); 80. (C); 81. (E)

(75) Very few histologic patterns of liver injury are pathognomonic for given disease process. However, many causes of liver injury do predictably produce patterns that suggest the diagnosis. Hepatic duct obstruction, for example, characteristically produces cholestasis in the liver. Cholestasis is first seen in centrilobular zones, and, if the obstruction persists, progressively involves the peripheral zones of the lobule and portal bile ducts. Although cholestasis may occur in other forms of liver disease, extrahepatic bile duct obstruction occasionally produces an additional unique feature called bile lakes or bile infarcts. These are produced by leakage of bile from small portal bile ducts with necrosis of surrounding liver cells. Bile infarcts are diagnostic of extrahepatic duct obstruction but occur in only 20% of cases *(p. 891)*.

(76) Drug-induced hepatic injuries fall into two basic categories: toxic injury and hypersensitivity reactions. In general, toxic injuries produce predictable pathologic changes. Hypersensitivity reactions are much less consistent in the pattern of injury they produce. They may result in cholestasis, nonspecific eosinophilic inflammation, granuloma formation, or injury resembling viral hepatitis ranging in severity from focal to massive hepatocellular necrosis. A few drugs tend to be more predictably associated with a specific type of hypersensitivity response than others. Reactions to sulfonamides, for example, most frequently produce a granulomatous hepatitis *(pp. 912–915)*.

(77 and 78) Anovulatory steroids and high-dose corticosteroids are examples of agents that produce toxic liver injury. They produce cholestasis and fatty change respectively *(pp. 18–19)*.

(79) Yellow fever is an acute viral disease that classically causes focal coagulative necrosis of liver cells. The dead hepatocytes become small, rounded, eosinophilic masses called Councilman bodies, after the renowned pathologist who first described them. This feature is not specific for yellow fever, however. It occurs in numerous other types of liver disease as well *(p. 290)*. **(80)** Acute viral hepatitis caused by any of the hepatotrophic viruses, for example, produces focal random necrosis of liver cells with Councilman body formation *(p. 906)*. **(81)** Cardiogenic shock typically produces marked centrilobular congestion in the liver and may result in centrilobular zonal necrosis. However, it is not characteristically associated with fatty change, cholestasis, Councilman body formation, or granulomas *(p. 897)*.

10

THE KIDNEY AND URINARY TRACT

DIRECTIONS: For Questions 1 to 8, choose the ONE BEST answer to each question

1. All of the following substances are components of the glomerular basement membrane EXCEPT:

   A. Fibronectin
   B. Heparin sulfate
   C. Laminin
   D. Type IV collagen
   E. Fibrin

2. Most forms of chronic renal failure produce *increased* serum levels of all of the following substances EXCEPT:

   A. Calcium
   B. Aldosterone
   C. Phosphate
   D. Parathormone
   E. Renin

3. Uremia is associated with all of the following abnormalities EXCEPT:

   A. Peripheral neuropathy
   B. Gastritis
   C. Polycythemia
   D. Pericarditis
   E. Diffuse alveolar damage

4. Glomerular injury caused by circulating complexes occurs with all of the following disorders EXCEPT:

   A. Bacterial endocarditis
   B. Goodpasture's syndrome
   C. Hepatitis B
   D. Systemic lupus erythematosus
   E. Lung cancer

5. Diabetes mellitus is associated with all of the following renal disorders EXCEPT:

   A. Diffuse glomerulosclerosis
   B. Nodular glomerulosclerosis
   C. Renal atherosclerosis
   D. Acute tubular necrosis
   E. Acute pyelonephritis

6. Clinical manifestations associated with the kidney tumor pictured in Figure 10–1 include all of the following EXCEPT:

   A. Hyperlipidemia
   B. Cushing's syndrome
   C. Polycythemia
   D. Hypercalcemia
   E. Femininization

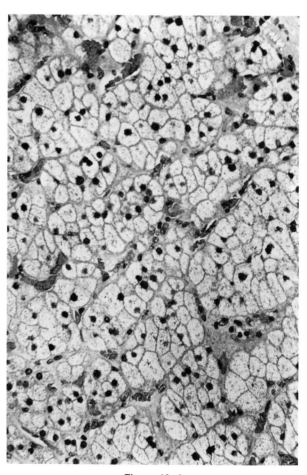

Figure 10–1

7. All of the following conditions predispose to urolithiasis EXCEPT:

A. Hypokalemic nephropathy
B. Hyperparathyroidism
C. Leukemia
D. Proteus infections
E. Analgesic abuse nephropathy

8. Conditions that predispose to acute pyelonephritis include all of the following EXCEPT:

A. Pregnancy
B. Vesicoureteral reflux
C. Catheterization of the bladder
D. Prostatism
E. Septicemia

DIRECTIONS: For Questions 9 to 21, ONE or MORE of the completions given correctly finishes the incomplete statement. Choose:

A—if only *1,2, and 3* are correct
B—if only *1 and 3* are correct
C—if only *2 and 4* are correct
D—if only *4* is correct
E—if all are correct

9. Mesangial cells:

1. Ingest macromolecules
2. Connect with Lacis cells
3. Are contractile
4. Receive sympathetic innervation

A. 1,2,3   B. 1,3   C. 2,4   D. 4 Only   E. All

10. In immunologically mediated glomerulonephritis, which of the following factors contribute(s) to glomerular injury?

1. Substances secreted by macrophages
2. Loss of glomerular polyanion
3. Neutrophilic enzymes
4. Cytotoxic T cells

A. 1,2,3   B. 1,3   C. 2,4   D. 4 Only   E. All

11. Systemic lupus erythematosus (SLE) gives rise to glomerular lesions that are histologically identical to which of the following primary glomerular diseases?

1. Focal sclerosis
2. Membranous glomerulonephritis
3. Lipoid nephrosis
4. Membranoproliferative glomerulonephritis

A. 1,2,3   B. 1,3   C. 2,4   D. 4 Only   E. All

12. Renal papillary necrosis usually occurs in the ABSENCE of infection in:

1. Urinary tract obstruction
2. Analgesic abuse nephropathy
3. Diabetes mellitus
4. Sickle cell anemia

A. 1,2,3   B. 1,3   C. 2,4   D. 4 Only   E. All

13. Chronic pyelonephritis (CPN):

1. Characteristically causes symmetrically scarred kidneys
2. Accounts for half of all end-stage kidney disease
3. Occurs in the absence of infection in chronic reflux nephropathy
4. Is associated with thyroidization of tubules

A. 1,2,3   B. 1,3   C. 2,4   D. 4 Only   E. All

14. Analgesic abuse nephropathy:

1. Occurs only after ingestion of about a kilogram of analgesic per year
2. Is most commonly caused by aspirin alone
3. Commonly causes sterile pyuria
4. Predisposes to the development of renal cell carcinoma

A. 1,2,3   B. 1,3   C. 2,4   D. 4 Only   E. All

15. Substances produced by the kidney that raise blood pressure include:

1. Neutral lipid factor
2. Kininogen
3. Prostacyclin
4. Renin

A. 1,2,3   B. 1,3   C. 2,4   D. 4 Only   E. All

16. Factors predisposing to essential hypertension include:

1. Genetic predisposition
2. Oral contraceptive use
3. High sodium intake
4. Pheochromocytoma

A. 1,2,3   B. 1,3   C. 2,4   D. 4 Only   E. All

17. Histologic features of malignant nephrosclerosis include:

1. Arteriolar necrosis
2. Hyperplastic arteriolitis
3. Necrotizing glomerulitis
4. Fibromuscular dysplasia of the renal artery

   A. 1,2,3 B. 1,3 C. 2,4 D. 4 Only E. All

18. Renal artery stenosis:

1. Is the most common curable form of hypertension
2. Is usually caused by atherosclerotic plaque
3. Has a favorable prognosis when high renin levels are present in the renal vein blood of the ischemic kidney
4. Is treated by surgical removal of the ischemic kidney

   A. 1,2,3 B. 1,3 C. 2,4 D. 4 Only E. All

19. Obstetric complications carry an increased risk of developing:

1. Diffuse cortical necrosis
2. Adult hemolytic uremic syndrome
3. Acute tubular necrosis
4. Hydronephrosis

   A. 1,2,3 B. 1,3 C. 2,4 D. 4 Only E. All

20. Hematuria is a characteristic clinical feature of:

1. Glomerulonephritis
2. Nephrolithiasis
3. Renal cell carcinoma
4. Bladder papilloma

   A. 1,2,3 B. 1,3 C. 2,4 D. 4 Only E. All

21. Transitional cell carcinoma of the bladder is associated with:

1. Exposure to azo dyes
2. *Schistosoma haematobium* infection
3. Cigarette smoking
4. Von Hippel–Lindau disease

   A. 1,2,3 B. 1,3 C. 2,4 D. 4 Only E. All

DIRECTIONS: For Questions 22 to 26, you are to decide whether EACH choice is TRUE or FALSE.

For each of the following statements about acute tubular necrosis (ATN), choose whether it is TRUE or FALSE.

22. Ischemic ATN commonly occurs after massive hemorrhage

23. Nephrotoxic ATN is associated with thiazide diuretics

24. In toxic ATN, distal tubules are most severely damaged

25. Measurement of Tamm-Horsfall protein in the urine aids in the diagnosis of ischemic ATN

26. Recovery depends upon the compensatory hypertrophy of tubules that have escaped injury

DIRECTIONS: For Questions 27 to 33 the set of lettered headings is followed by a list of numbered words or phrases. For each numbered word or phrase choose:

    A—if the item is associated with (A) only
    B—if the item is associated with (B) only
    C—if the item is associated with *both* (A) and (B)
    D—if the item is associated with *neither* (A) nor (B)

For each of the conditions associated with kidney disease listed below, choose whether it is a cause of rapidly progressive glomerulonephritis, the nephrotic syndrome, both, or neither.

A. Rapidly progressive glomerulonephritis (RPGN)
B. Nephrotic syndrome
C. Both
D. Neither

27. Streptococcal infection
28. Henoch-Schönlein purpura
29. Penicillamine therapy
30. Synthetic penicillin (e.g., methicillin) therapy
31. Wegener's granulomatosis
32. Goodpasture's syndrome
33. Systemic lupus erythematosus (SLE)

DIRECTIONS: Questions 34 to 50 are matching questions. For each numbered item, choose the most likely associated lettered item from those provided. Each numbered item has ONLY ONE answer. Within each group, each lettered item may be the answer to one, more than one, or none of the numbered items.

For each of the following statements about cystic disease of the kidney, choose whether it describes childhood polycystic disease, adult polycystic disease, medullary sponge kidney, all of these, or none of these.

    A. Childhood polycystic disease
    B. Adult polycystic disease
    C. Medullary sponge kidney
    D. All of these
    E. None of these

34. The disease is inherited as an autosomal dominant trait
35. Renal function is usually normal
36. Berry aneurysms are associated anomalies
37. Cysts arising from collecting ducts are present in the medulla
38. Cysts arising from proximal tubules are present in the cortex

For each of the characteristics of primary glomerular disease listed below, choose whether it describes lipoid nephrosis, membranous glomerulonephritis, membranoproliferative glomerulonephritis, IgA nephropathy, or none of these.

    A. Lipoid nephrosis
    B. Membranous glomerulonephritis
    C. Membranoproliferative glomerulonephritis (MPGN)
    D. IgA nephropathy
    E. None of these

39. The most common cause of the nephrotic syndrome in children
40. The most common cause of the nephrotic syndrome in adults
41. Normal-appearing glomeruli by light microscopy
42. Basement membrane splitting in glomeruli by light microscopy
43. Cellular "crescents" in glomeruli by light microscopy
44. Subendothelial electron-dense deposits in glomeruli
45. Mesangial electron-dense deposits in glomeruli
46. Association with malignant epithelial tumors
47. Association with prophylactic immunizations
48. Association with thyroiditis
49. Association with primary activation of the alternate complement pathway
50. Very good long-range prognosis

10

THE KIDNEY AND URINARY TRACT

ANSWERS

1. (E) The glomerular basement membrane is the structure that is primarily responsible for the molecular size–dependent permeability barrier in the glomerulus. Its normal biochemical components include fibronectin, heparan sulfate (the most important of the polyanionic proteoglycans responsible for the charge-glomerular filtration barrier), laminin, and type IV collagen, which gives structural support to the capillary wall. Fibrin is *not* a normal component of the glomerular basement membrane; its presence would indicate a pathologic alteration of glomerular permeability such as occurs in glomerulonephritis (*pp. 993, 1006*).

2. (A) Chronic renal disease of any etiology manifests the same major physiologic consequences and clinical abnormalities. Hyperaldosteronism is produced as a consequence of increased renin production and compounds the problem of salt and water retention that results from impaired glomerular filtration. Phosphate begins to be retained as soon as the glomerular filtration rate drops below 25% of normal and overt uremia develops. Increased serum phosphate leads to increased entry of calcium into bone and a *fall* in serum calcium levels. The failing kidney further contributes to hypocalcemia by its inability to synthesize 1,25-dihydroxyvitamin D_3, the active metabolite of vitamin D, which stimulates calcium absorption from the gut (see Chapter 3, Question 4). Hypocalcemia, in turn, stimulates the production of parathormone by the parathyroid glands, producing secondary hyperparathyroidism and renal osteodystrophy (*pp. 996–997*).

3. (C) Uremia is a clinical syndrome of metabolic and endocrine abnormalities resulting from chronic renal failure. Although the severity of the clinical manifestations of uremia correlates roughly with blood urea nitrogen levels, the primary etiologic agent in uremia is as yet unknown. It does not appear to be urea alone, however. Uremia causes neurologic abnormalities, including peripheral neuropathy, myopathy, and encephalopathy. In the gastrointestinal tract, gastritis, esophagitis, and colitis are the major abnormalities. Cardiopulmonary abnormalities commonly include uremic pericarditis and less commonly diffuse alveolar damage with hyaline membrane formation known as uremic pneumonitis. Although uremia is associated with an increase in one major endocrine function of the kidney—renin production—the second major endocrine function—erythropoietin production—is diminished. Thus, anemia (not polycythemia) is the major hematopoietic manifestation of uremia (*pp. 996–997*).

4. (B) Nephritis caused by trapping of circulating antigen-antibody complexes within glomeruli is known to occur in a variety of diseases. Those in which the antibody is formed against exogenous antigens of microbial origin include bacterial endocarditis and hepatitis B antigenemia. Diseases characterized by the production of antibodies against endogenous substances include systemic lupus erythematosus and lung cancer; the antigenic components of the circulating immune complexes are DNA and tumor-specific or tumor-associated antigen, respectively. The glomerular injury produced in Goodpasture's syndrome is not the result of circulating immune complexes. Rather, antibodies against intrinsic components of the glomerular basement membrane form immune complexes *in situ* as the antibodies are filtered through the glomerulus (*pp. 1004–1005*).

5. (D) Diabetes mellitus is the systemic disease that produces the widest variety of renal lesions. The spectrum of diabetic nephropathy includes glomerular, vascular, and tubulointerstitial disease. Diabetic glomerulosclerosis may be either diffuse or nodular, the latter known as the Kimmelstiel-Wilson syndrome. The accelerated atherosclerosis associated with diabetes is often more pronounced in the kidney than in other organs. Acute pyelonephritis also occurs more frequently in diabetics than nondiabetics and may be associated with papillary necrosis (see Question 12), a consequence of the coincidence of acute bacterial infection and impaired papillary circulation. Acute tubular necrosis, however, is produced either by direct toxic or *acute* ischemic damage to the tubules and is not associated with diabetes mellitus (*pp. 1022–1025*).

6. (A) The photomicrograph illustrates the typical "clear cell" appearance of renal cell carcinoma, the most common renal cancer in adults. It is known as one of the great "mimics" in medicine, since it is capable of manufacturing a wide variety of hormones that produce a number of diverse systemic syndromes. For example, Cushing's syndrome may result from the secretion of glucocorticosteroids by the tumor. Polycythemia may result from the production of erythropoietin. Secretion of a parathyroid-like hormone leads to hypercalcemia. Femininization or masculinization may occur if gonadotropins are elaborated by the tumor. Although renal cell carcinomas are known to contain a large amount of lipid, giving them a clear cell appearance on histologic section, they do not secrete lipid and are not associated with hyperlipidemia (*pp. 1055–1056*).

7. (A) Although stones may be formed at any level in the urinary tract, most originate in the kidney. The majority of urinary stones (75% to 85%) are composed of calcium salts and occur in association with conditions producing hypercalcemia and/or hypercalciuria such as hyperparathyroidism. Conditions that increase serum urate levels, such as leukemia (especially chemotherapeutically treated) with its rapid cell turnover or gout predispose to the formation of urate stones. Infections by urea-splitting bacteria such as Proteus, which convert urea to ammonia and create an alkaline urine, predispose to precipitation of magnesium ammonium phosphate salts in the urine; the result is the formation of some of the largest urinary stones (most staghorn calculi). Analgesic abuse nephropathy (see Question 14) produces an acquired distal renal tubular acidosis and diminished citrate secretion, which predispose to the development of renal stones. Hypokalemic nephropathy characteristically causes vacuolization of renal tubules and impaired renal concentrating ability with polyuria and nocturia but, unlike the above disorders, does not predispose to stone formation (*pp. 1037–1039, 1052–1053*).

8. (E) Bacterial infection with acute inflammation of the renal pelvis, tubules, and interstitium is known as acute pyelonephritis. It is usually acquired by ascending infection of the urinary tract and is associated with specific predisposing conditions. Urinary tract obstruction such as that occurring in pregnancy or prostatism predisposes to ascending bacterial infection. Instrumentation of the urinary tract, most commonly catheterization of the bladder, predisposes to acute pyelonephritis in the absence of obstruction or preexisting renal lesions. Septicemia alone, however, does not predispose to acute pyelonephritis since the kidney is remarkably resistant to bloodborne infection. Hematogenous infection of the kidney is far more likely to occur in the presence of urinary tract obstruction or previous renal injury (*pp. 1030–1035*).

9. (A) In addition to forming a branching cellular framework that supports the glomerular capillary tufts, mesangial cells have other important functions. They ingest macromolecules that have leaked across the glomerulus. They are also contractile and may thereby serve to regulate intraglomerular blood flow. They are connected with the Lacis cells of the juxtaglomerular apparatus, the organelle that senses changes in afferent arteriolar pressure and is the principal source of renin production. Although mesangial cells contract in response to neurohormonal agents, they are not innervated by fibers from the autonomic nervous system. Nerve endings are present in the smooth muscle of the vascular tree near the tubules, but the glomeruli are not innervated (*pp. 993–994*).

10. (B) Most glomerulonephritis is caused by antibody-mediated mechanisms of damage. Once immune complexes, either circulating and passively trapped or formed *in situ*, are localized in the glomerulus, glomerular injury is produced by a number of secondary phenomena. Activation of the complement pathway produces neutrophil chemotactic agents. Neutrophils in turn release proteases and other enzymes that cause cellular and basement membrane damage. Macrophages and monocytes also infiltrate the glomerulus and release a large number of biologically active molecules, which contribute to glomerular damage. There is no evidence, however, that cytotoxic T cells produce glomerular injury. Although loss of glomerular polyanion is an important form of glomerular injury, it principally occurs in glomerular disorders that are not immunologically mediated, such as congenital nephrosis, diabetic nephropathy, and lipoid nephrosis (*pp. 1006–1007*).

11. (C) Systemic lupus erythematosus (SLE) gives rise to a number of forms of glomerular injury, including renal lesions that are indistinguishable from idiopathic membranous glomerulonephritis (diffuse membranous GN of SLE) or membranoproliferative glomerulonephritis (diffuse proliferative GN of SLE). Other patterns include typical crescentic GN (see Question 27) and focal proliferative GN, but lesions morphologically identical to focal sclerosis or lipoid nephrosis are not produced by SLE (*pp. 1009, 1012–1016, 1021–1022*).

12. (C) Renal papillary necrosis (necrotizing papillitis) is a distinctive, dramatic form of tubulointerstitial disease resulting in necrosis and sloughing of renal papilli. It occurs only in well-defined sets of circumstances. Most notably, it occurs in the absence of infection in analgesic abuse nephropathy and sickle cell anemia. In these conditions, the necrosis is a direct result of toxic or anoxic damage, respectively. Although papillary necrosis may occur with urinary tract obstruction or diabetes mellitus, it is rarely produced in the absence of superimposed infection in these conditions (*pp. 1032–1033, 1037, 1050*).

13. (D) Chronic pyelonephritis (CPN) refers to irreversible renal injury caused by chronic bacterial infection superimposed on vesicoureteral reflux or urinary obstruction. Renal scarring is the result. CPN characteristically causes asymmetrical, irregular renal scarring in contrast to the symmetrically scarred kidneys of chronic glomerular disease. Although an important cause of end-stage kidney disease, CPN accounts for at most 20% of cases of renal failure. The great majority of renal failure is caused by chronic glomerulonephritis. Although the diagnosis is best made from gross examination of the kidneys, typical microscopic changes include patchy tubular atrophy and dilatation with interstitial inflammation and fibrosis. Dilated tubules may be filled with colloid casts and resemble thyroid follicles; thus, the pattern is referred to as "tubular thyroidization" (pp. 1034–1035).

14. (B) Analgesic abuse nephropathy is a form of chronic tubulointerstitial nephritis, with renal papillary necrosis caused by excessive intake of analgesic mixtures that include phenacetin. Although mixtures of aspirin and phenacetin readily induce papillary necrosis, aspirin alone does not produce this lesion. The minimum requirements for the development of renal damage range between 2 and 3 kilograms of a phenacetin-containing analgesic over a period of 3 years. Although often sterile, pyuria is an early clinical manifestation and occurs in virtually every patient. If the drug abuse is continued, renal failure often ensues. If discontinued, renal failure may be averted, but transitional papillary carcinoma of the renal pelvis has been found to occur with increased frequency in long-term survivors of this disorder. Increased risk of development of renal cell carcinoma, however, has not been noted (pp. 1037–1038).

15. (D) In addition to its central role in the regulation of fluids and electrolytes that maintain extracellular fluid and blood volume, the kidney further participates in the control of blood pressure by secretion of some substances that have a pressor effect and others that lower blood pressure. Secretion of renin in response to decreased pressure in afferent arterioles, decreased sodium or chloride load delivered to the macula densa, or adrenergic stimulation is the major renal mechanism for increasing blood pressure. Renin raises blood pressure in two ways: (1) It catalyzes the first step in the enzymatic conversion of angiotensinogen to angiotensin II, a potent vasoconstrictor; and (2) it stimulates aldosterone secretion by the adrenal cortex, thereby producing sodium retention. Neutral lipid factor, kininogen, and prostacyclin are all anti-hypertensive agents secreted by the kidney (pp. 1042–1043).

16. (B) Essential hypertension by definition occurs in the absence of any condition known to produce increases in systemic blood pressure. Thus, hypertension occurring in association with pheochromocy-

toma or oral contraceptive use would be considered a secondary form. It seems clear, however, that essential hypertension has both genetic and environmental contributory factors. In those with the genetic predisposition, a high sodium intake contributes to the generation of hypertension (p. 1044).

17. (A) Malignant nephrosclerosis refers to disease produced in the kidney by accelerated hypertension. Characteristic histologic alterations are produced that include fibrinoid necrosis of arterioles (necrotizing arteriolitis), intimal proliferation in larger interlobular arteries (hyperplastic arteriolitis), and glomerular thrombosis and necrosis (necrotizing glomerulitis). Fibromuscular dysplasia of the renal artery is a cause of nephrogenic hypertension rather than an effect of accelerated systemic hypertension. It refers to a heterogeneous group of lesions of unknown etiology characterized by fibrous or fibromuscular thickening of the artery producing renal artery stenosis (see Question 18) (pp. 1046–1047).

18. (A) Although its occurrence is relatively uncommon, renal artery stenosis is the most common curable form of hypertension. It is most frequently caused by an atheromatous plaque at the origin of the renal artery. The resultant reduction in blood flow to the kidney stimulates the renin-angiotensin system, which in turn elevates blood pressure. It has been shown that increased renin activity in blood obtained from the renal vein on the stenotic side and a fallen blood pressure in response to the administration of angiotensin antagonists favor a good outcome after surgical correction. About 75% of patients with atherosclerotic renal artery stenosis are cured after removal of the kidney on the nonstenotic side and surgical correction of the stenosis. The kidney on the stenotic side is protected from the arteriolosclerotic effects of hypertension, which takes its toll on the contralateral kidney (pp. 1047–1048).

19. (A) Obstetric complications are associated with a number of renal disorders, including diffuse cortical necrosis and acute tubular necrosis, both believed to be ischemic in nature, and the adult hemolytic uremic syndrome. The latter is a disorder characterized by widespread thrombosis in interlobular arteries, afferent arterioles, and glomeruli with patchy or widespread renal cortical necrosis and a microangiopathic hemolytic anemia. Hydronephrosis—dilatation of the renal pelvis and calyces due to obstruction to the outflow of urine, is a complication of normal pregnancy rather than an obstetric complication (pp. 1027, 1049–1051).

20. (E) Hematuria is an important but nonspecific indicator of renal disease. It occurs in a large number of renal disorders, including glomerulonephritis, nephrolithiasis, or urinary tract tumors (benign or malignant), to name only a few. Although red blood cells in the urine may originate from anywhere in the urinary tract, red blood cell casts formed in the renal tubules are indicative of glomerular disease and are useful in the differential diagnosis of hematuria (*pp. 1007, 1053, 1055, 1070*).

21. (B) Transitional cell carcinoma of the bladder constitutes about 90% of bladder cancer; 5% are squamous cell carcinomas, and 5% are mixed. Transitional cell carcinoma of the bladder has been shown to be related to a number of environmental carcinogenic agents. It has been clearly established that azo dyes contain a number of chemical compounds that dramatically increase the incidence of bladder cancer in exposed individuals. Tobacco smoking has also been identified as a potential factor contributing to bladder carcinogenesis, along with other substances such as food preservatives, artificial sweeteners, and alcohol. *Schistosoma haematobium* infection has long been known to increase the risk of bladder cancer. However, the vast majority of schistosoma-induced cancers are squamous cell carcinomas rather than transitional cell carcinomas. Von Hippel–Lindau disease is associated with dramatically increased risk of developing renal cell carcinoma, often bilaterally, but is not associated with an increased risk of bladder cancer (*pp. 139, 1055, 1071–1072*).

22. (False); 23. (False); 24. (False); 25. (False); 26. (False)

Acute tubular necrosis (ATN) is a syndrome of renal tubular damage on a toxic or ischemic basis producing acute renal failure. It is particularly important because it represents a reversible cause of acute renal failure. **(22)** Ischemic ATN occurs most commonly after an episode of shock produced by severe bacterial infections, large cutaneous burns, massive crush injuries, or any acute event complicated by peripheral circulatory insufficiency. It is of note, however, that ATN rarely occurs when the shock is due to massive hemorrhage alone. Therefore, it seldom complicates arterial rupture or laceration.

(23) Nephrotoxic ATN is caused by a wide variety of agents, including heavy metals, organic solvents, antibiotics, anesthetics, and other chemicals. Thiazide diuretics are not included in the list of drugs known to cause ATN; instead, they are associated with acute drug-induced (hypersensitivity) interstitial nephritis. **(24)** Histologically, toxic ATN can be differentiated from the ischemic pattern by its characteristic involvement of the proximal tubules, generally sparing the distal tubular segments of the nephron. Ischemic ATN, in contrast, is characterized by focal tubular necrosis at multiple points along the entire nephron. **(25)** Tamm-Horsfall protein is a specific urinary glycoprotein normally secreted by the cells of the thick ascending and distal tubules. This protein is the major constituent of the hyaline intratubular casts typically seen in ATN. It does not, however, constitute a useful clinically diagnostic feature in this process. **(26)** Recovery from ATN occurs with *regeneration* of injured tubules, since tubular cells have the capacity to divide. Tubular regeneration is compatible with full recovery from this disorder (*pp. 1027–1029, 1036*).

27. (A); 28. (C); 29. (B); 30. (D); 31. (A); 32. (A);33. (C)

Rapidly progressive glomerulonephritis (RPGN) is a syndrome of glomerular damage characterized clinically by hematuria with a rapid and progressive decline in renal function and pathologically by a marked accumulation of cells in Bowman's space, forming "crescents." The nephrotic syndrome is characterized clinically by massive proteinuria, hypoalbuminemia, edema, and hyperlipidemia, but the glomerular pathology is variable.

(27) Immunologically mediated glomerular damage occurring in association with nephritogenic stepto-coccal infection typically takes the form of an acute nephritis rather than the nephrotic syndrome. In a small proportion of patients with poststreptococcal glomerulonephritis, however, rapid renal failure develops, and the classic clinical and pathologic features of RPGN are seen.

(28 and 33) Henoch-Schönlein purpura and systemic lupus erythematosus are two noteworthy examples of systemic diseases that may produce either a nephritic or nephrotic syndrome and are well-known causes of rapidly progressive glomerulonephritis. Henoch-Schönlein purpura is a syndrome of immune complex–induced necrotizing vasculitis principally involving the skin, the GI tract, the joints, and the kidney. The renal disease is quite variable, ranging from mesangial proliferation with the nephrotic syndrome to typical crescentic glomerulonephritis. Systemic lupus erythematosus is even more variable in its renal manifestations, which range from normal renal function with minimal proteinuria and hematuria to an overt nephrotic syndrome or RPGN with corresponding differences in the associated histologic lesions.

(29) Penicillamine is one of several drugs including gold and "street heroin" that are known to cause glomerular damage productive of the nephrotic syndrome. **(30)** Synthetic penicillin (e.g., methicillin), on the other hand, is one of a long list of drugs that are more apt to cause tubular damage or interstitial inflammation. Methicillin is a well-known cause of both nephrotoxic acute tubular necrosis and acute drug-induced "hypersensitivity" interstitial nephritis but is not associated with glomerular disease.

(31 and 32) Both Wegener's granulomatosis, a syndrome of necrotizing vasculitis, and Goodpasture's syndrome, a disease produced by autoantibodies directed against basement membranes, typically in volve both the lung and kidney as their primary targets of injury. They are both well-known causes of crescentic glomerulonephritis (RPGN), which can be differentiated only on the basis of their immunofluorescent and electron microscopic characteristics. The antiglomerular basement membrane antibodies of Goodpasture's syndrome produce a diagnostic pattern of linear immunofluorescence and uniform basement membrane thickening not seen in Wegener's granulomatosis (*pp. 523, 527–528, 1007–1012, 1022, 1028, 1030, 1036*).

34. (B); 35. (C); 36. (B); 37. (D); 38. (B)

Diseases that produce cystic changes in the kidneys vary widely in their etiologies and clinical consequences. (34, 36, 37, 38) Adult polycystic disease is an inherited autosomal dominant disorder in which cysts arise from tubules throughout the nephron. Thus, in contrast to childhood polycystic disease and medullary sponge kidney in which cysts develop only from collecting tubules, adult polycystic disease produces proximal and distal tubular cysts in addition to those of collecting tubule origin. Although a third of the patients with this disease die with chronic renal failure, as many as 10% succumb to the rupture of a berry aneurysm, an associated congenital anomaly present in one sixth of patients.

(35) In contrast to the adult and childhood polycystic diseases, which produce profound abnormalities in renal function and ultimately lead to renal failure, medullary sponge kidney rarely causes any abnormality in renal function and is usually discovered incidentally or in relation to secondary complications such as infection or stone formation (*pp. 1000–1001*).

39. (A); 40. (B); 41. (A); 42. (C); 43. (E); 44. (C); 45. (D); 46. (B); 47. (A); 48. (B); 49. (C); 50. (A)

The majority of the primary forms of glomerular disease produce the nephrotic syndrome and are differentiated on the basis of their clinical manifestations and morphologic patterns of injury. (39, 41, 47, 50) Lipoid nephrosis (minimal change disease) is the most common cause of the nephrotic syndrome in children. Clinically, it is associated with prophylactic immunizations and respiratory infections, sug-

gesting an immunologic basis for the disease. However, affected glomeruli do not contain immunoglobulins or complement and appear normal by light microscopy. The only morphologic lesion is the fusion of glomerular epithelial cell foot processes, a nonspecific change also present in other proteinuric disorders. In contrast to the other forms of idiopathic glomerular diseases, which frequently go on to chronic glomerulonephritis and renal failure, lipoid nephrosis is responsive to steroid therapy and has an excellent long-term prognosis.

(40, 46, 48) Membranous glomerulonephritis (GN) is the most common cause of the nephrotic syndrome in adults. It is associated with certain malignant epithelial tumors (particularly carcinoma of the lung) and metabolic disorders such as thyroiditis. Immune complexes formed from tumor- or thyroid-derived antigens respectively localize in the glomerulus in the form of subepithelial electron-dense deposits, a characteristic ultrastructural feature of membranous GN.

(42, 44, 49) Membranoproliferative glomerulonephritis accounts for 5% to 10% of cases of idiopathic nephrotic syndrome in children and adults. It is characterized morphologically by basement membrane "splitting," the result of protrusion of mesangial cell processes into the basement membrane of the capillary loops (mesangial interposition). In two thirds of cases, subendothelial electron-dense deposits are seen by electron microscopy (Type I) MPGN). A second variant of MPGN is characterized by the deposition of electron-dense material in the lamina densa of the glomerular basement (Type II MPGN or dense-deposit disease). Most patients with Type II MPGN have abnormalities that suggest primary activation of the alternate complement pathway; neither C1q nor C4 is present in the glomeruli.

(45) IgA nephropathy, or Berger's disease, a recently recognized cause of proteinuria and the nephrotic syndrome, is characterized by the presence of prominent IgA deposits in the mesangial regions of affected glomeruli. (43) Although a rare patient with IgA nephropathy may present with rapidly progressive crescentic glomerulonephritis, none of these idiopathic forms of glomerulonephritis typically produce crescentic GN (*pp. 1012–1015*).

11

THE REPRODUCTIVE SYSTEM

DIRECTIONS: For Questions 1 to 7, choose the ONE BEST answer to each question.

1. In gonococcal pelvic inflammatory disease, which part of the female genital tract is most likely to be spared from infection?

   A. Vulva
   B. Endocervix
   C. Endometrium
   D. Fallopian tubes
   E. Ovaries

2. Which of the following lesions of the female genital tract is considered precancerous?

   A. Condyloma acuminatum
   B. Endocervical polyp
   C. Microglandular endocervical hyperplasia
   D. Endometrial polyp
   E. Endometrial adenomatous hyperplasia

3. Leiomyomas:

   A. Usually occur singly
   B. Are well encapsulated
   C. Require progesterone for growth
   D. Usually grow rapidly during pregnancy
   E. Give rise to most leiomyosarcomas of the uterus

4. Which of the following factors is NOT associated with an increased risk of developing endometrial carcinoma?

   A. Diabetes mellitus
   B. Infertility
   C. Oral contraceptive steroid use

   D. Hypertension
   E. Obesity

5. Factors that predispose to the development of ectopic pregnancy include all of the following EXCEPT:

   A. Previous appendicitis
   B. Endometriosis
   C. Intrauterine contraceptive devices
   D. Gonorrheal salpingitis
   E. Fetal chromosomal abnormalities

6. Seminoma and dysgerminoma share all of the following features EXCEPT:

   A. Origin from primordial germ cells
   B. Peak incidence in the fourth decade
   C. Lack of endocrine function
   D. Lymphocytic infiltration of the tumor stroma
   E. High degree of radiosensitivity

7. Which of the following statements about benign prostatic hypertrophy is INCORRECT?

   A. It originates in the periurethral portion of the prostate
   B. Hyperplasia of both glands and stroma is seen histologically
   C. It occurs in over 95% of males over 70 years of age
   D. Less than 10% of those with this condition require surgical treatment for symptoms
   E. It increases the risk of developing prostatic adenocarcinoma

DIRECTIONS: For Questions 8 to 13, ONE or MORE of the completions given correctly finishes the incomplete statement. Choose:

A—if only *1,2 and 3* are correct
B—if only *1 and 3* are correct
C—if only *2 and 4* are correct
D—if only *4* is correct
E—if all are correct

8. Risk factors for cervical carcinoma include:

   1. Low socioeconomic status
   2. Use of oral contraceptive steroids
   3. Large number of sexual partners
   4. Postmenopausal estrogen rise

   A. 1,2,3   B. 1,3   C. 2,4   D. 4 Only   E. All

9. Invasive cervical carcinoma:

   1. Originates from cervical dysplasia in the majority of cases
   2. Is on the decline as a cause of cancer death
   3. Is decreasing in incidence among young women
   4. Is the end result of the majority of cervical dysplasias

   A. 1,2,3   B. 1,3   C. 2,4   D. 4 Only   E. All

10. Causes of dysfunctional uterine bleeding include:

    1. Inadequate luteal phase
    2. Irregular shedding syndrome
    3. Anovulatory cycle
    4. Endometrial hyperplasia

    A. 1,2,3   B. 1,3   C. 2,4   D. 4 Only   E. All

11. Factors that contribute to the etiology of hypertension in toxemia of pregnancy include:

    1. Release of placental tissue thromboplastin
    2. Decreased placental prostaglandin production
    3. Increased maternal catecholamine production
    4. Increased placental renin production

    A. 1,2,3   B. 1,3   C. 2,4   D. 4 Only   E. All

12. Circumcision protects against:

    1. Balanoposthitis
    2. Erythroplasia of Queyrat
    3. Penile carcinoma
    4. Bowenoid papulosis

    A. 1,2,3   B. 1,3   C. 2,4   D. 4 Only   E. All

13. Which of the following conditions is/are associated with an increased risk of testicular cancer?

    1. Testicular irradiation
    2. Testicular dysgenesis
    3. Semen outflow obstruction
    4. Cryptorchidism

    A. 1,2,3   B. 1,3   C. 2,4   D. 4 Only   E. All

DIRECTIONS: For Questions 14 to 34, you are to decide whether EACH choice is TRUE or FALSE.

For each of the following statements about the normal menstrual cycle, choose whether it is TRUE or FALSE.

14. The basal third of the endometrium does not respond to ovarian steroids
15. The endometrium in the lower uterine segment does not respond to ovarian steroids
16. Following ovulation, endometrial glands contain numerous mitotic figures
17. Following ovulation, estrogen levels rise to their highest peak
18. The length of the postovulatory phase of the menstrual cycle is the same in all women

For each of the following statements about herpes simplex virus type 2 (HSV2) infection, choose whether it is TRUE or FALSE.

19. It is the most common cause of sexually transmitted disease in the United States
20. Following exposure, lesions usually appear after a symptom-free interval of about a month
21. Relapsing infection often leads to infertility
22. Relapse of latent infection is usually prevented by acyclovir
23. Herpetic cervicitis is associated with an increased risk of cervical carcinoma

For each of the following statements about gestational trophoblastic neoplasms, choose whether it is TRUE or FALSE.

24. Hydatidiform moles are usually accompanied by a developing fetus
25. Most hydatidiform moles have a normal female karyotype
26. The entire chromosome complement of most hydatidiform moles comes from the sperm
27. Moles are the most common precursors of choriocarcinoma
28. Moles are usually associated with higher serum levels of gonadotropin than choriocarcinomas
29. Chemotherapy is curative in most cases of gestational choriocarcinoma

For each of the following statements about prostate cancer, choose whether it is TRUE or FALSE.

30. About 30% of men over age 50 have a stage A prostate cancer
31. Prognosis correlates well with the histologic grade of the tumor
32. Most tumors originate from the periurethral region of the gland
33. Serum chemistry for acid phosphatase is a useful screening tool for localized disease
34. Osteoblastic bone lesions in men with prostatic cancer are virtually diagnostic of metastatic disease

DIRECTIONS: For Questions 35 to 52, the set of lettered headings is followed by a list of numbered words or phrases. For each numbered word or phrase choose:

A—if the item is associated with (A) only
B—if the item is associated with (B) only
C—if the item is associated with *both* (A) and (B)
D—if the item is associated with *neither* (A) nor (B)

For each of the features listed below, choose whether it describes adenomyosis, endometriosis, both, or neither.

A. Adenomyosis
B. Endometriosis
C. Both
D. Neither

35. Characterized by endometrial tissue in an abnormal location
36. Almost never occurs in women over age 50
37. Often produces dysmenorrhea
38. Often results in infertility
39. Caused by increased estrogen exposure

For each of the characteristics listed below, choose whether it describes serous ovarian tumors, mucinous ovarian tumors, both, or neither.

A. Serous tumors of the ovary
B. Mucinous tumors of the ovary
C. Both
D. Neither

40. The incidence is higher in black than in white women
41. Oral contraceptive steroid use is a predisposing factor
42. The majority of tumors exhibit cystic growth

43. The benign variant occurs much more frequently than the malignant variant
44. The majority of tumors are bilateral
45. Endometrial carcinoma occurs simultaneously in 15 to 30% of cases
46. Malignant variants tend to spread by direct seeding throughout the peritoneal cavity
47. Psammoma bodies are a common histologic feature
48. Serum alpha-fetoprotein levels provide a useful clinical tumor marker

For each of the characteristics of gonadal stromal tumors listed below, choose whether it describes granulosa cell tumors, Leydig cell tumors, both, or neither.

A. Granulosa cell tumors
B. Leydig cell tumors
C. Both
D. Neither

49. Usually causes virilization in women
50. Greatly predisposes to endometrial carcinoma in women
51. Characterized histologically by cytoplasmic crystalloids of Reinke
52. Seldom exhibits malignant biologic behavior

DIRECTIONS: Questions 53 to 62 are matching questions. For each numbered item, choose the most likely associated lettered item from those provided. Each numbered item has ONLY ONE answer. Within each group, each lettered item may be the answer to one, more than one, or none of the numbered items.

For each of the descriptions below, decide whether it refers to a Gartner's duct cyst, a Nabothian cyst, a Bartholin's cyst, a hydatid cyst of Morgagni, or none of these.

A. Gartner's duct cyst
B. Nabothian cyst
C. Bartholin's cyst
D. Hydatid cyst of Morgagni
E. None of these

53. Inflamed vulvovaginal gland with blocked duct
54. Mesonephric duct remnant of the vagina
55. Inflamed endocervical gland with a blocked duct
56. Endometriosis of the ovary
57. Wolffian duct remnant of the fallopian tube

For each of the characteristics of germ cell tumors listed below, choose whether it describes teratoma, choriocarcinoma, embryonal carcinoma, yolk sac tumor, or none of these.

A. Teratoma
B. Choriocarcinoma
C. Embryonal carcinoma
D. Yolk sac tumor
E. None of these

58. Most common malignant germ cell tumor in men
59. Most common benign germ cell tumor in women
60. Struma ovarii is a specialized variant
61. Produces only alpha-fetoprotein
62. Produces only human chorionic gonadotropin

11

THE REPRODUCTIVE SYSTEM

ANSWERS

1. (C) Gonococcal inflammation usually begins within the glands of the vulvar mucosa and spreads upward over the mucosal surfaces of the female genital tract to involve the tubes and the tubo-ovarian region. Often, however, the endometrium is remarkably spared. The reason for this relative resistance of the endometrium to gonococcal infection is still obscure (*p. 1114*).

2. (E) Endometrial hyperplasia, excessive proliferation of endometrial glands and stroma, is caused by high and prolonged levels of estrogenic stimulation, with diminished or absent progesterone production. Although it may occur as a result of adrenal or ovarian pathology, it is commonly the result of iatrogenic administration of estrogenic substances. In its mildest form, endometrial hyperplasia is not associated with an increased risk of endometrial carcinoma. However, in its more severe form, known as adenomatous hyperplasia, particularly when accompanied by atypia, the disorder is considered precancerous. In one study of untreated endometrial hyperplasia, it has been demonstrated that nearly 60% of women with atypical adenomatous hyperplasia progressed to endometrial carcinoma within 2 to 18 years. The greater the degree of atypia, the greater the risk appears to be.

Condyloma acuminatum is a venereal wart produced by the human papilloma virus. Since condylomata are diploid or polyploid (rather than aneuploid like precancerous cells), they are not believed to be precancerous lesions. Although condylomata may coexist with areas of cervical dysplasia or carcinoma *in situ*, their biologic relationship to these lesions is as yet unclear. Endocervical polyps are completely benign lesions consisting of hypertrophied endocervical glands in a loose fibromyomatous stroma cured by simple curettage. Microglandular endocervical hyperplasia is a benign cervical lesion seen in women ingesting progesterone-containing oral contraceptive agents. Its importance lies in its possible histologic confusion with endocervical adenocarcinoma, to which it is biologically unrelated.

Endometrial polyps are benign lesions consisting of hyperplastic endometrium, mostly of the mild, cystic variety. Although malignant change in an initially benign endometrial polyp may occur, it is extremely rare. Thus, endometrial polyps are not considered precancerous lesions (*pp. 1116–1117, 1128–1129, 1133–1136*).

3. (D) Leiomyomas are the most common tumors in women, occurring in about 25% of women in active reproductive life. These benign smooth muscle tumors are well circumscribed but not encapsulated. In the great majority of cases, multiple leiomyomas are present. Although the role of hormones in their pathogenesis is controversial, leiomyomas are known to be hormone-dependent tumors that require estrogen for growth. Thus, during pregnancy they tend to increase rapidly in size and tend to atrophy following menopause or castration. Malignant transformation of leiomyomas is extremely rare. The malignant counterpart of this tumor, the leiomyosarcoma, almost always arises directly from the myometrium (*pp. 1136–1137, 1140*).

4. (C) Endometrial carcinoma is rising in incidence and now accounts for close to 10% of all cancer in women. A number of important risk factors for this disease have been defined: diabetes mellitus, infertility, hypertension, and obesity. Overt diabetes mellitus is present in 5 to 11% of patients with endometrial carcinoma and abnormal glucose tolerance in over 60%. Infertility and a clinical history of menstrual irregularities consistent with anovulatory cycles tend to be common among those who develop this disease. Fifty per cent of patients with endometrial carcinoma have hypertension, and 50% weigh more than 180 pounds.

Oral contraceptive steroids do not increase the risk for development of endometrial carcinoma. In the past, an increased risk was reported only with sequential contraceptive regimens consisting of potent estrogens in high dose and weak progestins, but these have since been withdrawn from prescription use (*pp. 1135, 1138*).

5. (E) Ectopic pregnancy refers to implantation of the fetus in any site other than the normal uterine location. It occurs most commonly as a result of acquired abnormalities of the fallopian tubes. Inflammatory conditions (most commonly, chronic salpingitis of gonococcal origin; less commonly, previous appendicitis or endometriosis) produce peritubal fibrous adhesions that interfere with tubal function. Intrauterine contraceptive devices also predispose to ectopic pregnancy; in the event of contraceptive failure in women using IUD's, almost 5% of the pregnancies are ectopic.

In contrast to these maternal abnormalities, fetal

abnormalities do not contribute appreciably to the development of ectopic pregnancy. They are, however, responsible for the majority of spontaneous abortions (*p. 1158*).

6. (B) Seminoma and dysgerminoma are the most common type of malignant germ cell tumors in men and women respectively. Despite their different names, these tumors represent the same biologic type of germ cell tumor—that which presumably arises from primordial germ cells. They are both composed of sheets of uniform, undifferentiated germ cells that are divided into poorly demarcated lobules by lymphocyte-laden, fibrous tissue septa. The tumor cells themselves lack endocrine function. Occasionally, however, syncytiotrophoblastic cells, which produce human chorionic gonadotropin, may occur within the tumor.

In addition to their histologic similarities, seminomas and dysgerminomas share biologic traits as well. They have an excellent prognosis when excised while still localized within the gonad. Furthermore, since they are both highly radiosensitive, neoplasms that extend beyond the gonad can be well controlled or even eradicated by radiation therapy in most cases.

The greatest biologic difference between these tumors is the age group in which they are most likely to occur. On the one hand, 75% of dysgerminomas occur in the second and third decades. On the other hand, seminomas peak in the fourth decade, distinctly later than the peak occurrence of dysgerminoma and somewhat later than the collective peak for other testicular germ cell tumors (*pp. 1092–1093, 1151*).

7. (E) Benign prostatic hypertrophy refers to a process of stromal and glandular hyperplasia that originates from and is most severe within the periurethral portion of the prostate. It is an extremely common disorder in men over the age of 50 and increases in frequency with increasing age. Thus, greater than 95% of men over age 70 develop this condition. However, in the great majority of cases the disorder is clinically insignificant. Only about 5 to 10% of men with this condition require surgical treatment for relief of urinary tract obstruction. Although it was once held that benign prostatic hypertrophy was a precursor to prostatic carcinoma, it is no longer believed that the two conditions are causally related. The coexistence of the two lesions is felt to be a reflection of the ubiquitous occurrence of benign prostatic hypertrophy in older men (*pp. 1101–1103*).

8. (B) A great deal of data defining risk factors of cervical carcinoma has now been collected from clinical and epidemiologic studies. A high incidence (indicative of increased risk) of cervical carcinoma has been noted among those of low socioeconomic status, which is usually associated with early marriage and increased parity. The risk of cervical carcinoma is also increased with large numbers of sexual partners, early age of onset of sexual relations, early age at first pregnancy, and high frequency of coitus.

The use of oral contraceptive steroids or estrogenic supplements after menopause is not associated with increased risk of cervical carcinoma. Use of estrogenic supplements postmenopausally, however, may be associated with an increased risk of endometrial carcinoma through its induction of endometrial hyperplasia, a premalignant lesion (see Question 2) (*pp. 1124, 1138*).

9. (A) The realization that epithelial malignancies could arise from precursor lesions of increasingly disordered epithelial growth and differentiation (dysplasia) came from studies of cervical carcinoma. It is now recognized that cervical carcinoma is the end stage of a continuum of progressive cervical dysplasia in the vast majority of cases. Thus, early diagnosis and treatment of premalignant lesions and *in situ* neoplasms have greatly improved the cure rate for this disease and resulted in a dramatic decline in the death rate from cervical carcinoma, a trend that appears to be continuing.

Although most cervical carcinomas arise from cervical dysplasia, cervical dysplasia does not inevitably progress to carcinoma in all cases. In fact, most cervical dysplasias followed over time remain static, without progression, or may even regress, although this is debatable. Although the likelihood of developing carcinoma increases with dysplasias of increasing severity, less than a third of severe dysplasias appear to go on to carcinoma *in situ*.

The peak incidence of carcinoma *in situ* is in the fourth decade. However, with the sexual revolution, the lesion has been appearing more frequently in younger women. Whereas the overall incidence of invasive cervical carcinoma is declining because of early detection and treatment of precursor lesions, the frequency of cervical carcinoma in young women has recently risen significantly (*pp. 1124–1126*).

10. (A) Dysfunctional uterine bleeding encompasses a group of disorders that produce abnormal uterine bleeding in the absence of an organic lesion in that organ. These disorders are caused by various abnormalities of ovarian function, including anovulatory cycles, inadequate progesterone production by the corpus luteum (inadequate luteal phase), and the irregular shedding syndrome. The latter is caused by a delay in the involution of the corpus luteum and persistent elevation of progesterone levels for a number of days after the onset of menstrual flow. In contrast to dysfunctional uterine bleeding, bleeding due to endometrial hyperplasia is accompanied by an organic lesion of the endometrium, namely a variety of disordered glandular and stromal growth patterns. Other organic lesions that cause abnormal uterine bleeding include leiomyomata, endometrial polyps, adenomyosis, and endometrial carcinoma (*pp. 1132–1133*).

11. (C) Toxemia of pregnancy (preeclampsia) refers to a syndrome of hypertension, proteinuria, and edema that occurs in about 6% of pregnant women. A subset of these patients become seriously ill, developing coma or convulsions, a situation known as eclampsia. Many but not all patients with eclampsia develop disseminated intravascular coagulation (DIC).

The pathogenesis of toxemic hypertension appears to involve abnormalities in the physiologic adaptations of the renin-angiotensin system, which usually occur during pregnancy. The normal pregnant woman develops a resistance to the vasoconstrictive and hypertensive effects of angiotensin through the protective effect of prostaglandin E produced in the uteroplacental vascular bed. In toxemia of pregnancy, the placenta produces less prostaglandin E and more renin than in normal pregnancy, and hypertension is the result. Catecholamines are not known to contribute to the pathogenesis of toxemia.

DIC is a separate and variable feature of toxemia of pregnancy and has a distinct pathogenesis. In contrast to its role in the pathogenesis of hypertension, the placenta contributes to the pathogenesis of DIC by the slow release of thromboplastic substances (*p. 1156*).

12. (A) A number of important diseases of the penis, both inflammatory and neoplastic, occur with much greater frequency in uncircumcised than in circumcised males. By definition, some pathologic conditions such as phimosis occur only in the presence of a foreskin. Others, such as balanoposthitis (bacterial infection of the glans penis and/or prepuce) are encountered predominantly among the uncircumcised. Circumcision also confers protection against penile squamous cell carcinoma. Although fortunately an uncommon disease in the United States, penile carcinoma is far more common among the uncircumcised. Erythroplasia of Queyrat refers to squamous cell carcinoma *in situ* (Bowen's disease) of the glans penis, a disorder seen almost exclusively in uncircumcised men. Progression to an invasive squamous cell carcinoma usually occurs in about 5 to 10% of patients with this disease.

Bowenoid papulosis is a penile lesion that appears clinically as a venereal wart and histologically as a squamous cell carcinoma *in situ* (Bowen's disease). Despite their malignant histologic appearance, these lesions are clinically benign. They are believed to be viral in origin, almost always occur in individuals under the age of 40, and are usually located on the shaft of the penis or on the scrotum. Circumcision is not known to confer protection against this disease (*pp. 1082–1085*).

13. (C) Testicular germ cell tumors occur with greatly increased frequency in certain pathologic conditions of the male genital tract that result in germ cell maldevelopment. Testicular dysgenesis and cryptor-

chidism are the most important disorders in this category. Cryptorchidism increases the risk of developing testicular carcinoma as much as 10- to 40-fold over the normal male population. In this disorder, there is also an increased risk of carcinogenesis in the contralateral, normally positioned testis. Surgical correction does not reduce these risks.

Testicular irradiation and obstruction to the outflow of semen are examples of conditions that, like cryptorchidism, cause testicular atrophy but are not associated with an increased risk of testicular carcinoma (*pp. 1088, 1092*).

14. (True); 15. (True); 16. (False); 17. (False); 18. (True)

The cyclic rise and fall of ovarian hormones normally produces a regular sequence of histologic changes in the endometrium. **(14)** Since the basal third of the endometrium does not respond to ovarian steroids, it remains behind after the menstrual flow and gives rise to the regenerated surface epithelium during the next cycle. **(15)** Not all regions of the endometrium participate in this phenomenon, however. The endometrium in the lower uterine segment, an ill-defined zone located just above the endocervix, is not responsive to ovarian hormones and does not participate in the cyclic changes of the functional endometrium. **(16)** During the *preovulatory*, proliferative phase of the cycle, the regenerating endometrial glands contain numerous mitotic figures. **(17)** Endometrial growth is stimulated by the estrogen production of the enlarging ovarian follicle. Estrogen rises progressively, reaches a peak just prior to ovulation, and then falls. Following ovulation, estrogen levels again rise briefly at the end of the first postovulatory week, but the level is never as high as the preovulatory peak. **(18)** Although the preovulatory phase of the menstrual cycle varies in length from woman to woman or even in the same woman during different cycles, postovulatory events occur according to a fixed physiologic schedule 14 days in length. Thus, glandular secretions, stromal predecidualization, and menstruation all normally occur in a highly predictable fashion and temporal sequence after ovulation (*pp. 1110–1113*).

19. (False); 20. (False); 21. (False); 22. (False); 23. (True)

(19) Although for centuries the leading causes of venereal disease have been spirochetes and bacteria, sexually transmitted viral diseases have been rising dramatically in incidence over the past 10 years and in some areas of the United States have reached epidemic proportions. Herpes simplex virus type II (HSV2) infection, in particular, is at the time of this writing second only to gonorrhea in incidence.

(20) Following exposure, lesions consisting of painful red papules usually appear within 3 to 7 days. The papules progress to vesicles and coalesce to form ulcers. During the latter two stages, the lesions contain numerous viral particles, and a high transmission rate is the rule. (**21**) Unlike gonorrhea, which may produce infertility as one of its most feared complications, HSV2 infection is usually limited to the vulva, vagina, and cervix and does not compromise reproductive function.

(**22**) Unfortunately, there is no known cure or prevention for HSV2 infection. Topical or intravenous treatment with the new antiviral agent acyclovir shortens the duration of viral shedding and accelerates healing of lesions but does not prevent relapse of latent infection. (**23**) Perhaps even more important than the problem of relapse of latent HSV2 infection is the association of cervical cancer or dysplasia with viral infection of the genital tract. Currently, two classes of viruses are suspected to play a role in the causation of cervical cancer: HSV2 and the human papilloma virus (HPV). At the moment, the data linking viral infection to the pathogenesis of cervical cancer are inconclusive. It is observed, however, that women with herpes infection have a much higher incidence of cervical dysplasia or cancer (23% in one study) compared with those without this infection (2.6%). It has been estimated that herpetic cervicitis increases the risk of cervical cancer by as much as 4- to 16-fold. Cervical tumor cells have been shown to express herpes virus messenger RNA and a variety of other viral proteins. Viral DNA sequences corresponding to about 40% of the genome have been found in cervical cancer. Whether these represent epiphenonema or a cause and effect relationship between viral infection and neoplasia remains to be proven (*pp. 284, 1114, 1124–1125*).

24. (False); 25. (True); 26. (True); 27. (True); 28. (False); 29. (True)

Gestational trophoblastic neoplasms encompass a spectrum of tumors of varying malignant potential that originate from trophoblastic tissue. (**24**) The hydatidiform mole is the benign variety and is composed of hydropic chorionic villi. In the great majority of cases, an embryo or fetus is not present. (**25**) Cytogenetic studies have shown that over 90% of hydatidiform moles have a 46XX (normal female) karyotype. (**26**) Furthermore, chromosome banding studies suggest that the entire chromosome complement of moles comes from the sperm, a phenomenon known as androgenesis. (**27**) Although most moles are benign neoplasms, those that are cytologically atypical have a greater malignant potential. In general, the greater the atypia, the greater the biologic aggressiveness of the tumor. Indeed, the fully malignant gestational choriocarcinoma arises from a mole in the majority of cases. It has been estimated that about 1 in 40 hydatidiform moles may be expected to give rise to a choriocarcinoma, whereas only 1 in approximately 150,000 normal pregnancies result in choriocarcinoma. (**28**) Serum levels of human chorionic gonadotropin are often helpful in distinguishing

between a benign mole and a choriocarcinoma, since the latter usually produces higher serum levels of this hormone. (**29**) Although gestational choriocarcinoma was once a highly lethal disease, it is now completely curable with chemotherapy in all but the most refractory cases (*pp. 1159–1162*).

30. (True); 31. (True); 32. (False); 33. (False); 34. (True)

Carcinoma of the prostate is the second most common form of cancer and the third leading cause of cancer deaths in males. (**30**) Although it can be a lethal disease, prostate cancer occurs most frequently in a clinically insignificant form that is often discovered as an incidental finding at postmortem examination or within a surgical specimen removed for other reasons. In fact, it has been estimated that about 30% of men over the age of 50 harbor a stage A (confined to the prostate) prostatic carcinoma.

(**31**) In prostate cancer, the grade of the tumor is of particular importance in determining the prognosis, since the correlation between histologic grade and biologic behavior is very good.

(**32**) In contrast to benign prostatic hypertrophy, which originates from the periurethral portion of the prostate gland, nearly all carcinomas arise from the peripheral zone of the gland. (**33**) While still localized within the prostate, serum tumor markers, such as prostatic acid phosphatase, cannot be detected with standard assays. Only when the cancer has extended beyond the prostate capsule or has metastasized or both are serum elevations of prostatic acid phosphatase detectable by traditional biochemical assays. (**34**) Metastatic spread of prostate cancer occurs chiefly to bones, particularly the vertebral bodies. Metastatic lesions are characteristically osteoblastic in contrast to most other forms of metastatic carcinoma, which are osteolytic. Therefore, osteoblastic bone lesions in men with known prostate cancer are virtually diagnostic of metastatic disease (*pp. 1104–1107*).

35. (C); 36. (B); 37. (C); 38. (B); 39. (D)

(**35**) Adenomyosis refers to a pathologic process within the uterus characterized by the presence of endometrial tissue deep within the myometrial wall. Although endometriosis also refers to the presence of endometrial tissue in an abnormal location, it involves extrauterine sites such as the ovaries, uterine ligaments, rectovaginal septum, or pelvic peritoneum. The two processes are biologically and clinically distinct.

(**36**) Adenomyosis may occur at any stage of adult life. It can be quite common among postmenopausal women and has been reported to occur in 10 to 50% of uteri examined at autopsy. In contrast, endometriosis is a disease of women in active reproductive life and virtually never occurs in women over the age of 50. (**37**) In the premenopausal age group, however, women with either of these processes frequently have dysmenorrhea and other functional pain. (**38**) Although both disorders may produce significant discomfort, only endometriosis is associated with serious complications. In long-standing disease with tubal and ovarian involvement, repeated bleeding of the ectopic endometrium with menstrual cycles leads to progressive scarring and, eventually, sterility.

(**39**) Although the pathogenesis of both of these conditions is still somewhat controversial, neither of these processes is believed to be related to increased estrogen exposure. Adenomyosis is believed to represent an abnormal growth activity of the endometrium even in the presence of normal or low estrogen levels. Endometriosis is believed to occur for unknown reasons by regurgitation of endometrial tissue through the fallopian tubes and implantation on adjacent structures; an alternate theory proposes lymphatic spread (*pp. 1130–1131*).

40. (D); 41. (D); 42. (C); 43. (B); 44. (A); 45. (D); 46. (C); 47. (C); 48. (D)

Tumors of the surface epithelium of the ovary are the most common types of ovarian neoplasms and among these, serous and mucinous tumors are the two most common variants. (**40**) Although rates for germ cell and gonadal stromal cancers are slightly higher in blacks than in whites, black women have a *lower* incidence of epithelial carcinomas. (**41**) Although the risk factors for ovarian carcinoma are much less clear than for other genital malignancies, it is at least apparent that the use of oral contraceptive steroids is not associated with ovarian carcinoma and may even decrease the risk of developing this malignancy.

(**42**) Both mucinous and serous carcinomas are cystic tumors in the majority of cases and cannot be definitively differentiated from one another by gross examination. (**43**) One of the most important reasons to differentiate between the two tumor types is that mucinous tumors are much more commonly benign than malignant, whereas serous tumors are seldom benign. (**44**) Furthermore, serous tumors are far more likely than mucinous tumors to be bilateral. About 20 to 30% of benign serous tumors involve both ovaries, whereas only 5% of benign mucinous tumors are bilateral. Malignant serous tumors are bilateral in about two thirds of cases, in striking contrast to the 20% bilaterality rate of mucinous malignancies. (**45**) Simultaneous occurrence of an endometrial carcinoma in a significant number of cases is a property associated with endometrioid carcinomas of the ovary rather than serous or mucinous neoplasms.

(**46**) Despite the difference in frequency of occurrence, malignant variants of both serous and mucinous tumors have certain similarities in biologic behavior, the strongest being their tendency to spread by direct seeding throughout the peritoneal cavity. For both tumors, metastasis by lymphatic or hematogenous routes is much less common. (**47**) Another feature common to both serous and mucinous tumors is a histologic one: the presence of psammoma bodies within the tumor or its metastases. Psammoma bodies are not pathognomonic of ovarian carcinoma, however, since they may occur in any type of papillary malignancy, including those of the thyroid or pancreas. (**48**) In contrast to the malignant germ cell tumor of the ovary, epithelial tumors are not associated with increased serum levels of embryonic proteins such as alpha-fetoprotein or gonadotrophic hormones (*pp. 1144–1146*).

49. (B); 50. (A); 51. (B); 52. (C)

Gonadal stromal tumors, either ovarian or testicular, are of particular interest because of their ability to elaborate hormones. (**49**) Since Leydig cell tumors predominantly synthesize androgens, they usually cause virilization in females. In adult males, the only clinically detectable hormonal influence is gynecomastia, occurring only in rare cases of estrogen-producing Leydig cell tumors. (**50**) Granulosa cell tumors, in contrast, are predominantly estrogen-producing and greatly predispose to endometrial carcinoma in women (see Question 2). About 10 to 15% of patients with estrogen-producing granulosa cell tumors eventually develop endometrial carcinoma.

(**51**) A pathognomonic histologic feature of Leydig cell neoplasms is the rod-shaped crystalloids of Reinke, which appear in the cytoplasm of about half of these tumors.

(**52**) Although occasionally troublesome or even dangerous (see Question 50) because of their hormone-producing capacity, both of these tumor types tend to be benign in their biologic behavior. Granulosa cell tumors in women exhibit malignant behavior in 5 to 25% of cases, and in males about 10% of these tumors are malignant. Leydig cell tumors are almost always benign in women, and in men they exhibit malignant behavior in about 10% of cases (*pp. 1097–1098, 1152–1153*).

53. (C); 54. (A); 55. (B); 56. (E); 57. (D)

(**53**) Benign cystic lesions are extremely common in the female genital tract. They are commonly the result of cystic dilatation of either an inflamed normal gland or a remnant of an embryologic structure. Bartholin's cysts are examples of the former. They arise from vulvovaginal glands and are often associated with gonorrheal infections.

(**55**) Similarly, Nabothian cysts originate from inflamed endocervical glands. In contrast to Bartholin's cysts, however, these lesions are not usually the result of gonococcal infection. They usually occur as a result of so-called "nonspecific cervicitis," a commonplace inflammatory process thought to be caused by a variety of bacteria, including streptococci, *E. coli,* and staphylococci.

(**54**) Among the developmental structures that may

persist as remnants and undergo cystic change are the Gartner's duct cysts of the vagina, which represent mesonephric ductal structures, and (57) hydatid cysts of Morgagni of the fallopian tube, which arise from Wolffian duct remnants.

(56) Endometriosis of the ovary (see Question 38) may, with repeated bleeding, undergo cystic change. These cysts have a distinctive gross appearance characterized by a brown, hemosiderin-laden wall and turbid hemorrhagic cyst fluid. On the basis of this appearance, they have become known as "chocolate cysts" (pp. 1114, 1119, 1122, 1131, 1141).

58. (E); 59. (A); 60. (A); 61. (D); 62. (B)

Whereas germ cell tumors represent only 15 to 20% of all ovarian cancers, they comprise the vast majority (about 95%) of testicular malignancies. (58) Among the malignant germ cell tumors in both sexes, the most biologically primitive (the dysgerminoma in the female and the seminoma in the male) are the most common (see Question 6). (59) Whereas testicular germ cell tumors are almost always malignant, ovarian germ cell tumors are almost always benign. Benign cystic teratomas or "dermoid cysts" constitute about 95% of ovarian germ cell tumors. These teratomas are very well differentiated. Although they contain primarily ectodermal structures, mesodermal and endodermal elements are also encountered and are also well differentiated. (60) Occasionally, a single histologic element of a teratoma will comprise the entire ovarian tumor, a phenomenon known as "monodermal" or specialized teratoma. One of the most interesting of these is a tumor composed entirely of mature thyroid tissue known as struma ovarii. Since these tumors may hyperfunction, they may be a rare cause of hyperthyroidism.

(61) Like fetal tissues arising from germ cells, germ cell tumors synthesize embryonic and trophoblastic polypeptides, which serve as useful tumor markers. Alpha-fetoprotein, the major serum protein of the early fetus, is synthesized by the yolk sac as well as the fetal intestine and liver. Analogously, yolk sac tumors synthesize alpha-fetoprotein (AFP) exclusively. Embryonal carcinoma and teratomas may both synthesize AFP, but these tumors usually produce both AFP and human chorionic gonadotropin (HCG) simultaneously. (62) At the other end of the spectrum, choriocarcinoma produces only HCG like its normal counterpart, the trophoblast (pp. 1090–1097, 1149–1152).

12

THE BREAST

DIRECTIONS: For Questions 1 to 8 choose the ONE BEST answer to each question.

1. The most important prognostic feature in breast cancer is:

   A. The histologic type of the tumor
   B. The histologic grade of the tumor
   C. The absolute size (diameter) of the tumor
   D. The status of the draining lymph nodes
   E. Involvement of the overlying skin

2. Which of the following lesions is LEAST likely to occur as a lump in the axilla of a 40-year-old woman?

   A. Metastatic breast cancer
   B. Hidradenitis suppurativa
   C. Primary site of a breast carcinoma
   D. Lymphoma
   E. Intraductal papilloma

3. Which one of the following statements about breast cancer in young women (age 30 or less) is true?

   A. The incidence of carcinoma is highest in this age group
   B. The overall prognosis is better in this age group than for older women
   C. An increased incidence is related to use of oral contraceptive steroids with high estrogen content
   D. The proportion of lobular carcinomas is increased in this age group
   E. None of the above

4. All of the following microscopic features are characteristic of gynecomastia EXCEPT:

   A. Lobular hyperplasia
   B. Ductal ectasia
   C. Stromal hyperplasia

   D. Ductal hyperplasia
   E. Lymphoplasmacytic infiltrates

5. All of the following conditions are causes of gynecomastia EXCEPT:

   A. Alcoholic cirrhosis
   B. Prostatic carcinoma
   C. Cimetidine administration
   D. Leydig cell tumors
   E. Klinefelter's syndrome

6. All of the following statements about sclerosing adenosis are true EXCEPT:

   A. It is a component of fibrocystic disease
   B. It often resembles carcinoma clinically
   C. It is often unilateral
   D. Florid cases resemble carcinoma histologically
   E. It is considered a premalignant condition

7. All of the following are risk factors for mammary carcinoma EXCEPT:

   A. Jewish ancestry
   B. Late menarche
   C. Nulliparity
   D. History of endometrial carcinoma
   E. Obesity

8. All of the following statements about cystosarcoma phyllodes are true EXCEPT:

   A. It is the malignant counterpart of fibroadenoma
   B. It is a bulky, locally expansive tumor
   C. It tends to metastasize early
   D. Stromal rather than epithelial anaplasia is the major histologic characteristic
   E. It has a characteristically rapid growth rate

DIRECTIONS: For Questions 9 to 19, ONE or MORE of the completions given correctly finishes the incomplete statement. Choose:

A—if only *1,2, and 3* are correct
B—if only *1 and 3* are correct
C—if only *2 and 4* are correct
D—if only *4* is correct
E—if all are correct

9. Which of the following statements about the normal breast is/are true?

1. The breast is a group of modified eccrine glands
2. A single layer of epithelial cells comprises the wall of the mammary ducts
3. Mitotic activity in the ductal epithelium is stimulated by estrogens
4. The mammary ducts form a complex network of branching and anastomosing channels throughout the breast

A. 1,2,3   B. 1,3   C. 2,4   D. 4 Only   E. All

10. Which of the following histologic patterns of breast carcinoma is/are associated with a better prognosis than infiltrating duct carcinoma?

1. Tubular carcinoma
2. Carcinoma arising in a fibroadenoma
3. Colloid (mucinous) carcinoma
4. Medullary carcinoma

A. 1,2,3   B. 1,3   C. 2,4   D. 4 Only   E. All

11. Which of the following statements about carcinoma of the male breast is/are true?

1. The incidence is about 100 times less than that of carcinoma of the female breast
2. The overall prognosis is better than for cancer of the female breast
3. Paget's disease of the breast is relatively more common in males
4. There is usually a coexistent history of gynecomastia

A. 1,2,3   B. 1,3   C. 2,4   D. 4 Only   E. All

12. Which of the following statements about Paget's disease of the breast is/are true?

1. It is caused by dermal lymphatic invasion from an underlying ductal carcinoma
2. It is accompanied by an osteolytic-osteoblastic process in bone
3. It has a worse prognosis than infiltrating ductal carcinoma of comparable stage
4. It often appears clinically in the absence of a palpable breast mass

A. 1,2,3   B. 1,3   C. 2,4   D. 4 Only   E. All

13. Which of the following histologic lesions is/are considered to increase the risk of subsequent development of carcinoma?

1. Ductal hyperplasia
2. Florid papillomatosis
3. Lobular hyperplasia
4. Apocrine metaplasia

A. 1,2,3   B. 1,3   C. 2,4   D. 4 Only   E. All

14. Estrogen receptor protein positivity in breast cancer is likely to be associated with which of the following factors?

1. Advanced age of the patient
2. Previous exposure to estrogenic drugs
3. Increased therapeutic response of the tumor to tamoxifen
4. Increased therapeutic response of the tumor to adriamycin

A. 1,2,3   B. 1,3   C. 2,4   D. 4 Only   E. All

15. Lesions of the breast that are characteristically PAINFUL include:

1. Galactocele
2. Mammary duct ectasia
3. Cystic disease
4. Infiltrating ductal carcinoma

A. 1,2,3   B. 1,3   C. 2,4   D. 4 Only   E. All

16. Which of the following statements about fibroadenoma is/are TRUE?

1. It represents both a stromal and a glandular proliferation
2. It is rare before age 30
3. It is a sharply circumscribed lesion
4. It often harbors a carcinoma

A. 1,2,3   B. 1,3   C. 2,4   D. 4 Only   E. All .

17. Which of the following features is/are characteristic of fibrocystic disease?

1. Stromal degeneration (atrophy)
2. Proliferation of small ductules
3. Acute inflammation
4. Proliferation of ductal epithelium

A. 1,2,3   B. 1,3   C. 2,4   D. 4 Only   E. All

18. A 35-year-old woman notices a lump in the upper outer quadrant of the left breast that fluctuates in size with her menstrual cycles. This clinical behavior would be compatible with which of the following lesions?

1. Fibroadenoma
2. Cystic disease
3. Stromal fibrosis
4. Ductal carcinoma

   A. 1,2,3   B. 1,3   C. 2,4   D. 4 Only   E. All

19. A 50-year-old woman has a brownish discharge from the nipple but has no palpable mass in the breast. This clinical situation describes:

1. Intraductal papilloma
2. Duct ectasia
3. Paget's disease
4. Galactocele

   A. 1,2,3   B. 1,3   C. 2,4   D. 4 Only   E. All

DIRECTIONS: For Questions 20 to 37, the set of lettered headings is followed by a list of numbered words or phrases. For each numbered word or phrase choose:
   A—if the item is associated with (A) only
   B—if the item is associated with (B) only
   C—if the item is associated with *both* (A) and (B)
   D—if the item is associated with *neither* (A) nor (B)

For each of the characteristics listed below, choose whether it describes ductal carcinoma, lobular carcinoma, both, or neither.

   A. Ductal carcinoma
   B. Lobular carcinoma
   C. Both
   D. Neither

20. Occurs most frequently in the upper outer quadrant of the breast
21. Is often in the *in situ* state
22. Commonly produces scirrhous tumors
23. Produces Paget's disease in the nipple
24. Tends to arise multicentrically in the same breast
25. Occurs bilaterally in approximately 20% of cases
26. Constitutes the most common type of breast malignancy in children

For each of the characteristics listed below, choose whether it describes medullary carcinoma, colloid (mucinous) carcinoma, both, or neither.

   A. Medullary carcinoma
   B. Colloid (mucinous) carcinoma
   C. Both
   D. Neither

27. Represents a variant of lobular carcinoma
28. Occurs bilaterally twice as frequently as usual ductal carcinoma
29. Typically feels soft on palpation
30. Composed of anaplastic tumor cells with a high mitotic rate
31. Characterized histologically by an accompanying lymphocytic infiltrate
32. Frequently occurs in combination with other histologic types of mammary carcinoma

For each of the characteristics listed below, choose whether it describes inflammatory carcinoma of the breast, acute mastitis, both, or neither.

   A. Inflammatory carcinoma of breast
   B. Acute mastitis
   C. Both
   D. Neither

33. The involved breast is usually red and hot
34. The process is usually unilateral
35. Skin retraction is a common clinical finding
36. The process is more common in women over age 50
37. Neutrophils are found in affected ducts

12

THE BREAST

ANSWERS

1. (D) Overall, the status of the draining lymph nodes of the breast containing malignancy is the most important prognostic factor in breast cancer, largely determining the stage of the tumor and the corresponding survival rate. The absolute number of lymph nodes involved by metastatic carcinoma, the size (transverse diameter) of involved nodes, and the fixation of nodes to the skin or deeper structures of the axilla are all factors considered in the assessment. Although the histologic type of the tumor, its grade, size, and involvement of the overlying skin are all significant prognostic factors, none as accurately reflects the clinical course and survival rates of breast cancer patients as the degree of nodal involvement (*p. 1188*).

2. (E) Because the axilla contains the lymph nodes that drain the upper outer quadrant of the breast (the most common location for development of a breast carcinoma), metastatic breast cancer may present as an axillary lump. A mass in the axilla may also represent a primary breast tumor, since the glandular tissue of the female breast often extends deep into the axilla (a common anatomic variant). Hidradenitis suppurativa is a chronic suppurative folliculitis affecting the axillary and anogenital regions. Hidradenitis suppurativa often produces deep-seated abscesses that extend into the subcutaneous tissue and present as a tender axillary mass. Axillary lymph nodes may also be the site of a primary neoplastic process; a lymphoma arising in an axillary node would present as a nontender axillary lump. Intraductal papillomas, however, are benign tumors of the major excretory ducts of the breast. Since the excretory ducts are located beneath the nipple, a papillary adenoma would not be found in the axillary region (*pp. 1165–1177*).

3. (E) Cancer of the breast is relatively uncommon in women aged 30 or less. The disease has a poorer prognosis in women of this age group than in older women with cancers of comparable stage. Contributing to this poor prognosis is the fact that malignant tumors arising in young women tend to be estrogen receptor protein negative. Although there is some epidemiologic evidence to suggest that the "pill" increases the risk of developing breast cancer, the association has been made only with combination-type oral contraceptive steroids with high progesterone (not estrogen) content. Lobular carcinoma of the breast tends to be a disease of older women and is relatively rare in women aged 30 or less (*pp. 1179, 1184, 1188*).

4. (A) Gynecomastia is a term referring to enlargement of the male breast in response to hyperestrogenism or increased prolactin. The major histologic component of the normal male breast is fibrostromal tissue. The epithelial element is composed of major mammary ducts and secondary branches, but lobular elements are not found. As in the female, breast elements in the male are responsive to estrogenic stimulation and will undergo hyperplasia when excessive estrogens are present. Microscopically, gynecomastia is characterized by proliferation of ductal elements with ductal ectasia, stromal hyperplasia, and a periductal lymphocytic and plasma cell infiltrate. Since lobules are not a component of the male breast, lobular hyperplasia is not a feature of gynecomastia (*p. 1189*).

5. (B) Elevated serum levels of either estrogen or prolactin in the male may cause gynecomastia. Conditions that cause hyperestrogenism in males are diverse and include metabolic, and iatrogenic (drug-induced) etiologies. The hepatic parenchymal destruction of cirrhosis leads to decreased catabolism of estrogenic compounds. A small percentage of patients treated with cimetidine for peptic ulcer disease develop gynecomastia as a consequence of elevated serum levels of prolactin caused by the drug. Leydig (interstitial) cell tumors of the testis are often hormonally active and may secrete a large variety of steroid hormones, including estrogens. Patients with Klinefelter's syndrome have atrophic testes and primary hypogonadism. The levels of circulating androgens in these patients are drastically reduced, and relative hyperestrogenism with gynecomastia results. Carcinoma of the prostate does not itself cause gynecomastia. Rather, it is the therapy for this disease involving hormonal manipulations such as estrogen administration or castration that is associated with the development of gynecomastia (*p. 1189*).

6. (E) Sclerosing adenosis is a benign condition characterized by proliferation of both intralobular connective tissue and small ductules or acini. Although sclerosing adenosis is considered a component of fibrocystic disease, it is important to recognize it as a separate entity, since it often resembles carcinoma both clinically and histologically. Like carcinoma, it most often occurs unilaterally in the upper outer quadrant of the breast as a hard, localized mass. The histologic picture of florid proliferation of small glandular structures as well as nests and cords of cells within a fibrous stroma closely resembles infiltrating carcinoma. Sclerosing adenosis, however, is benign in its biologic behavior and is not associated with increased risk of developing carcinoma (pp. 1172–1173).

7. (B) Although the etiology of human breast cancer is still unknown, epidemiologic studies have shown that certain clinical factors are associated with development of the disease and are now considered risk factors for breast carcinoma. Major categories of risk factors include: (1) genetic background (race and family history); (2) endogenous hormonal factors related to reproductive history; and (3) premalignant pathologic lesions in the breast tissue, specifically epithelial hyperplasia. Compared with gentiles, Jews are at twice the risk of developing breast carcinoma. Women with a strong family history (carcinoma developing in first-degree female relatives) are at exceptionally high risk.

In general, the longer the uninterrupted exposure to endogenous estrogens, the greater the risk of developing breast carcinoma. Nulliparity, early menarche, and late menopause, therefore, are all risk factors. Endometrial carcinoma is also known to be associated with uninterrupted estrogen stimulation (of endometrial glands). Because the two tumors share this common risk factor, the development of endometrial carcinoma is often accompanied by the development of a breast malignancy in the same patient, and a history of endometrial carcinoma represents a risk factor for breast cancer.

Less well understood is the relationship of obesity to increased risk of breast cancer. Clearly, estrogen metabolism is altered in obese women, and synthesis of estrone is increased. Some investigators have hypothesized that increased fat in the diet may augment steroid (estrogen) hormone production by providing increased amounts of precursor substrate molecules.

Furthermore, it is known that adipose tissue directly contributes to increased estrogen production by converting androstenedione of adrenal origin to estrone. The local effects of this may be highly significant, since breast tissue (especially in obese women) is composed largely of fat (pp. 426, 1179).

8. (C) The unfortunate term cystosarcoma phyllodes refers to a lesion that is rarely cystic and is not a true sarcoma. It is considered the malignant counterpart of the fibroadenoma, which it resembles histologically. Phyllodes is a Greek term that refers to the "leaf-like," scalloped appearance of these locally expansive tumors. Cystosarcoma phyllodes are tumors of low virulence and unlike most true sarcomas

remain localized for long periods of time. Although they may metastasize, this usually occurs late in the course of the disease. Clinically, malignant transformation is usually heralded by a rapid increase in size, but the definitive prognosis of cystosarcoma phyllodes rests with the histologic findings of stromal anaplasia, increased stromal cellularity, and high mitotic rate. Simple mastectomy is usually the treatment of choice (p. 1177).

9. (B) Embryologically, the breast derives from the epidermis and represents a group of modified eccrine glands. Like eccrine ducts elsewhere in the body, the mammary ducts are lined by a *double* layer of epithelial cells—an inner layer of cuboidal secretory epithelial cells and an outer layer of flattened myoepithelial cells. Mixed with these ductal elements is a densely collagenized connective tissue stroma admixed with fat. Breast tissue is hormonally responsive and undergoes cyclic changes with the menses. During the first half of the cycle, estrogens stimulate proliferative activity in the epithelium of the ducts and gland buds, whereas progesterone causes stromal growth in the latter half of the cycle. The overall architectural organization of the mammary ducts is strictly compartmentalized. Each of the seven to nine major excretory ducts drains a single, wedge-shaped compartment of the breast. Each compartment is discrete, and the ductal channels within it do not anastomose with the ducts of adjacent segments. This architectural arrangement is a fundamental concept in breast pathology, since lesions arising within a duct in a single segment cannot spread to other breast segments via the ductal system (pp. 1165–1166).

10. (E) Tubular carcinoma of the breast is a form of ductal carcinoma displaying a high degree of differentiation. It behaves less aggressively than infiltrating ductal carcinoma and has a low incidence of axillary lymph node metastasis. Carcinoma arising within a fibroadenoma, although rare, is also associated with a good prognosis. This may be related to the fact that the carcinoma is brought to clinical attention early by the discovery of the fibroadenoma. Thus, these carcinomas are frequently found in the *in situ* stage and are completely limited to the fibroadenoma. Colloid (mucinous) carcinoma of the breast and medullary carcinoma are variants of ductal carcinoma that have a relatively good prognosis, because they tend to metastasize to axillary lymph nodes less frequently than the usual infiltrating ductal carcinoma. The reason for this difference in behavior is unknown, however (pp. 1180–1181, 1188).

11. (B) Carcinoma of the male breast is a very rare entity and, compared with carcinoma of the female breast, has an incidence ratio of 1:100. When it does occur, however, carcinoma of the male breast has a worse prognosis than carcinoma of the female breast. Because males have a small amount of breast tissue, tumors can rapidly infiltrate the underlying chest wall or the overlying skin. Thus, skin involvement by fixation, ulceration, and microscopic Paget's disease is relatively much more common in males than in females. Although the predisposing factors for carcinoma in the male breast remain obscure, there is no evidence that gynecomastia is related to the development of carcinoma. Carcinoma does not develop with increased frequency in patients with gynecomastia, and conversely, patients with carcinoma rarely have a history of preceding or coexisting gynecomastia (*p. 1189*).

12. (D) Paget's disease of the breast is a form of ductal carcinoma arising in the major excretory ducts beneath the nipple and extending outward along the duct toward the skin surface, directly invading the nipple epidermis. The primary tumor may or may not show stromal invasion and may often appear in the absence of a palpable breast mass. Skin involvement is, however, considered a grave finding in any breast carcinoma, and patients with Paget's disease have the same prognosis as patients with usual infiltrating ductal carcinoma of similar stage (stage C). When comparing Paget's disease arising from an *in situ* lesion (no evidence of penetration through the duct basement membrane or invasion of periductal stroma) with other *in situ* ductal carcinomas, Paget's disease has a distinctly worse prognosis, with a 30 to 40% incidence of metastasis at the time of surgery. Although the eczematoid appearance of the skin in Paget's disease may resemble inflammatory carcinoma of the breast clinically, the two lesions can be differentiated from one another by their histologic appearance. Inflammatory carcinoma of the breast corresponds to dermal lymphatic invasion from an underlying breast carcinoma (see Question 33), whereas Paget's disease refers to epidermal involvement. Paget's disease of the breast is not to be confused with Paget's disease of bone, a totally unrelated disorder. Paget's disease of bone is a benign disorder of unknown etiology that is characterized by an osteolytic-osteoblastic process in the bones of affected individuals (*pp. 1181–1182, 1331*).

13. (A) Epithelial hyperplasias of either ductal or lobular origin are the two forms of benign breast disease that are associated with increased risk of development of carcinoma. The more severe and atypical the hyperplasia, the greater the risk of carcinoma is considered to be. Florid papillomatosis is a histologic subtype of ductal hyperplasia in which the epithelial projections grow into the lumen. Apocrine metaplasia is a very frequent finding in fibrocystic disease of the breast and is virtually always a benign lesion (*pp. 1172–1174*).

14. (B) There is a direct relationship between the amount of estrogen receptor protein found in a breast carcinoma and its response to hormonal manipulation. Age of the patient appears to be the single most important determinant of estrogen receptor protein positivity in breast carcinomas: in general, the greater the age of the patient, the greater the probability of estrogen receptor protein positivity in the tumor. Previous exposure to exogenous estrogen, although known to be related epidemiologically to the development of breast carcinoma, appears to have no influence on the estrogen receptor positivity of tumors developing in this setting. Although there is a high correlation between estrogen receptor positivity of a tumor and its response to anti-estrogenic drugs such as tamoxifen, estrogen receptor positivity has no predictive value in the response of the tumor to nonhormonal chemotherapeutic agents such as adriamycin (*p. 1188*).

15. (A) Pain is a symptom more often associated with benign rather than malignant diseases of the breast and is characteristic of such lesions as galactocele, mammary duct ectasia, and cystic disease. Although infiltrating ductal carcinoma may present as a painful lesion in certain patients, the tumor most often comes to the patient's or physician's attention as a firm but painless mass in the breast (*pp. 1168–1169, 1172, 1186*).

16. (B) The fibroadenoma is the most common benign tumor of the female breast and is found most frequently in women under the age of 30. It is believed to arise from breast lobules representing a proliferation of both the stromal and glandular elements. It is an encapsulated, sharply circumscribed lesion that has a rubbery consistency. Although it may be confused clinically with a cyst, a fibroadenoma is usually easy to differentiate clinically from carcinoma. Although the overwhelming majority of fibroadenomas are completely benign, the epithelial element, like the epithelial elements elsewhere in the breast, may give rise to a carcinoma. This, however, is an extremely rare event (*pp. 1175–1176*).

17. (C) Fibrocystic disease of the breast is a very common condition caused by an exaggeration of the response of stromal and glandular breast elements to the cyclic hormonal cycles of menses. Stromal elements are rather unidirectional in their response, undergoing proliferative rather than degenerative changes. Stromal hyperplasia with increased collagen production (stromal sclerosis or fibrosis) may be the predominant feature in fibrocystic disease or may be accompanied by various degrees of epithelial hyperplasia. Types of hyperplastic epithelial responses that occur in fibrocystic disease include the proliferation of small ductules or acinar structures (adenosis), the proliferation of ductal lining cells (intraductal hyperplasia), and cyst formation. Fibrocystic disease is not an inflammatory condition and is not characteristically associated with the presence of acute inflammation histologically unless infection has been superimposed on the process. Nonspecific chronic inflammation in the form of stromal lymphocytic infiltrates, on the other hand, is a common finding in fibrocystic disease (*pp. 1169–1173*).

18. (A) In the varying hormonal environment produced by the normal menstrual cycle, there may be fluctuation in the size of hormonally responsive proliferative lesions of the breast, including fibroadenomas, cystic disease, and stromal fibrosis.

Malignant processes, in contrast, tend to relentlessly increase in size without fluctuation in response to hormonal cycles (*pp. 1170, 1172, 1176, 1186–1187*).

19. (A) Nipple discharge in a middle-aged woman may be the result of either a benign or neoplastic process involving the major excretory ducts of the breast. Intraductal papilloma of the nipple is a lesion that usually affects women of middle age and often causes nipple discharge. It consists of a benign neoplastic growth of the epithelium of the lactiferous ducts that forms multiple delicate papillae. Duct ectasia, an inflammatory disorder principally involving the major excretory ducts, tends to occur in the fifth decade of life. It often causes discharge from the nipple as well as pain and induration. Paget's disease of the breast is the principal malignant disease causing nipple discharge and must be differentiated from benign conditions producing this symptom. Paget's disease represents a form of ductal carcinoma involving the major excretory ducts and the skin of the overlying nipple. In addition to an oozy, bloody discharge, the nipple often shows ezcematous changes and fissuring or ulceration with surrounding inflammatory hyperemia and edema. A galactocele is a cystic dilatation of an obstructed duct occurring during lactation and would not correspond to the described situations (*pp. 1167–1168, 1177, 1181–1184*).

20. (C); 21. (D); 22. (A); 23. (A); 24. (B); 25. (B); 26. (D)
(20) Both ductal and lobular carcinomas of the breast occur with greatest frequency in the upper outer quadrant, which is the region of greatest concentration of glandular tissue in the breast. **(21)** In general, neither ductal carcinoma nor lobular carcinoma is palpable *in situ*. It is the infiltrating tumor with its sclerotic stromal response that presents clinically as a firm lump. **(22)** Infiltrating tumors of ductal origin classically induce marked stromal sclerosis. Such tumors have a hard, cartilaginous consistency on palpation and are known as scirrhous tumors.

Although the great majority of scirrhous tumors are infiltrating ductal carcinomas, any given scirrhous malignancy may be of either ductal or lobular origin. Most invasive lobular carcinomas, however, are rubbery and typically are not scirrhous.

(23) Paget's disease of the breast is produced only by ductal carcinoma that arises in a major excretory duct and extends to involve the skin of the nipple.

Lobular carcinoma is associated with two clinically important features: **(24)** a tendency to be multicentric within the same breast and **(25)** a high incidence of bilaterality (approaching 20% as compared with 10 to 12% bilaterality in ductal carcinomas). Bilaterality and multicentricity are not unique to lobular carcinoma but occur about twice as frequently with lobular carcinomas as ductal carcinoma.

(26) Carcinoma of the breast is exceedingly rare in children, but when it occurs, it is usually of the so-called juvenile type. Because of its extreme rarity, this type of carcinoma has been poorly described, but it is associated with a distinctive tubulopapillary histologic growth pattern and an indolent clinical course. The precise cell of origin has not yet been determined. Juvenile carcinoma is not comparable, either histologically or clinically, with the adult carcinomas of ductal or lobular origin (*pp. 1181–1184*).

27. (D); 28. (D); 29. (C); 30. (A); 31. (A); 32. (B)
(27) Both medullary carcinoma and colloid carcinoma of the breast arise from ductal epithelial cells and represent variants of ductal carcinomas.

(28) The incidence of bilaterality in patients with either of these tumor types is not significantly different from that in patients with usual ductal carcinoma.

(29) Unlike usual ductal carcinomas, medullary carcinoma and colloid carcinoma induce little stromal response. They typically feel soft on palpation and may resemble each other clinically. **(30)** Histologically, however, the two variants are distinctly different. Medullary carcinomas are characterized by a high degree of anaplasia and a high mitotic rate **(31)** and are typically accompanied by an abundant lymphocytic infiltrate. **(32)** Furthermore, medullary carcinoma most often occurs as an isolated entity, and colloid carcinoma frequently occurs in combination with other histologic types of ductal carcinoma (*p. 1181*).

33. (C); 34. (C); 35. (C); 36. (A); 37. (B)
(33) Although inflammatory carcinoma of the breast shares some clinical features with mastitis, it is not truly an inflammatory process. Inflammatory carcinoma is actually an infiltrating ductal carcinoma of the breast with a characteristic tendency to extensively invade the lymphatics of the breast and overlying skin. Acute mastitis is a true inflammatory process caused by bacteria (usually *Staphylococcus aureus*), which gain access to the breast substance

through cracks in the nipple skin created during nursing. The involved breast in both inflammatory carcinoma and acute mastitis is usually reddened, swollen, and warm to touch. (34) In both processes, the involvement is usually unilateral and (35) produces skin retraction or nipple retraction as a result of marked edema. (36) Inflammatory carcinoma is more common in women over 50 because infiltrating ductal carcinoma of the breast is more common in this age group. Mastitis, although relatively rare, is a disease of young lactating women. (37) Histologically, the presence of numerous neutrophils within affected ducts is characteristic only of acute mastitis (*pp. 1167, 1185*).

13

THE SKIN

DIRECTIONS: For Questions 1 to 12, choose the ONE BEST answer to each question.

1. All of the following statements about basal cell carcinoma are true EXCEPT:

   A. It is the most common malignant tumor of skin in Caucasians
   B. It tends to spare the hands and forearms
   C. It rarely metastasizes
   D. It is associated with arsenic exposure
   E. The morphea-like variant is characterized by more aggressive growth

2. A 20-year-old woman develops hives when she eats nuts. All of the following statements about this patient are true EXCEPT:

   A. The development of the lesions is mediated by IgE
   B. Mast cell degranulation occurs in the lesions
   C. Complement activation is important in the pathogenesis of the lesions
   D. She probably has relatives with asthma
   E. Aspirin administration is contraindicated

3. All of the following statements about the excised lesion shown in Figure 13–1 are true EXCEPT:

   A. It is the most common benign tumor of mankind
   B. The cells originate from the neural crest
   C. Infiltration of the deep dermis corresponds to locally aggressive biologic behavior
   D. Mitoses are rarely found in these lesions
   E. This histologic type is least likely to undergo malignant transformation

4. A patient notices a deeply pigmented, slightly raised nodule with indefinite borders on the upper extremity. Although a nodular melanoma is suspected, none of the following lesions can be ruled out on clinical inspection EXCEPT:

   A. Pigmented basal cell carcinoma
   B. Pigmented seborrheic keratosis
   C. Blue nevus
   D. Dermatofibroma
   E. Lentigo simplex

5. Malignant melanoma is associated with all of the following situations EXCEPT:

   A. Occurrence in congenital hairy nevi
   B. Histologic appearance resembling a sarcoma
   C. Occurrence of lesions with no melanin present
   D. Spontaneous regression of primary lesions
   E. High cure rate with chemotherapy

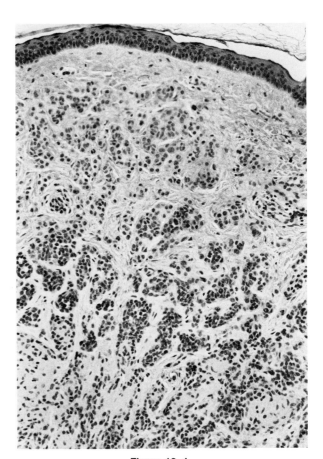

Figure 13–1

6. Which of the following statements about mycosis fungoides is TRUE?

    A. Early lesions resemble superficial fungal infection both clinically and histologically

    B. The causative agent is an atypical mycobacterium

    C. Suppressor T cells with highly convoluted nuclei are often present in the lesions

    D. Hematogenous involvement is known as Sézary's syndrome

    E. Munro's microabscesses are diagnostic

7. Which one of the following lesions has the best prognosis?

    A. Lentigo maligna

    B. Lentigo maligna melanoma

    C. Superficial spreading melanoma

    D. Nodular melanoma

    E. Melanoma arising in a congenital nevus

8. Which of the following would be the LEAST likely cause of thrombocytopenia-induced purpuric lesions developing in a patient with promyelocytic leukemia?

    A. Hypersplenism

    B. Bone marrow replacement

    C. Intercurrent infection

    D. Disseminated intravascular coagulation

    E. Administration of drugs

9. A Langerhans' cell is

    A. Seen in tubercular granulomas in the skin

    B. An endocrine cell resembling those in pancreas islets

    C. A melanocyte precursor

    D. An epidermal macrophage

    E. A transformed lymphocyte in the dermis

10. Which of the following statements regarding actinic keratosis is TRUE?

    A. It is a premalignant skin condition

    B. It is more common in India than in Australia

    C. The essential diagnostic features are hyperplasia and hyperkeratosis of the epidermis

    D. The proliferating cells infiltrate the epidermal basement membrane

    E. The superficial cell layers of the epidermis are most severely involved

11. Which of the following skin disorders is LEAST likely to occur in an individual with diffuse B-cell lymphoma?

    A. Xanthoma

    B. Acanthosis nigricans

    C. Squamous cell carcinoma

    D. Cutaneous necrotizing vasculitis

    E. Mycosis fungoides

12. Which of the following statements about nevus flammeus is TRUE?

    A. It is a rare congenital lesion

    B. It has a tendency to involute spontaneously

    C. The extremities are the most common sites of occurrence

    D. Histologically, it resembles a halo nevus

    E. It is often associated with congenital heart disease

DIRECTIONS: For Questions 13 to 23, ONE or MORE of the completions given correctly finishes the incomplete statement. Choose:

    A—if only *1,2 and 3* are correct

    B—if only *1 and 3* are correct

    C—if only *2 and 4* are correct

    D—if only *4* is correct

    E—if all are correct

13. Mitosis occurs in cell layers more than one cell layer above the basal layer of the epidermis in which of the following?

    1. Normal skin

    2. Bowen's disease

    3. Lentigo maligna

    4. Psoriasis

    A. 1,2,3 B. 1,3 C. 2,4 D. 4 Only E. All

14. A 40-year-old man develops a 1-cm brownish nodule on the skin of the thigh. Biopsy reveals dermatofibroma. Which of the statements regarding this lesion is/are true?

    1. It is a tumor of histiocytes

    2. It is biologically identical to a sclerosing hemangioma

    3. Hyperpigmentation of the overlying epidermis causes the brown color

    4. Its superficial location makes malignancy highly unlikely

    A. 1,2,3 B. 1,3 C. 2,4 D. 4 Only E. All

15. Palpable purpura developing in patients treated for chronic myelogenous leukemia is caused by:

1. Malignancy-associated vasculitis
2. Drug sensitivity
3. Intercurrent infection
4. Leukemic infiltration of skin

   A. 1,2,3   B. 1,3   C. 2,4   D. 4 Only   E. All

16. Squamous cell carcinoma:

1. Is the most common malignant tumor of skin with significant metastatic potential
2. Is uncommon on the backs of the hands
3. Usually appears as leukoplakia when occurring in mucous membranes
4. Has a more aggressive biologic behavior when arising on sun-exposed skin than on genitalia

   A. 1,2,3   B. 1,3   C. 2,4   D. 4 Only   E. All

17. A patient with new skin lesions is found to have a gastric carcinoma. Which of the following cutaneous lesions is/are consistent with this situation?

1. Seborrheic keratosis
2. Acanthosis nigricans
3. Erythema nodosum
4. Paget's disease

   A. 1,2,3   B. 1,3   C. 2,4   D. 4 Only   E. All

18. Which of the following statements about seborrheic keratosis is/are true?

1. The characteristic cell is a keratinocyte with a basaloid appearance
2. Extension into the dermis usually indicates transition into a squamous cell carcinoma
3. Keratin-filled horn cysts are a typical histologic feature
4. Excisional biopsy is the recommended treatment

   A. 1,2,3   B. 1,3   C. 2,4   D. 4 Only   E. All

19. Cutaneous horns are produced by which of the following skin disorders?

1. Actinic keratosis
2. Verruca vulgaris
3. Squamous cell carcinoma
4. Basal cell carcinoma

   A. 1,2,3   B. 1,3   C. 2,4   D. 4 Only   E. All

20. A patient taking sulfonamides has an increased probability of developing which of the following cutaneous lesions?

1. Erythema multiforme
2. Erythema nodosum
3. Urticaria
4. Rosacea

   A. 1,2,3   B. 1,3   C. 2,4   D. 4 Only   E. All

21. Which of the following statements regarding glomus cells is/are true?

1. They are smooth muscle cells
2. They function in regulation of blood pressure by the skin
3. They are controlled by sympathetic innervation
4. They occasionally give rise to highly aggressive malignant tumors

   A. 1,2,3   B. 1,3   C. 2,4   D. 4 Only   E. All

22. Xeroderma pigmentosa is associated with an increased incidence of which of the following neoplasms?

1. Cutaneous malignant melanoma
2. Acute granulocytic leukemia
3. Basal cell carcinoma
4. Colon cancer

   A. 1,2,3   B. 1,3   C. 2,4   D. 4 Only   E. All

23. Characteristics of keratoacanthoma include which of the following?

1. Histologic resemblance to squamous cell carcinoma
2. Slow development and chronic progression
3. Extension of the lesion into the dermis
4. Etiologic association with solar exposure

   A. 1,2,3   B. 1,3   C. 2,4   D. 4 Only   E. All

DIRECTIONS: For Questions 24 to 47, the set of lettered headings is followed by a list of numbered words or phrases. For each numbered word or phrase choose:

A—if the item is associated with (A) only
B—if the item is associated with (B) only
C—if the item is associated with *both* (A) and (B)
D—if the item is associated with *neither* (A) nor (B)

For each of the characteristics listed below, choose whether it describes Spitz nevus (juvenile melanoma), nodular malignant melanoma, both, or neither.

A. Spitz nevus (juvenile melanoma)
B. Nodular malignant melanoma
C. Both
D. Neither

24. The lesion represents a pleomorphic proliferation of melanocytes with a high mitotic rate
25. Deep infiltration of the dermis by the tumor cells is a prominent feature
26. Infiltration of the epidermis by the tumor cells is a common feature
27. The lesions occur only in adults
28. Lesions are most often deeply pigmented

For each of the following statements, choose whether it describes molluscum contagiosum, verruca vulgaris, both, or neither.

A. Molluscum contagiosum
B. Verruca vulgaris
C. Both
D. Neither

29. The etiologic agent is a pox virus
30. Children and young adults are most commonly affected
31. The process spares mucous membranes
32. Intracytoplasmic inclusions are seen in infected cells
33. Lesions are highly contagious

For each of the following characteristics, choose whether it is associated with psoriasis vulgaris, parapsoriasis en plaques, both, or neither.

A. Psoriasis vulgaris
B. Parapsoriasis en plaques
C. Both
D. Neither

34. The epidermal mitotic rate is increased
35. Other organ systems are often involved
36. Lesions are sometimes precipitated by infection
37. Epidermal microabscesses are seen histologically
38. Treatment with ultraviolet light is often effective
39. The disorder is usually self-limited
40. The condition predisposes to lymphoid malignancy

For each of the statements listed below, decide whether it describes lentigo maligna, level I superficial spreading melanoma, both, or neither.

A. Lentigo maligna
B. Level I superficial spreading melanoma
C. Both
D. Neither

41. An intraepithelial proliferation of atypical melanocytes characterizes lesions
42. Dermal invasion develops in almost all lesions
43. Lesions occur on mucous membranes
44. Lesions occur in any age group
45. Lesions often measure 5 cm or more
46. Borders are characteristically irregular
47. Surgical excision is curative

DIRECTIONS: Questions 48 to 61 are matching questions. For each numbered item, choose the most likely associated lettered item from those provided. Each numbered item has ONLY ONE answer. Within each group, each lettered item may be the answer to one, more than one, or none of the numbered items.

For each of the following features of blistering disease of the skin, choose whether it describes pemphigus vulgaris (PV) *only*, bullous pemphigoid (BP) *only*, dermatitis herpetiformis (DH) *only*, both BP *and* PV, or both BP *and* DH.

    A. Pemphigus vulgaris only
    B. Bullous pemphigoid only
    C. Dermatitis herpetiformis only
    D. Both bullous pemphigoid *and* pemphigus vulgaris
    E. Both bullous pemphigoid *and* dermatitis herpetiformis

48. Subepidermal blisters are characteristic
49. Acantholysis is the predominant histologic feature
50. Injury is mediated by IgG and C3
51. Nontropical sprue is an associated disorder
52. The disease has a high mortality rate
53. Treatment with corticosteroids is indicated
54. Affected individuals are usually more than 60 years of age

For each of the characteristics listed below, choose whether it describes acne vulgaris, rosacea (acne rosacea), lichen planus, pityriasis rosea, or pityriasis lichenoides et varioliformis acuta (PLEVA)

    A. Acne vulgaris
    B. Rosacea (acne rosacea)
    C. Lichen planus
    D. Pityriasis rosea
    E. Pityriasis lichenoides et varioliformis acuta (PLEVA)

55. Corynebacteria are involved in the pathogenesis
56. An eruption of scaling plaques typically occurs on the trunk of a young adult in a "Christmas tree" pattern
57. Papules and vesicles typically erupt on the trunk of a young adult
58. Histologically, a band-like lymphohistiocytic infiltrate fills the upper dermis along the dermal'-epidermal junction
59. Erythema and pustular lesions of the mid-face typically occur in a middle-aged adult
60. Treatment with broad-spectrum antibiotics is useful
61. Squamous cell carcinoma develops in 1 to 4% of lesions occurring on the oral mucosa

13

THE SKIN

ANSWERS

1. (E) Basal cell carcinoma is the most common malignant epidermal tumor in the light-skinned races, although blacks and Orientals are sometimes affected. Although common on most other sun-exposed skin surfaces, basal cell carcinoma rarely appears on the backs of the hands and forearms. Besides actinic radiation, another factor associated with an increased risk of basal cell carcinoma (and squamous cell carcinoma as well) is exposure to arsenicals.

Histologically, the tumors are composed of small, dark "basaloid" cells with scant cytoplasm usually growing in nests with peripheral palisading. Although numerous histologic variants do occur, all exhibit similar biologic behavior; they are aggressively infiltrative locally but rarely metastasize. The morphea-like (sclerosing) variant is notable only because its borders are more difficult to define. It may therefore be incompletely excised at surgery and give rise to a troublesome, locally recurrent tumor *(pp. 1265–1266)*.

2. (C) Urticaria, commonly known as hives, is a very common skin disorder resulting from transient localized increases in vascular permeability, producing dermal edema. Clinically these lesions appear as pruritic pink or white wheals. The lesions are produced through a variety of mechanisms, which include immunologic, nonimmunologic, and idiopathic mechanisms. In IgE-mediated immunologic urticaria (allergic type), specific antigen sensitivity to foods, pollens, or drugs produces a Type I hypersensitivity immune response with mast cell degranulation and a histamine-induced increase in venular permeability. A family history of atopy (reagin sensitivity) is common, and patients often suffer from other atopic maladies such as allergic rhinitis, asthma, or eczema.

Complement activation is *not* involved in the pathogenesis of allergic urticaria; this contrasts with the other known form of immunologic urticaria in which an immune complex–mediated, complement-activating reaction (Type III immune response, p. 164) is the underlying mechanism.

Agents that act as arachidonic acid metabolism inhibitors, such as aspirin, tend to potentiate IgE-mediated urticaria by impairing prostaglandin synthesis. Prostaglandins would be beneficial in this patient, since they retard IgE-dependent release of mast cell granules. Therefore, prostaglandin inhibitors such as aspirin would complicate or perhaps exacerbate the clinical situation described here *(p. 1284)*.

3. (C) The lesion pictured is an intradermal nevocellular nevus. Nevocellular nevi are extremely common. Nearly every human being has one or more of these lesions, and the average number per individual in fair-skinned populations is 15. Nevi represent proliferations of melanocytic cells that originate from the neural crest and may appear congenitally or later in life. Neval cells grow in nests, which may be present at the dermal-epidermal junction alone (junctional nevus), only within the dermis (intradermal nevus), or in both places simultaneously (compound nevus). Neval cells tend to become progressively more spindle-shaped ("neuralize") at the edge of the lesion where they may deeply penetrate the dermis, but this has no biologic significance. Mitoses can rarely be seen but in increased numbers may suggest malignant transformation. Junctional nevi or nevi with a junctional component are most often associated with transformation to melanoma *(pp. 1275–1278)*.

4. (E) Marked hyperpigmentation can be a feature of basal cell carcinoma, seborrheic keratosis, or dermatofibroma, all of which are *nodular* lesions. When deeply pigmented, these lesions or the darkly pigmented blue nevus may be confused clinically with malignant melanoma. Lentigines, however, are never nodular; they are macular lesions that are usually tan-brown. Even if deeply pigmented, lentigo simplex is always small (5 to 10 mm) and has smooth, well-demarcated borders, unlike its premalignant cousin, the lentigo maligna (see Question 7) *(pp. 1263, 1265, 1268, 1275, 1277)*.

5. (E) Although the relationship of other forms of nevocellular nevi with malignant melanoma is still debated, it is well known that giant congenital hairy (pigmented) nevi give rise to malignant melanoma in 10 to 20% of cases. Because of its wide variety of histologic appearances, from epithelioid to sarcomatoid to anaplastic, melanoma is included in the differential diagnosis of a wide variety of malignant tumors. Diagnosis of melanoma can be further complicated by the occurrence of amelanotic tumors or by metastatic disease without an identifiable primary lesion. The latter may occur either because a primary cutaneous tumor has undergone spontaneous regression, as they are known to do, or because the melanoma has arisen in an unrecognized atypical site such as the uveal tract in the eye, the mucous membranes, or the gastrointestinal tract. Because there is, at present, no effective form of chemotherapy, radiation therapy, or immunotherapy, the treatment of melanoma is dependent upon adequate surgical resection. Prognosis correlates best with the stage (size of tumor and depth of penetration) of the malignancy at the time of resection *(pp. 1279–1282)*.

6. (D) Mycosis fungoides is a cutaneous T-cell lymphoma of unknown etiology that sometimes evolves into generalized systemic disease with involvement of lymph nodes and viscera. The development of a leukemia-like picture with spillage of the malignant cells into the peripheral blood is known as Sézary's syndrome.

Although the name is suggestive of fungal infection, mycosis fungoides bears no relation or resemblance to mycotic infection of the skin. Early lesions resemble eczema clinically and histologically, with epidermal hyperplasia, spongiosis, exocytosis, and a polymorphous inflammatory infiltrate of the upper dermis. Plaque-like lesions develop as the disease progresses and are characterized by an intensification of the features of the eczematous phase with the addition of Pautrier's microabscesses (collections of mycosis cells, see below) in the epidermis. These are not to be confused with the Munro's microabscesses of psoriasis, which are collections of neutrophils in the stratum corneum. The diagnosis of mycosis fungoides depends upon the identification of mycosis cells within the dermal inflammatory infiltrate. Mycosis cells are atypical lymphocytes with hyperchromatic, highly convoluted nuclei. Marker studies and functional studies have shown that these cells are actually T lymphocytes belonging to the *helper-cell* subset of T cells *(pp. 665, 1272–1273)*.

7. (A) Although all of these lesions represent proliferations of atypical, pleomorphic melanocytes, lentigo maligna is not considered a true malignancy. It is regarded as a premalignant condition, since despite its name, up to half of these lesions never become invasive. In 30 to 50% of cases, however, malignant melanoma does develop, and the invasive lesion is known as lentigo maligna melanoma. The development of nodules in a lentigo maligna, a brown-black macule, usually indicates invasion. The course is usually extremely indolent, with a latent period of 10 to 15 years between appearance of lentigo maligna and development of invasive melanoma. Once invasion occurs, the prognosis is determined by the depth of invasion exactly as it is for other forms of melanoma. Deep invasion is likely to occur more rapidly in nodular melanomas than in superficial spreading melanoma or in lentigo maligna melanoma. Melanomas arising in congenital nevi tend to be nodular and

carry the same unfavorable prognosis as nodular melanoma *(pp. 1279–1282)*.

8. (A) A reduction in the platelet count is the most common cause of generalized bleeding and is most commonly manifested by petechial skin lesions. Thrombocytopenia will result from any condition causing either decreased platelet production, increased platelet destruction, sequestration of platelets, or dilution of platelets (massive transfusions). Patients with acute leukemia have an increased risk of developing thrombocytopenia from several of these causes. Leukemic infiltration of the bone marrow replaces normal hematopoietic elements and causes decreased production of platelets. Administration of drugs, particularly chemotherapeutic agents, will further reduce normal hematopoiesis. Immunologic mechanisms associated with drugs or intercurrent infection may also cause increased platelet destruction. Patients with promyelogenous leukemia are especially prone to increased platelet destruction from disseminated intravascular coagulation (DIC), since the cytoplasmic granules that characterize the neoplastic promyelocytes are rich in a thromboplastin-like substance capable of activating the coagulation cascade.

Although patients with *chronic* myelogenous leukemia may develop massive splenomegaly leading to platelet sequestration (hypersplenism), splenomegaly is usually *not* a feature of the acute forms of leukemia *(pp. 679–684)*.

9. (D) Along with keratinocytes and melanocytes, Langerhans' cells are one of the three basic cell types of the epidermis. They are dendritic cells with clear cytoplasm and are characterized by distinctive tennis racquet–shaped cytoplasmic granules seen by electron microscopy. Since they contain hydrolytic enzymes and exhibit cell surface markers characteristic of monocytes and macrophages, it is likely that they are descendents of this cell line. Although the terminology is confusing, Langerhans' cells have nothing to do with the pancreatic islets of Langerhans or with the Langhans' giant cells of tubercular granulomata *(pp. 64, 972, 1259)*.

10. (A) Actinic (solar) keratosis is a premalignant lesion in which squamous cell carcinoma may develop. Since its incidence increases with increasing dosage of ionizing radiation, proximity to the equator is an important factor in its pathogenesis. Only fair-skinned individuals are susceptible to this effect, however. For both these reasons, then, actinic keratosis is much more common in fair-skinned Australians than in darker-skinned Indians living farther from the equator.

Although the lesions are often hyperplastic and hyperkeratotic, epidermal atrophy may also be seen. The essential microscopic feature of actinic keratosis, then, is *atypia* of the epidermal keratinocytes. This atypia may involve all but the most superficial cell layers, since by definition, involvement of the full thickness of the epidermis would constitute squamous cell carcinoma *in situ* (Bowen's disease). Likewise, the atypical cells of actinic keratosis never penetrate the underlying basement membrane, a feature that would be diagnostic of invasive squamous cell carcinoma (*p. 1265*).

11. (E) Xanthomas, lesions composed of foamy histiocytes, may occur in association with hyperlipidemic disorders (either acquired or familial), in normal individuals, or in association with malignancies. Acanthosis nigricans may arise in normal individuals but can also occur in association with malignancies. Both xanthoma and the malignant type of acanthosis nigricans are most frequently associated with the lymphoproliferative and myeloproliferative malignancies. Patients with lymphoma are also prone to develop second malignancies, especially cutaneous squamous cell carcinomas. Numerous conditions are associated with *cutaneous vasculitis:* lymphomas, leukemias, carcinomas, infections, drug sensitivities, C2 deficiency, and collagen vascular diseases. In contrast to the above disorders, mycosis fungoides is *itself* a T-cell lymphoma originating in the skin and is not a paraphenomenon of a lymphoproliferative disorder (*pp. 665, 1270, 1272, 1274, 1286*).

12. (B) Nevus flammeus, or port-wine stain, is a very *common* congenital lesion. Not to be confused with a nevocellular nevus, nevus flammeus is a developmental malformation of telangiectatic vessels (a congenital hemangioma). It commonly involutes spontaneously but may persist into adulthood. Nevus flammeus bears no resemblance to a halo nevus, which is a true nevocellular nevus with an associated lymphocytic infiltrate. Early lesions, although recognizable clinically, may show no apparent histopathologic changes and may resemble normal skin microscopically, but older lesions will contain dilated, thin-walled vessels.

Nevus flammeus occurs most commonly on the face and neck, although it may occasionally be found on one or more extremities (see below). Although there is no known association with congenital heart disease, associations with vascular malformations are well recognized and are known as: (1) the Sturge-Weber syndrome, when a nevus flammeus occurs in the fifth cranial nerve area of the face and is accompanied by ipsilateral retinal and meningeal angiomas; or (2) the Klippel-Trenaunay syndrome, when the nevus occurs on an extremity, and vascular malformations are found in the underlying soft tissues and bone (*pp. 1269–1270*).

13. (C) Mitosis occurring above the suprabasal cell layer of the epidermis indicates a pathologic process; in normal skin, it occurs only in the basal layer itself or at most one cell layer above the basal layer. In some inflammatory processes and in cell tumors of the epidermis, mitotic figures may be found in more superficial locations. Although lentigo simplex is characterized by a benign proliferation of melanocytes in the epidermis, the proliferating cells are limited to the basal layer. Mitoses are uncommon in this condition; their presence higher in the epidermis with superficial migration of melanocytes would indicate melanocytic malignancy rather than lentigo simplex. Bowen's disease is an intraepithelial squamous cell malignancy. In all epidermal malignancies, mitotic figures may be seen at any level from the deepest to the most superficial layers. Psoriasis is a disease characterized by very rapid turnover of epidermal keratinocytes, and mitoses commonly occur as high as two cell layers above the basal zone but rarely higher (*pp. 1258, 1266–1267, 1275, 1292*).

14. (E) A dermatofibroma is a vascular intradermal tumor of histiocytes acting as facultative fibroblasts. The lesion has many synonyms, including sclerosing hemangioma, fibrous xanthoma, and nodular subepidermal fibrosis. It is a benign variant in a family of histiocytic lesions called fibrous histiocytomas. The dermal lesions have poorly demarcated borders and are accompanied by hyperplasia and hyperpigmentation of the overlying epidermis, which can cause confusion with melanoma clinically. Hemosiderin deposition within the lesion itself may contribute to its pigmented appearance. The superficial fibrous histiocytomas of the dermis are almost always benign. Malignant fibrous histiocytomas do occur; however, they are usually large and located in deeper soft tissues and bone. They are recognized by their pleomorphism and high mitotic rate (*pp. 1267–1268, 1364*).

15. (E) Purpura represents hemorrhage into the skin, and when caused by inflammatory damage to the vessel wall, will produce palpable induration. An important cause of palpable purpura is cutaneous necrotizing vasculitis. This disorder produces fibrinoid necrosis of venular walls with extravasation of red blood cells and serum; neutrophils and nuclear debris are present in and around the walls of the damaged vessels. The lesions are believed to be produced by an immune complex–mediated mechanism (Type III hypersensitivity, p. 164) in which complement is activated.

Numerous diverse conditions are associated with this type of vasculitis. For some, the inciting antigen is well known; sensitivities to drugs, foreign proteins (e.g., serum sickness), viruses, and bacteria (intercurrent infections) are common examples. For others, the precise antigen is unknown; malignancies (leukemias, lymphomas, and carcinomas) collagen vascular diseases, Henoch-Schönlein purpura, and C2 deficiency are included in this group.

Although it is not mediated by immune complexes,

leukemic infiltration of the skin can be purpuric in nature and must always be included in the differential diagnosis of palpable purpura in this setting. The histopathology of these lesions is not that of a necrotizing vasculitis but of a dense dermal infiltrate of myeloid cells, including numerous immature forms (*pp. 683, 1285–1286*).

16. (B) Squamous cell carcinoma is the most common malignant tumor of skin, having significant potential for metastasis. Basal cell carcinoma is more common but virtually never metastasizes. In further contrast to basal cell carcinoma, squamous cell carcinomas most often arise from dysplastic premalignant lesions, including those induced by chronic sun exposure (actinic keratosis). Because they are sun-exposed, the backs of the hands and the face are common sites of occurrence. Only basal cell carcinomas, tumors that are also related to sun exposure, are curiously uncommon on the backs of the hands. For unknown reasons, squamous cell carcinomas arising in sun-damaged skin are about 10 to 20 times *less* likely to metastasize than those arising in other types of preexisting lesions (chronic ulcers or radiation-damaged skin), those arising on mucosal surfaces, or those occurring on genitalia. Whereas only about 2% of actinic-associated squamous cell carcinomas metastasize, 20 to 50% of those not associated with sun damage metastasize.

On mucous membranes, squamous cell carcinoma usually appears as white patches called leukoplakia, although leukoplakia is seen in benign conditions as well (*pp. 1265–1267*).

17. (A) Seborrheic keratosis, acanthosis nigricans, and erythema nodosum are all benign dermal lesions that can be associated with underlying malignancy. Seborrheic keratoses suddenly appearing in association with a gastrointestinal malignancy is called the sign of Leser-Trélat. The majority of malignancies associated with acanthosis nigricans are adenocarcinomas, most commonly of gastric origin. Erythema nodosum, although most often idiopathic or associated with infections or drugs, can also be associated with visceral malignancy. In contrast to the above disorders, Paget's disease presents actual invasion of the epidermis by malignant cells usually originating in an underlying or adjacent structure. It most often refers to nipple involvement by an underlying ductal carcinoma of breast (*pp. 1262, 1273, 1274, 1288*).

18. (B) Seborrheic keratosis is a common benign tumor of basaloid keratinocytes growing in cords and sheets and focally forming keratin-filled cysts ("horn cysts"). It is usually exophytic but occasionally grows inward, extending into the dermis (inverted follicular keratosis). When irritated, the lesion may develop groups of keratinized squamous cells and a lymphocytic inflammatory infiltrate in the dermis. The le-

sions are completely benign, however, and do not undergo malignant degeneration. They usually require no treatment and are excised only for itching, painful inflammation, cosmesis, or uncertain diagnosis. As they are frequently pigmented, they can resemble pigmented basal cell carcinoma or malignant melanoma clinically (*p. 1262*).

19 (A) Exuberant conical excrescences of keratin known as cutaneous horns may be the presenting clinical feature of numerous skin disorders. Viral lesions, actinic lesions, and squamous cell carcinomas may all appear clinically as cutaneous horns and require biopsy for definitive diagnosis. The gross appearance of basal cell carcinoma is usually that of a pearly, semitranslucent papule. Less common variations include brown or black nodules, plaques, or ulcerated lesions but not cutaneous horns (*pp. 1265–1266, 1298*).

20. (A) Erythema multiforme is an uncommon self-limited dermatosis believed to be a hypersensitivity response usually to an infection or drug. Its association with certain specific types of drugs is well established. Sulfonamides, for example, are among the primary offenders. Erythema nodosum, an acute inflammatory lesion of the subcutaneous fat, is also commonly associated with infections or the administration of certain drugs, especially sulfonamides. A nonimmunologic urticaria can also result from exposure to drugs such as antibiotics that act as direct mast cell–releasing agents. Rosacea is a common inflammatory dermatosis involving the central face whose etiology is unknown. Although rosacea may be exacerbated by alcohol, it has no other known drug associations (*pp. 1284–1285, 1288–1289*).

21. (B) Glomus bodies are smooth muscle cells regulating blood flow in the arteriovenous shunts in the skin and elsewhere in the body. Their function in the skin—temperature control—is mediated by the hypothalamus and the sympathetic nervous system. Tumors of these cells commonly occur on the distal portions of the fingers and toes where glomus bodies are most numerous. Tumors of glomus cells are exquisitely painful and bothersome but have virtually no malignant potential (*pp. 540–541*).

22. (B) Xeroderma pigmentosa is an autosomal recessive disorder characterized by a predisposition to chromosomal breakage secondary to a defect in enzyme-mediated DNA repair. The defect is manifested by an inability to repair acquired cellular mutations in the skin induced by ultraviolet irradiation and, hence, by an increased susceptibility to cutaneous malignancies. All epidermal malignancies (carcinomas and melanomas) as well as benign epidermal lesions that are known to be associated with the ionizing radiation of the sun (e.g., actinic keratosis) occur with greater frequency in individuals with xeroderma pigmentosa. In addition, even primary dermal tumors such as sarcomas, angiomas, and fibromas are increased in these patients. There is no evidence that patients with xeroderma pigmentosa are at increased risk of developing malignancies in noncutaneous sites, however. In fact, patients with xeroderma pigmentosa typically die at a young age from one of their many cutaneous malignancies and do not survive long enough to develop visceral or hematogenous malignancies (pp. 241, 1265, 1266, 1279).

23. (B) Keratocanthoma is a rapidly growing but benign tumor of keratinocytes. Its etiology is unknown, and the once popular theory of viral genesis has not been confirmed. There is no proven association with solar exposure. These lesions may closely resemble a squamous cell carcinoma histologically. They may deeply penetrate the underlying dermis but never beyond the depth of adjacent hair follicles. Differentiation from squamous cell carcinoma depends on the overall symmetrical, smooth contour of the lesion and the mature, homogenous "glassy" appearance of its component squamous cells (p. 1263).

24. (C); 25. (C); 26. (B); 27. (D); 28. (B)
(24 to 28) The Spitz nevus, once termed "juvenile melanoma," is an uncommon nevocellular nevus that is not often seen in children but can also occur in adults. Spitz nevi are benign in their biologic behavior but paradoxically are characterized by histologic features usually associated with malignancy. The cells are often highly infiltrative, extending deep into the dermis. Large atypical cells, multinucleate cells, and mitoses may be numerous among the spindle-shaped and epithelioid neval cells that compose the lesion. Pigmentation is usually sparse, and the nevus appears clinically as a pink-tan papule or nodule.

Dermal infiltration is not an innocuous feature in nodular malignant melanoma, however; its extent is the most important factor in determining the prognosis in this disease. Melanoma can occur in any age group, although it is most common between the ages of 40 and 60. In contrast to Spitz nevus, malignant melanoma is most often a heavily pigmented, brown-black lesion. Histologically, both have markedly atypical neoplastic melanocytes and frequent mitoses. Helpful features in differentiating the two lesions include the involvement of the overlying epidermis and the presence of atypical mitoses; these are seen in nodular melanoma but are lacking in Spitz nevi (pp. 1277–1282).

29. (A); 30. (C); 31. (D); 32. (C); 33. (D)
(29 to 33) Molluscum contagiosum and verruca vulgaris are the two most common viral lesions of skin. Molluscum contagiosum is caused by a pox virus, whereas verruca vulgaris is caused by a papovavirus. Both occur most frequently in children and young adults and are characterized by epidermal hyperplasia. Both may occur on mucous membranes. Virally infected keratinocytes in both conditions exhibit some of the same histologic changes: verruca cells show eosinophilic cytoplasmic inclusions and cytoplasmic vacuolization; nuclei are deeply basophilic and contain viral particles. Molluscum bodies (virally infected cells) are uniquely characterized by large, homogenous eosinophilic cytoplasmic inclusions containing replicating virions that compress the nucleus to one side of the cell. Although direct contact is implicated in transmission of both these diseases, neither one is highly contagious (pp. 1298–1299).

34. (A); 35. (A); 36. (A); 37. (C); 38. (A); 39. (D); 40. (B)
Despite the unfortunate similarity in their names, psoriasis and parapsoriasis are totally unrelated diseases, both clinically and pathologically. Psoriasis vulgaris is the most common type of a group of chronic skin disorders known collectively simply as psoriasis, all of which are characterized by epidermal proliferation.

(34) The itchy, scaly plaques of psoriasis are caused by the extremely rapid turnover time of the epidermal keratinocytes (3 or 4 days as compared with 28 days in normal skin). Parapsoriasis en plaques, in contrast, typically produces epidermal thinning.

(35) Whereas parapsoriasis en plaques is a disorder limited to the skin, psoriasis is often associated with disease in other organ systems, especially the joints (psoriatic arthritis), skeletal muscles, myocardium, and gastrointestinal tract.

(36) Factors known to precipitate the development of psoriasis include infection, trauma, and endocrine changes such as pregnancy. Precipitating factors in parapsoriasis are unknown.

(37) The most distinctive histologic feature of psoriasis is the epidermal neutrophilic microabscesses found in the subcorneal region (spongiform pustule of Kogoj) as well as intracorneally (Munro's microabscesses). Epidermal microabscesses also occur in parapsoriasis en plaques (see below).

(38 and 39) Psoriasis vulgaris is chronic and unremitting. It cannot be cured but can be treated with ultraviolet light and topical steroids. Parapsoriasis is also a chronic disorder but is usually asymptomatic and requires no treatment.

(40) Unlike psoriasis, parapsoriasis en plaques evolves into a lymphoreticular malignancy (usually mycosis fungoides) in a small number of cases. With evolution to malignancy, increasing numbers of atypical, hyperchromatic lymphoid cells with convoluted nuclei (mycosis cells) appear in the dermis (pp. 1291–1293).

41. (C); 42. (B); 43. (B); 44. (B); 45. (A); 46. (C); 47. (C)

(41) Lentigo maligna and superficial spreading melanoma (SSM) are both proliferative lesions of atypical melanocytes characterized by intraepithelial growth. Lentigo maligna, however, is considered a benign lesion with the *potential* for transformation to melanoma and subsequent invasion.

(42) Superficial spreading melanoma is a type of malignant melanoma with a propensity for lateral (horizontal) intraepithelial growth (Level I or *in situ* stage). Although SSM does eventually penetrate the basement membrane and invade deeply (vertical growth), the invasive phase is delayed as compared with nodular melanomas. Lentigo maligna does not penetrate the basement membrane unless it has undergone malignant transformation; it is then termed lentigo maligna melanoma.

(43) Although most common on sun-exposed areas, SSM may occur on any cutaneous site or on mucous membranes. Lentigo maligna occurs almost exclusively on sun-exposed cutaneous surfaces (usually the face) and does not arise in mucous membranes.

(44) SSM occurs in all age groups, although it is most common in middle-aged persons. Lentigo maligna, in contrast, occurs only in older adults (age 50 and older).

(45) The lesions of superficial spreading melanoma average 2 to 3 cm in diameter; those of lentigo maligna are commonly twice that size or even larger. **(46)** Similarities between the two lesions include their irregular borders and **(47)** the curative potential of surgical excision while the lesions remain localized to the epidermis *(pp. 1280–1282)*.

48. (E); 49. (A); 50. (D); 51. (C); 52. (A); 53. (D); 54. (B)

(48 to 54) Pemphigus vulgaris (PV), bullous pemphigoid (BP), and dermatitis herpetiformis (DH) are all blistering diseases of unknown etiology mediated by immune mechanisms. They are associated with autoantibodies directed against cutaneous antigens.

Bullous pemphigoid is characterized by linear deposits of complement-fixing IgG along the epidermal basement membrane. The basement membrane is destroyed, leading to the formation of subepidermal bullae. BP is a disease of the over-60 age group; it runs a chronic but self-limited course and often responds to steroid therapy.

Subepidermal blisters also characterize dermatitis herpetiformis. In this disease the immunoglobulin involved is IgA, which forms granular deposits along the dermal-epidermal junction. An additional microscopic feature is microabscess formation within the dermal papillae adjacent to the large vesicles, which helps to differentiate DH from BP. Furthermore, DH is a disease of younger adults and, interestingly, is usually associated with a gluten-sensitive enter-

opathy. The skin lesions respond to therapy with sulfonamides; they may also clear upon treatment of the associated enteropathy with a gluten-free diet.

In contrast to the above, pemphigus vulgaris is characterized not by subepidermal blistering but by acantholysis (lysis of the desmosomal junctions between epidermal keratinocytes) and suprabasal, intraepidermal blisters. The immunoglobulin responsible for the acantholytic lesion in pemphigus is an IgG autoantibody. PV most frequently affects individuals between ages 40 to 60. Extensive denudation of the skin and mucous membranes is a characteristic clinical feature and can lead to serious problems with electrolyte balance or infection. Before the advent of corticosteroid therapy, patients usually died of these complications. Even with therapy, this disease has a mortality rate of 40% *(pp. 1294–1296)*.

55. (A); 56. (D); 57. (E); 58. (C); 59. (B); 60. (A); 61. (C)

(55 and 60) Acne vulgaris is unique among the dermatoses listed in that its pathogenesis is known to be mediated by a bacterium. *Corynebacterium acnes*, although part of the normal skin flora, appears to be the major source of lipolytic enzymes that hydrolyze triglycerides of the sebum to form irritating free fatty acids that induce inflammation. The treatment of acne with broad-spectrum antibiotics is aimed at reducing the population of *C. acnes* *(p. 1289)*.

(56) Pityriasis rosea is a common self-limited dermatosis of unknown etiology affecting older children and young adults. It is characterized by an eruption of oval, salmon-colored patches in a "Christmas tree" distribution over the trunk. Resolution occurs in 2 to 14 weeks. Focal, "skipping" parakeratosis with a mixed acute and chronic inflammatory infiltrate in the superficial dermis, exocytosis, and spongiosis are the characteristic histologic features of the scaling plaques *(p. 1291)*.

(57) Pityriasis lichenoides et varioliformis acuta (PLEVA) is an uncommon papulovesicular disorder of unknown etiology. Any age group can be affected, but the disease occurs most commonly in young adults. Papules and vesicles arising in successive crops over the trunk and extremities characterize the disorder. The histologic features of the lesions include spongiosis, dyskeratosis, exocytosis, extravasated red cells, and parakeratosis. PLEVA has a course that varies from weeks to years but eventually remits spontaneously *(p. 1291)*.

(58 and 61) Lichen planus is a common inflammatory dermatosis that also affects mucous membranes in 70% of cases. Lesions appear as itchy, violaceous, flat-topped papules flecked with white dots or lines (Wickham's striae). The cardinal histologic feature is a band-like infiltrate of lymphocytes and histiocytes in the upper dermis hugging the epidermal border.

Basal vacuolization and hypergranulosis are also prominent. The disease is self-limited and will resolve spontaneously one to two years after its onset. Oral lesions, however, last longer and evolve into squamous cell carcinoma in 1 to 4% of cases (*p. 1290*).

(**59**) Rosacea (acne rosacea) is a common inflammatory skin disorder of unknown cause occurring in middle-aged adults. It usually involves the central face but, in contrast to acne vulgaris, spares the trunk. Lesions begin as erythematous areas in which papules and pustules later arise. In males, rhinophyma (telangiectasia and hyperplasia of the soft tissues of the nose) may occur and is exacerbated by alcohol abuse (the "W. C. Fields nose"). Microscopically, a loose perivascular lymphocytic infiltrate is seen around ectatic dermal vessels. Follicular pustules and perifollicular abscesses may also be present (*pp. 1289–1290*).

14

THE ENDOCRINE SYSTEM

DIRECTIONS: For Questions 1 to 11, choose the ONE BEST answer to each question.

1. After giving birth, a woman fails to lactate or menstruate. Which of the following is the most likely cause?

A. Pituitary infarction
B. A chromophobe adenoma
C. The empty sella syndrome
D. A hypothalamic glioma
E. A hypothalamic germ cell tumor

2. Thyroid gland enlargement is associated with all of the following conditions EXCEPT:

A. Ingestion of oral contraceptives
B. Puberty
C. Androgenic steroid therapy
D. Dietary iodine deficiency
E. Pregnancy

3. The most common cause of the syndrome of inappropriate antidiuretic hormone (SIADH) secretion is:

A. Subdural hematoma
B. Radiation injury to the hypothalamus
C. Meningitis
D. Oat cell carcinoma of lung
E. Pituitary adenoma

4. A goitrogen is a substance that:

A. Mimics the action of T_3
B. Mimics the action of T_4
C. Suppresses T_3 and T_4 synthesis
D. Mimics the action of TSH
E. Depletes the body of iodine

5. A 30-year-old female with infectious mononucleosis suddenly develops a painful enlarged thyroid. The most likely diagnosis is:

A. Subacute lymphocytic thyroiditis
B. Reidel's thyroiditis
C. Thyroid abscess
D. Subacute granulomatous thyroiditis
E. Hashimoto's thyroiditis

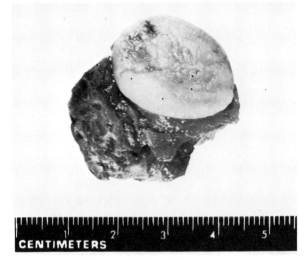

Figure 14–1

6. Thyroid enlargement is greatest in:

A. Grave's disease
B. Simple goiter
C. Hashimoto's thyroiditis
D. Multinodular goiter
E. de Quervain's thyroiditis

7. A lobe of thyroid removed from a male with thyrotoxicosis contained the 2.0-cm nodule pictured in Figure 14–1. It is most likely:

A. A medullary carcinoma
B. A papillary carcinoma
C. A multinodular goiter
D. A follicular carcinoma
E. A follicular adenoma

8. All of the following characteristics are associated with the thyroid lesion pictured in Figure 14–2 EXCEPT:

A. Aggressive biologic behavior and poor prognosis
B. Multifocality within the thyroid gland
C. Preference for lymphatic rather than hematogenous spread
D. Strong association with external irradiation
E. Appearance as a "cold" nodule on thyroid scan

9. Parathyroid hormone increases serum calcium by all of the following mechanisms EXCEPT:

A. Reduces renal calcium excretion
B. Increases intestinal absorption of calcium
C. Blocks calcitonin secretion from the thyroid
D. Produces an immediate efflux of calcium from bone
E. Produces a prolonged release of calcium from bone through osteoclast activation

10. On a check-up visit to his physician, a 50-year-old man who has noticed some muscular weakness and fatigability is found to have hypercalcemia by routine laboratory tests. Statistically, it is most likely that this man has:

A. Primary parathyroid hyperplasia
B. Secondary parathyroid hyperplasia
C. A parathyroid adenoma
D. A parathyroid carcinoma
E. A nonparathyroid carcinoma

11. Hyperaldosteronism associated with an adrenal adenoma is known as:

A. Bartter's syndrome
B. Nelson's syndrome
C. Conn's syndrome
D. Cushing's syndrome
E. None of these

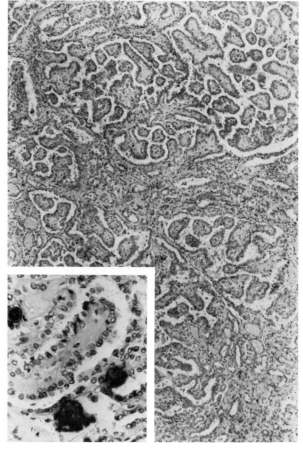

Figure 14–2

DIRECTIONS: For Questions 12 to 17, ONE or MORE of the completions given correctly finishes the incomplete statement. Choose:

A—if only *1,2, and 3* are correct
B—if only *1 and 3* are correct
C—if only *2 and 4* are correct
D—if only *4* is correct
E—if all are correct

12. Somatostatin exerts inhibitory control over:

1. Insulin
2. Glucagon
3. Gastrin
4. Growth hormone

A. 1,2,3   B. 1,3   C. 2,4   D. 4 Only   E. All

13. Which of the following characteristics describes the disease of the thyroid pictured in Figure 14–3?

1. Occurs predominantly in women

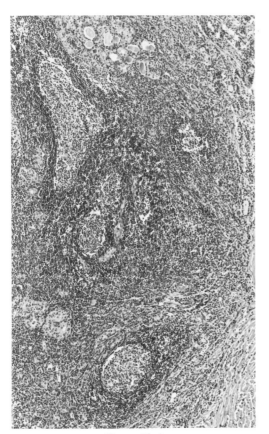

Figure 14–3

2. Is caused by a suppressor cell deficiency
3. Is characterized by TSH-receptor autoantibodies
4. Is characterized by antimicrosomal antibodies

A. 1,2,3   B. 1,3   C. 2,4   D. 4 Only   E. All

14. Features associated with medullary carcinoma of the thyroid include:

1. Neurosecretory granules
2. Amyloid stroma
3. Prostaglandin production
4. Calcitonin production

A. 1,2,3   B. 1,3   C. 2,4   D. 4 Only   E. All

15. Most females born with 21-hydroxylase deficiency would be expected to have:

1. Hypertension
2. Clitoral hypertrophy
3. Reduced aldosterone levels
4. Elevated ACTH levels

A. 1,2,3   B. 1,3   C. 2,4   D. 4 Only   E. All

16. The possible occurrence of pheochromocytoma should be expected in patients with which of the following disorders?

1. Medullary carcinoma of the thyroid
2. Pituitary adenoma
3. Parathyroid adenoma
4. Pancreatic islet cell adenoma

A. 1,2,3   B. 1,3   C. 2,4   D. 4 Only   E. All

17. Thymomas:

1. Are composed of neoplastic T cells
2. Are often associated with myasthenia gravis
3. Respond to treatment with thymosin
4. Rarely occur in children

A. 1,2,3   B. 1,3   C. 2,4   D. 4 Only   E. All

DIRECTIONS: For Questions 18 to 22, you are to decide whether EACH choice is TRUE or FALSE.

For each of the following statements about Graves' disease, choose whether it is TRUE or FALSE.

18. It can be distinguished from all other forms of thyrotoxicosis by the presence of proptosis
19. It is usually caused by toxic nodular goiter

20. Virtually all patients have anti-TSH autoantibodies
21. It has the same HLA genotype association as Hashimoto's thyroiditis
22. Localized myxedema is a characteristic clinical feature

DIRECTIONS: For Questions 23 to 51, the set of lettered headings is followed by a list of numbered words or phrases. For each numbered word or phrase choose:
    A—if the item is associated with (A) only
    B—if the item is associated with (B) only
    C—if the item is associated with *both* (A) and (B)
    D—if the item is associated with *neither* (A) nor (B)

For each of the following characteristics, choose whether it describes Cushing's syndrome, acromegaly, both, or neither.

    A. Cushing's syndrome
    B. Acromegaly
    C. Both
    D. Neither

23. Caused by basophilic adenoma of the pituitary
24. Caused by lung cancer
25. Rarely associated with visual field defects
26. Produces hyperglycemia
27. Produces hypertension
28. Produces osteoporosis
29. Produces hyperpigmentation

For each of the characteristics listed below, choose whether it describes myxedema, Addison's disease, both, or neither.

    A. Myxedema
    B. Addison's disease
    C. Both
    D. Neither

30. In adults, the disease is most commonly caused by an autoimmune process
31. Fatigability and constipation are common symptoms
32. Hypertension is frequently produced
33. Cardiomyopathy is characteristic
34. Hyperpigmentation is characteristic
35. Mental dysfunction is common
36. Candidiasis and hypoparathyroidism are associated disorders

For each of the characteristics listed below, choose whether it describes pheochromocytoma, neuroblastoma, both, or neither.

    A. Pheochromocytoma
    B. Neuroblastoma
    C. Both
    D. Neither

37. Characteristically elaborates catecholamines
38. Primarily affects children over the age of 5
39. Is virtually always malignant
40. Carries a worse prognosis when occurring in extra-adrenal sites
41. Occasionally regresses spontaneously

For each of the statements below, choose whether it describes insulin-dependent diabetes mellitus, non–insulin-dependent diabetes mellitus, both, or neither:

    A. Insulin-dependent diabetes mellitus (IDDM)
    B. Non–insulin-dependent diabetes mellitus (NIDDM)
    C. Both
    D. Neither

42. Underutilization of glucose is characteristic
43. Cellular insulin resistance is a major feature
44. Obesity is a major pathogenetic factor
45. Autoantibodies against pancreatic islet cells are characteristic
46. Strong associations with specific HLA types exist
47. Viral infection of the islet cells is causally related in some cases
48. Hyperglucagonemia is usually present
49. Most treated individuals do not develop retinopathy
50. Most treated individuals now enjoy a normal life expectancy
51. Ketoacidosis is a major cause of death

DIRECTIONS: Questions 52 to 69 are matching questions. For each numbered item, choose the most likely associated lettered item from those provided. Each numbered item has ONLY ONE answer. Within each group, each lettered item may be the answer to one, more than one, or none of the numbered items.

For each of the endocrine organs listed below, choose whether its embryologic origin is from Rathke's pouch, the foramen cecum, pharyngeal pouches, or none of these.

    A. Rathke's pouch
    B. Foramen cecum
    C. Pharyngeal pouches
    D. None of these

52. Thyroid gland
53. Parathyroid glands
54. Thymus gland
55. Anterior pituitary gland
56. Posterior pituitary gland
57. Pineal gland

For each of the characteristics listed below, choose whether it describes prolactin, growth hormone, corticotropin, thyrotropin, or none of these.

    A. Prolactin
    B. Growth hormone
    C. Corticotropin
    D. Thyrotropin
    E. None of these

58. A hormone produced in the hypothalamus
59. The hormone most often secreted by chromophobes

60. Cause of the most common endocrinopathy produced by pituitary tumors
61. A hormone rarely elaborated by pituitary adenomas
62. A hormone frequently secreted by pituitary carcinomas
63. The most common hormone to be affected in an isolated pituitary hormone deficiency
64. First hormone to produce a clinically evident deficiency in panlobular pituitary destruction

For each of the characteristics listed below, choose whether it describes pituitary dwarfism, cretinism, achondroplastic dwarfism, or none of these.

    A. Pituitary dwarfism
    B. Cretinism
    C. Achondroplastic dwarfism
    D. None of these

65. Characterized by autosomal dominant inheritance
66. Produces mental retardation
67. Produces a large head and body relative to extremities
68. Associated with a broad flat nose and large tongue
69. Cannot be prevented with treatment

14

THE ENDOCRINE SYSTEM

ANSWERS

1. (A) Postpartum pituitary necrosis, also known as Sheehan's syndrome, is one of the three most common causes of pituitary hypofunction. Nonfunctioning (usually chromophobe) pituitary adenomas and the empty sella syndrome constitute the other two, but these are not related to pregnancy. It is believed that during pregnancy the pituitary enlarges to almost twice its normal size, compressing its own venous vasculature and causing relative ischemia. Thus, an episode of sudden systemic hypotension, such as that which may occur from blood loss during delivery, precipitates ischemic necrosis of the anterior lobe. The posterior pituitary, which is less vulnerable to anoxia, is spared.

Hypothalamic tumors such as gliomas or germ cell tumors are also known to occasionally cause anterior pituitary hypofunction but do so far less commonly than the disorders mentioned above. Furthermore, unlike Sheehan's syndrome, they have no known association with pregnancy (*pp. 1198–1200*).

2. (C) Thyroid function is determined by a complex set of physiologic stimuli and regulatory feedback mechanisms at the level of the hypothalamus and pituitary as well as within the thyroid gland itself (autoregulatory feedback loop). Physiologic stimuli that cause an increase in both glandular size and function include puberty, pregnancy, or stress from any source. Contributory physiologic mechanisms are often multiple in these circumstances. For example, pregnancy and other situations associated with increased estrogens (e.g., oral contraceptive steroid ingestion) increase serum levels of thyroid-binding globulin (TBG). Increased TBG levels increase the amount of T_3 and T_4, which are bound and concomitantly reduce the unbound (active) fractions. Decreased serum concentrations of free hormones, in turn, reduce feedback inhibition of the anterior pituitary, resulting in thyroid stimulating hormone (TSH) release and thyroid stimulation.

Lack of iodine in the diet also leads to thyroid stimulation. Since iodine is the critical element in the synthesis of both T_3 and T_4, iodine deficiency leads to decreased synthesis of these hormones and a compensatory increase in TSH. Thus, the thyroid is stimulated to increase the number of follicular cells and hormone output to achieve a euthyroid state. In addition, through autoregulation within the thyroid

gland itself, follicular cells become more efficient in extracting and concentrating iodine.

In contrast to the effects of increased estrogens, androgenic steroids produce the converse effect on thyroid activity by lowering serum levels of TBG (*pp. 1202, 1212*).

3. (D) The syndrome of inappropriate antidiuretic hormone (SIADH) secretion is a condition characterized by independent elaboration and secretion of ADH irrespective of plasma osmolarity. Although under normal conditions the posterior lobe of the pituitary is the source of ADH, this is not often the case in syndromes of inappropriate ADH secretion. Far more commonly, the source of inappropriate ADH secretion is a nonendocrine tumor. Approximately 80% of all cases are caused by bronchogenic carcinoma, especially oat cell carcinoma. Although subdural hematoma, as well as other types of intracranial hemorrhage or infections in and around the central nervous system (e.g., meningitis), may occasionally underlie this syndrome, they do so far less commonly than nonendocrine malignancies.

In contrast to conditions causing an overproduction of ADH, inflammatory injury or neoplastic involvement of the hypothalamo-hypophyseal axis (e.g., by radiation or a pituitary adenoma) usually leads to ADH deficiency and diabetes insipidus. Although mentioned above as an uncommon cause of increased ADH secretion, meningitis is also known to occasionally result in decreased ADH secretion and produce diabetes insipidus (*p. 1200*).

4. (C) A goitrogen is any chemical agent that suppresses the synthesis of T_3 and T_4. With the suppression of thyroid hormone synthesis, feedback inhibition to the hypothalamus and pituitary is reduced. In turn, increased amounts of TSH are released, causing nodular hyperplastic enlargement of the thyroid gland, a condition known as goiter (*p. 1212*).

5. (D) The sudden development of an enlarged painful thyroid in association with some form of viral infection (e.g., infectious mononucleosis, mumps, or an upper respiratory tract infection) is characteristic of a self-limited inflammation of the thyroid gland known as subacute granulomatous thyroiditis, or de Quervain's thyroiditis. This entity is 3 to 6 times more common in females than in males, and its peak incidence is in the 2nd to 5th decades of life. In contrast to de Quervain's thyroiditis, subacute lymphocytic thyroiditis and Reidel's thyroiditis are painless processes and have no association with prior viral infections. Hashimoto's thyroiditis, which may occasionally be painful and usually occurs in females, has no known association with viral illness. Whereas thyroid abscesses may occur from direct extension of a local infectious process or even by metastatic spread, this is extremely uncommon and would not be expected in the setting of a viral illness such as infectious mononucleosis (*pp. 1206–1209*).

6. (**D**) Multinodular goiter is associated with the most extreme enlargement of the thyroid gland, which may achieve weights of over 2000 grams in this disorder. Although Graves' disease, simple goiter, Hashimoto's thyroiditis, and de Quervain's thyroiditis all produce thyroid enlargement, it is usually modest in comparison, perhaps 2- to 3-fold greater than normal (*pp. 1213–1214*).

7. (**E**) A discrete, encapsulated single nodule is apparent in the otherwise normal thyroid lobe pictured. Since the patient has thyrotoxicosis, it is most likely that this nodule representa s functioning thyroid adenoma. Although most adenomas do not function and appear as "cold" nodules on thyroid scan, some are associated with hyperfunction; these accumulate radioiodine and appear as "hot" nodules. Along with Graves' disease and toxic multinodular goiter, toxic adenomas are one of the three most common causes of thyrotoxicosis. Only rarely do well-differentiated thyroid carcinomas secrete sufficient thyroid hormone to cause clinical hyperthyroidism; moreover, in such instances, the tumor is usually widely metastatic. Medullary carcinoma of the thyroid originates from the neurosecretory parafollicular cell of the thyroid follicles. Multinodular goiter (toxic type), although a major cause of thyrotoxicosis, is characterized by multiple thyroid nodules with enlargement of the entire gland and would not correspond to the single nodule within a normal lobe that is pictured (*pp. 1204, 1214, 1216, 1223*).

8. (**A**) A papillary carcinoma of the thyroid with characteristic psammoma bodies is pictured in the photomicrograph. Papillary adenocarcinoma is the most common form of thyroid cancer, but the great majority of these are indolent in their biologic behavior and have an excellent prognosis. Among the salient features of this tumor are its tendency to be multifocal within the thyroid gland as a result of intraglandular spread and its preference for local lymphatic rather than hematogenous metastasis. Many cases of papillary thyroid carcinoma are associated with prior exposure to ionizing radiation, which is now known to cause thyroid carcinoma in 4 to 9% of exposed individuals. Although papillary tumors are not the only radiation-associated thyroid

cancers, they are the most common. Papillary carcinomas usually appear as cold nodules on thyroid scintiscans. Although a small number of papillary tumors may concentrate iodine and elaborate thyroglobulin, they are less likely to do so than well-differentiated follicular carcinomas (*pp. 1219–1221*).

9. (**C**) Parathyroid hormone, the most important physiologic regulator of serum calcium levels, has several modes of action. It acts to raise serum calcium by reducing renal excretion and increasing intestinal absorption of the element. It also modulates calcium stores in the bone by two separate mechanisms. It produces an immediate efflux of calcium from bone into the blood within minutes and subsequently produces a prolonged release of calcium from bone through an increase in the number and activity of osteoclasts. However, PTH has no known direct effect on the secretion of calcitonin, the calcium-lowering hormone produced by the C cells of the thyroid (*p. 1226*).

10. (**E**) Hypercalcemia is caused at least as frequently by nonparathyroid cancer as by all other forms of hyperparathyroidism combined. Parathyroid adenomas and primary parathyroid hyperplasia constitute 95% of cases of primary hyperparathyroidism. Secondary hyperparathyroidism is most commonly the result of renal insufficiency and, in contrast to the primary form, is characterized by *hypo*calcemia. Parathyroid carcinoma, although a cause of primary parathyroid hyperfunction, is indeed rare (*pp. 1226–1230*).

11. (**C**) Conn's syndrome is caused by an adrenal adenoma producing large amounts of aldosterone. This syndrome is characterized by sodium retention and potassium wasting, which in turn cause hypertension and neuromuscular abnormalities.

Bartter's syndrome is a form of secondary hyperaldosteronism caused by overproduction of renin by the kidneys. In contrast to other forms of secondary hyperaldosteronism, the blood pressure is often low in Bartter's syndrome instead of increased. Nelson's syndrome, in contrast, has little to do with the adrenals. It is caused by hypersecretion of ACTH from a pituitary tumor that cannot be eradicated and therefore necessitates removal of the end organs. Following bilateral adrenalectomy, the feedback inhibition of cortisol on the pituitary adenoma is removed, and intense hyperpigmentation related to excess production of ACTH and melanotropin ensues. Although Cushing's syndrome may be caused by a hyperfunctioning adrenal adenoma, it would be the result of a cortisol-producing rather than an aldosterone-producing tumor (*p. 1240*).

12. (**E**) Somatostatin is an intriguing inhibitory hormone that is produced in the hypothalamus as well

as in many other tissues throughout the body. It exerts inhibitory control over a number of other hormones, including insulin, glucagon, gastrin, and growth hormone. Thus, it plays a number of physiologic roles in addition to its well-known function as a release-inhibiting factor controlling growth hormone release from the anterior pituitary (*p. 1193*).

13. (E) The photomicrograph shows the typical microscopic features of Hashimoto's thyroiditis. Extensive infiltration of the thyroid by lymphoid cells in all stages of transformation and differentiation with the formation of germinal centers dominates the histologic picture. Clusters of thyroid follicles persist but are atrophic. This disease, which occurs 10 times more frequently in women than in men, is an organ-specific autoimmune disorder thought to be caused by a deficiency in thyroid antigen–specific suppressor T cells. The result is an uncontrolled immunologic attack on follicular cells by cytotoxic T cells and an unregulated T helper cell participation in the formation of autoantibodies. The autoantibodies most commonly isolated from patients with Hashimoto's thyroiditis are TSH-receptor antibodies and thyroid micrsomal antibodies. Some of the TSH-receptor autoantibodies appear to mimic the stimulatory action of TSH, whereas others simply block the hormone receptor site (*pp. 1206–1207*).

14. (E) Medullary carcinoma of the thyroid is a neuroendocrine tumor derived from the C cells of the thyroid. Histologically, one of its most distinctive features is amyloid stroma. As in other neuroendocrine neoplasms, neurosecretory dense core granules can be identified in the cytoplasm of medullary carcinoma cells when examined by electron microscopy. Approximately 80 to 90% of these tumors elaborate the major product of their cell of origin—the calcium-lowering hormone, calcitonin. Less frequently, medullary carcinomas produce prostaglandins which induce diarrhea in about 30% of patients (*pp. 1222–1223*).

15. (C) Ninety per cent of cases of virilizing congenital adrenal hyperplasia are caused by a 21-hydroxylase deficiency. This defect impairs the synthesis of cortisol and shunts the precursors into the alternate pathway of androgen production. As a result of increased androgens, females with this syndrome would be expected to show signs of virilization such as clitoral hypertrophy. Due to the block in cortisol synthesis, feedback inhibition to the pituitary is reduced and ACTH secretion is consequently increased. In this syndrome of simple virilizing congenital adrenal hyperplasia, however, aldosterone is produced normally. In contrast to 11-hydroxylase deficiency in which the mineralocorticoid 11-deoxycorticosterone is produced in excess and causes hy-pertension, 21-hydroxylase deficiency does *not* result in hypertension (*p. 1242*).

16. (B) Pheochromocytoma is a neoplasm of the adrenal medulla that usually occurs sporadically but is also known to occur in several different familial syndromes. The tumor has at least four hereditary patterns, two of which are part of a multiple endocrine neoplasia syndrome. In Sipple's syndrome (multiple endocrine neoplasia, type II$_a$), pheochromocytoma is associated with medullary carcinoma of the thyroid and parathyroid adenoma or hyperplasia. In this syndrome, which is transmitted by autosomal dominant inheritance, the pheochromocytomas are bilateral in 60 to 100% of cases. Other hereditary patterns of pheochromocytoma include: multiple endocrine neoplasia, type II$_b$ (MEN II$_b$), in which the pheochromocytoma is associated with mucosal neuromas and a marfanoid habitus; a simple autosomal dominant hereditary predisposition to pheochromocytomas; and a familial syndrome in which pheochromocytoma is associated with neurofibromatosis.

Pituitary adenomas and pancreatic islet cell adenomas are part of MEN I, in which they are associated with parathyroid and adrenocortical adenomas. They are not part of the constellation of endocrine adenomas associated with pheochromocytoma (*pp. 264, 1244*).

17. (C) Thymomas, although rare, are the most common neoplasm of the thymus gland and one of the most common anterior mediastinal tumors. The neoplastic element of a thymoma is not the thymic lymphocyte but rather the thymic *epithelial* cell. In the normal gland, this cell is the source of a humoral factor known as thymosin that influences the differentiation of thymocytes (T cells). Patients with thymomas have a striking predisposition to the development of myasthenia gravis, an autoimmune disorder characterized by autoantibodies to acetylcholine receptors in skeletal muscle motor end-plates. Approximately 45% of patients with thymoma develop myasthenia gravis, and conversely, thymic abnormalities are present in about 75% of patients with myasthenia gravis (thymic follicular hyperplasia in 60–65%; thymomas in 10–15%). The relationship between these two diseases is still unclear. However, it is thought that the thymoma leads to a derangement of T cell development with a loss of self-tolerance and the development of self-reactive clones. Furthermore, one of the structural elements of the normal thymus is a skeletal muscle-like cell, called a myoid cell, that may participate in the pathogenesis of myasthenia gravis.

The great majority of thymomas occur in adults; the average age of patients with thymomas is 50 years. The great majority of these neoplasms are benign and can be cured by surgical excision. Malignant thymomas are rare and have a poor prognosis despite surgical resection and postoperative irradiation. Thymosin, although used in the treatment of some lymphoid malignancies, would not be expected to have an effect on the epithelium-derived thymoma (*pp. 1250–1252, 1310–1312*).

18. (True); 19. (False); 20. (True); 21. (False); 22. (True)

Graves'disease is thyrotoxicosis caused by a hyperfunctioning diffuse hyperplastic goiter accompanied by ophthalmopathy and sometimes dermopathy.

(**18**) Although other forms of thyrotoxicosis may have eye changes such as retraction of the upper eyelid and lid lag, only in Graves' disease is there protrusion of the globe (proptosis) caused by autoimmune and inflammatory processes.

(**19**) In addition to Graves' disease and functioning thyroid adenomas, toxic nodular goiter is one of the three major causes of thyrotoxicosis. However, as stated above, Graves' disease refers only to *diffuse* hyperfunctioning goiter.

(**20**) Graves' disease is an autoimmune disorder in which anti–TSH-receptor antibodies mimic the action of TSH on thyroid follicular cells, inducing thyroid growth and hyperfunction. With sensitive assay techniques, anti-TSH antibodies can be identified in virtually all patients with Graves' disease.

(**21**) Although Graves' disease and Hashimoto's thyroiditis are both thyroid-specific autoimmune disorders, they have separate and distinctive genotype associations. Graves' disease is associated with the HLA-DR3 genotype, whereas Hashimoto's thyroiditis is associated with the HLA-DR5 genotype. Presumably, this difference in genotypic association is related to the difference in the type of TSH-receptor autoantibodies produced in each of these diseases. In Graves' disease the autoantibodies are predominantly stimulatory, whereas in Hashimoto's thyroiditis blocking antibodies may play a more important role.

(**22**) The dermopathy that is present in about 10 to 15% of patients with Graves' disease takes the form of localized areas of skin thickening (dermal edema) over the dorsum of the legs or feet. Despite the fact that this is a characteristic feature of Graves' disease, the change has been called localized "myxedema" (*pp. 1203–1204, 1210–1212*).

23. (A); 24. (A); 25. (A); 26. (C); 27. (C); 28. (C); 29. (A)

Cushing's syndrome and acromegaly are syndromes of hormonal excess caused respectively by cortisol and growth hormone. In the case of Cushing's syndrome, overproduction of cortisol may be caused either by a functioning neoplasm in the adrenal cortex or by adrenal response to elevated plasma levels of ACTH. (**23**) Thus, Cushing's syndrome is caused by functioning basophilic adenomas of the pituitary in about 60 to 70% of cases. (**24**) Less commonly (10 to

15% of cases), the disorder is produced by nonendocrine cancers that elaborate ACTH, producing Cushing's syndrome as a paraneoplastic phenomenon. The most common ACTH-producing tumors are bronchogenic carcinomas (particularly oat cell carcinoma), and altogether they account for about 60% of cases of ectopic Cushing's syndrome.

(**25**) Any functional pituitary tumor of sufficient size can cause manifestations of a space-occupying lesion in addition to hyperpituitarism. ACTH-producing adenomas, however, are usually small (microadenomas) and rarely cause the visual disorders associated with enlarging masses in the sella turcica. Visual field defects, usually homonymous hemianopsia, most commonly result from pituitary tumors, which tend to be large (e.g., growth hormone–secreting adenomas) and impinge on the immediately adjacent optic chiasm and optic nerve.

(**26**) Hyperglycemia and (**27**) hypertension are clinical characteristics of both Cushing's syndrome and acromegaly. In both of these conditions, in fact, glucose intolerance may be severe enough to produce overt diabetes mellitus. (**28**) Another feature common to both of these disorders is osteoporosis. (**29**) Only Cushing's syndrome of pituitary origin, however, is associated with hyperpigmentation. With increased secretion of ACTH, there is a concomitant overproduction of melanotropin, a melanocyte-stimulating hormone derived from cleavage of the polypeptide precursor of ACTH (*pp. 1194, 1196, 1238–1240*).

30. (C); 31. (C); 32. (D); 33. (A); 34. (B); 35. (A); 36. (B)

Myxedema and Addison's disease are endocrine deficiency syndromes caused by hypofunction of the thyroid and the adrenal cortex respectively. Both have profound systemic effects, some of which are similar in the two diseases.

(**30**) In adults, both myxedema and Addison's disease are most commonly caused by autoimmune processes. Hashimoto's thyroiditis, the archetype of organ-specific autoimmune diseases, is the most common cause of goitrous hypothyroidism in regions having a sufficiency of iodine. Although in the past tuberculosis was the most common cause of Addison's disease, at present the disorder is usually the result of so-called idiopathic adrenalitis, a condition believed to be autoimmune in origin. In addition, as part of a polyglandular autoimmune syndrome, the two conditions may be associated with one another or with another autoimmune disorder such as pernicious anemia or diabetes mellitus.

(**31**) Certain clinical manifestations such as fatigability and constipation are common in both diseases. (**32**) Hypertension, however, is a feature of neither myxedema nor Addison's disease. On the contrary, virtually all patients with Addison's disease are hypotensive. (**33**) Moreover, those with full-blown myxedema usually have symptoms of congestive heart failure, the result of a characteristic cardiomyopathy. The term "myxedema heart" refers to this pathologically distinctive process of interstitial mucopolysaccharide deposition and swelling of myofibers with loss of striations. A dilated, flabby heart is the typical end result.

(34) Hyperpigmentation is a distinguishing feature of Addison's disease. It results from increased secretion of ACTH as a result of lowered serum cortisol levels and reduced feedback inhibition to the hypothalamus and pituitary. Increased synthesis of both ACTH and melanotropin ensues, melanocytes are stimulated, and hyperpigmentation results.

(35) In contrast to cortisol insufficiency, lack of thyroid hormones produces a slowing of mental as well as physical processes. Thus, myxedema causes a reduction in intellectual function that is not seen in Addison's disease.

(36) As mentioned above, both myxedema and Addison's disease may be associated with other autoimmune diseases. It has recently become evident, however, that syndromes of multiple autoimmune disorders that include Addison's disease fall into two distinct subsets. Type I is characterized by at least two of the triad of Addison's disease, hypoparathyroidism, and mucocutaneous candidiasis. Type II, also known as Schmidt's syndrome, is characterized by Addison's disease, autoimmune thyroid disease, and/or insulin-dependent diabetes mellitus without hypoparathyroidism or candidiasis (pp. 1205–1206, 1235–1236).

37. (C); 38. (D); 39. (B); 40. (A); 41. (B)

Pheochromocytoma and neuroblastoma constitute the two most significant disease processes of the adrenal medulla. The pheochromocytoma originates from the adrenal medullary chromaffin cell, whereas the neuroblastoma is derived from autonomic ganglion cell precursors known as neuroblasts. (37) Both of these tumors characteristically elaborate catecholamines, predominantly norepinephrine in both cases. (38) Although both tumor types do occur in children over 5, this is not the primary age group in which either arises. The principal age group affected by neuroblastoma is children under the age of 5. Pheochromocytoma is most common in the 4th and 5th decades. (39) In sharp contrast to pheochromocytomas, which are usually benign, neuroblastomas are virtually always malignant and usually metastatic by the time the diagnosis is made. (40) Pheochromocytomas occurring in the adrenal are malignant in only 2 to 5% of cases. Thus, they have a better prognosis than their extra-adrenal counterparts, which are as much as 15 times more likely to be malignant. Neuroblastomas, although invariably malignant, carry a poorer prognosis when arising from the adrenal than when occurring in extra-adrenal sites. (41) One of the most intriguing and unpredictable behavioral features of neuroblastoma is occasional spontaneous

regression, presumably the result of an immunologic response to the tumor. Even more unusual, the highly malignant neuroblastoma may undergo differentiation into a benign ganglioneuroma. This unusual biologic behavior is associated only with neuroblastoma and is not known to occur with pheochromocytoma (pp. 1244–1248).

42. (C); 43. (B); 44. (B); 45. (A); 46. (A); 47. (A); 48. (C); 49. (D); 50. (D); 51. (D)

Diabetes mellitus is a chronic endocrine disorder characterized by an absolute or relative deficiency of insulin. Marked derangements in the metabolism of carbohydrate, fat, and protein are the result. The disease has two major variants: insulin-dependent diabetes mellitus (IDDM), constituting about 10% of cases, and non–insulin-dependent diabetes mellitus (NIDDM), accounting for the remaining 90%.

(42) Although the two variants have numerous distinctive features, they have in common an inability to utilize glucose. (43) In contrast to IDDM, which is the result of injury to the beta cells of the pancreatic islets producing an absolute and severe lack of insulin, only a relative lack of insulin is present in NIDDM. However, NIDDM has an additional pathogenetic feature: namely, resistance to the action of insulin at the cellular level. This universal feature of NIDDM is the result of both a decrease in cellular insulin receptors and an impairment of the postreceptor effects of insulin within the cell. (44) Obesity is a major contributing factor to the pathogenesis of NIDDM. Even in otherwise normal individuals, obesity is associated with an increased resistance to insulin. Its presence in those with an underlying genetic predisposition to insulin resistance fosters the expression of a diabetic state. It is significant that approximately 80% of patients with NIDDM are considerably overweight and that weight loss in the overweight diabetic notably improves the metabolic derangement.

(45) In contrast to NIDDM, IDDM is believed to be an organ-specific (more accurately in this case, a cell-specific) autoimmune disorder. Islet cell autoantibodies can be found in 60 to 90% of all newly diagnosed cases of IDDM. Some of these antibodies are known to be complement-fixing and are capable of causing pancreatic islet cell membrane damage in vitro. In some patients there is also evidence for a cellular immune response in the form of sensitized T cells reactive against beta cells. Indeed, lymphocytes are a characteristic histologic finding in the pancreatic islets of young diabetics with IDDM, a phenomenon known as "insulitis."

(46) Although there are no specific genetic markers for either form of diabetes, it is certain that diabetes mellitus is at least in part a genetic disorder. Epidemiologic studies indicate that genetic factors play a much larger role in the induction of NIDDM than in that of IDDM. In NIDDM, for example, the con-

cordance rate between identical twins is over 90%, as contrasted with only about 50% concordance in IDDM. However, IDDM shows a strong association with certain histocompatibility types, whereas it has not been possible to demonstrate a relationship between NIDDM and specific HLA types. Among IDDM patients there is a significant increase in the frequency of HLA-B8, B15, B18, Dw3, Dw4, DR3, and DR4 antigens. (47) There is also ample evidence that in a few cases IDDM may be caused by a direct, severe virus-induced injury of the pancreatic beta cells. In the majority of cases, however, IDDM is believed to result from a combination of factors that may include viral infection but also involve HLA-linked genetic factors as well as immunologic factors.

(48) Yet another contributory factor to the pathogenesis of diabetes mellitus is a concomitant overproduction of glucagon, which can be demonstrated in both major forms of diabetes. Since the metabolic effects of glucagon are directly opposite to those of insulin, absolute or relative insulin deficiency is exacerbated by glucagon excess.

(49) Despite the major etiologic differences between IDDM and NIDDM, their major systemic pathologic manifestations are remarkably similar. One of the most common and characteristic pathologic features of diabetes, regardless of type, is a group of retinal vascular changes known collectively as diabetic retinopathy. It has been estimated that a patient with a 25-year history of diabetes mellitus has a 90% chance of developing this complication. (50) Unfortunately, both major variants of diabetes also share a shortened life expectancy. On the average, life expectancy for male diabetics is reduced approximately 9 years and for female diabetics, approximately 7 years. (51) Happily, however, ketoacidosis is no longer a major cause of death in the diabetic population. In fact, with modern methods of treatment it has become rare as a cause of mortality (*pp. 972–986*).

52. (B); 53. (C); 54. (C); 55. (A); 56. (D); 57. (D)

The endocrine system is composed of numerous unique and complex organs with diverse functions and embryologic origins. A knowledge of the embryologic source of each organ is useful in understanding their respective developmental pathologies. (52) The thyroid gland develops from a tubular invagination at the root of the tongue called the foramen cecum. The tube, called the thyroglossal duct, elongates as the thyroid migrates to its final position in front of the trachea. Vestigial remnants of the thyroglossal duct may develop into midline cystic structures later in life and require surgical removal.

(53) Although at least one pair are intimately associated with the thyroid gland, the parathyroid glands originate from an altogether different embryologic source—the third (lower pair) and the fourth (upper pair) pharyngeal pouches. (54) Since the thy-

mus gland also originates from the third and sometimes fourth pair of pharyngeal pouches, one or two parathyroids occasionally become enclosed within the thymic capsule.

(55) The pituitary is actually a composite gland made up of an anterior, epithelium-derived portion and a neurally derived posterior portion. The anterior pituitary is derived from an evagination of the roof of the primitive oral canal called Rathke's pouch, whereas (56) the posterior pituitary arises from an outpouching of the floor of the third ventricle. Although in the course of normal development Rathke's pouch is detached from its origin by the growing sphenoid bone, rests of epithelial cells may occasionally be caught below the sphenoid and give rise to pharyngeal pituitary tissue.

(57) The pineal gland is a small structure located at the base of the brain that is derived from ependymal cells lining the third ventricle. Although its function is still somewhat obscure, the pineal gland is thought to play some role in maintaining diurnal awake/asleep rhythms and sexual cycles (*pp. 1192, 1201, 1225, 1249, 1253*).

58. (E); 59. (E); 60. (A); 61. (D); 62. (E); 63. (B); 64. (E)

Prolactin, growth hormone, corticotropin, and thyrotropin are all hormones produced in the anterior pituitary. (58) Hypothalamic hormones include oxytocin and vasopressin, which are stored in the posterior pituitary; in addition, the hypothalamus produces releasing factors for all six of the anterior pituitary hormones and release-inhibiting factors for at least two. (59) The cells of the anterior pituitary have classically been divided into three separate categories according to their staining properties with acidic and basic dyes. Acidophilic cells are now known to be lactotropes or somatotropes, whereas basophilic cells are either corticotropes, thyrotropes, or gonadotropes. Chromophobic cells, however, do not appear to contain any anterior pituitary hormones by immunohistochemical methods and are thought of as either degranulated or nonsecretory cells.

(60) For reasons that are poorly understood, the vast majority of functioning pituitary adenomas secrete either prolactin, growth hormone, or corticotropin. Hyperprolactinemia is now recognized as the most common pituitary tumor–related endocrinopathy. (61) Tumors secreting thyrotropin, luteinizing hormone, or follicle-stimulating hormone are very uncommon; it has been estimated that pituitary tumors elaborating thyrotropin constitute less than 1% of all pituitary adenomas. (62) In contrast to benign pituitary tumors, which are frequently secretory, pituitary carcinomas are not only exceedingly rare but only rarely elaborate hormones.

(63) Hypopituitarism usually arises from some destructive process involving the anterior pituitary and usually involves more than one hormone. Rarely,

however, pituitary insufficiency may manifest itself as an isolated hormone deficiency; in such cases, it usually takes the form of a growth hormone deficiency. (**64**) More commonly, anterior pituitary destruction leads to impaired production of *all* the tropic hormones. Clinically, loss of the gonadotropins (LH and FSH) is usually the first to become manifest, since it quickly produces derangements of reproductive function (*pp. 1194–1196*).

65. (C); 66. (B); 67. (C); 68. (B); 69. (C)

Dwarfism is not a discrete process but rather a retardation of growth that may occur in various diverse conditions. Hypopituitarism in the prepubertal child causes so-called pituitary dwarfism. Thyroid hypofunction in the infant is the cause of the growth-retarding condition known as cretinism. In contrast to these two conditions, achondroplastic dwarfism is not known to be associated with an endocrinologic deficit.

(**65**) Achondroplasia is an autosomal dominant disorder in which the exact pathogenetic mechanisms are unknown. The disease is characterized by a failure of cartilage cell proliferation and premature closure of the growth plates of bones preformed in cartilage. (**66**) Neither pituitary dwarfism nor achondroplastic dwarfism is associated with decreased intelligence. Cretinism, however, produces profound retardation of intellectual growth as well as physical growth.

(**67**) Achondroplastic dwarfism can be readily distinguished on the basis of its characteristic body habitus—a large head and small extremities. Head growth is not affected in this disorder, since many bones of the face and cranium are produced by membranous rather than endochondral bone formation.

(**68**) A broad flat nose and a very large protuberant tongue are characteristic features of cretinism.

(**69**) Since pituitary dwarfism and cretinism are the result of hormone deficiencies, they can be successfully treated if recognized early enough by iatrogenic replacement of the missing hormonal elements. There is at present, however, no known effective therapy for achondroplasia (*pp. 1197, 1205, 1321*).

15

THE MUSCULOSKELETAL SYSTEM

DIRECTIONS: For Questions 1 to 9, choose the ONE BEST answer to each question.

1. The pathologic feature most helpful in differentiating a muscular dystrophy from denervation changes in muscle is:

A. Random and irregular variation in muscle cell size
B. Dislocation and internalization of muscle cell nuclei
C. Accumulation of phagocytic macrophages around disintegrating muscle cells
D. Proliferation of endomysial and perimysial connective tissue
E. Accumulation of fat cells between muscle fibers

2. All of the following statements about myasthenia gravis are true EXCEPT:

A. The proximal muscles of the extremities are usually affected first
B. Muscle weakness progresses with persistent use
C. Muscle strength is recovered following periods of rest
D. The risk of developing diabetes mellitus is increased
E. Congenital myasthenia occurs in infants of affected mothers

3. All of the following statements about osteoblasts are true EXCEPT:

A. They are the precursors of osteocytes
B. They synthesize the collagen component of the osteoid matrix
C. They are rich in alkaline phosphatase
D. They synthesize calcium-binding proteins needed for osteoid mineralization
E. They participate in the rapid phase of calcium mobilization in bone resorption

4. Osteomyelitis most often arises:

A. As a primary infection in previously healthy individuals
B. In immunosuppressed individuals
C. As a consequence of local trauma
D. As a result of metastatic seeding from a distant infection
E. From local spread of a contiguous soft tissue infection

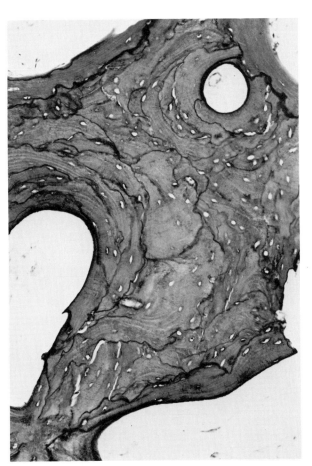

Figure 15–1

5. Which of the following lesions is the *least* common complication of osteomyelitis in adults?

A. A Brodie's abscess
B. A skin sinus
C. A sequestrum
D. An involucrum
E. Suppurative arthritis

6. All of the following characteristics are typical of the bone disease pictured in Figure 15–1 EXCEPT:

A. Children are virtually never affected
B. Involved bones appear thickened radiologically
C. Involved bones are characteristically extremely hard
D. Serum alkaline phosphatase levels are characteristically high
E. Affected individuals are at increased risk of developing osteosarcoma

7. The disease most commonly associated with hypertrophic osteoarthropathy is:

A. Pleural mesothelioma
B. Bronchogenic carcinoma
C. Infective endocarditis
D. Congenital heart disease
E. Ulcerative colitis

8. All of the following statements about giant cell tumors of bone are true EXCEPT:

A. Children are rarely affected
B. The lesions almost always arise in the epiphyses
C. The bones about the knee are most commonly involved
D. The giant cells are not the neoplastic element
E. Most lesions exhibit highly aggressive clinical behavior

9. Pathologic features of osteoarthritis include all of the following EXCEPT:

A. Cartilage fibrillation
B. Pannus formation
C. Eburnation
D. Heberden's node formation
E. Osteophyte formation

DIRECTIONS: For Questions 10 to 13, ONE or MORE of the completions given correctly finishes the incomplete statement. Choose:

A—if only *1,2, and 3* are correct
B—if only *1 and 3* are correct
C—if only *2 and 4* are correct
D—if only *4* is correct
E—if all are correct

10. Granular cell tumors:

1. Arise from Schwann cells
2. Occur most commonly in the tongue
3. Induce pseudoepitheliomatous hyperplasia in the overlying epithelium
4. Are almost always benign

A. 1,2,3   B. 1,3   C. 2,4   D. 4 Only   E. All

11. Osteoporosis:

1. Rarely occurs in males
2. Is caused by impaired osteoid mineralization
3. Primarily involves cortical bone
4. Predisposes to hip fractures

A. 1,2,3   B. 1,3   C. 2,4   D. 4 Only   E. All

12. An asymptomatic 10-year-old boy was discovered to have a single bone involved by the lesion pictured in Figure 15–2. The patient:

1. Most likely has an underlying endocrine disorder
2. Is at increased risk of developing more of these lesions in other bones
3. Has about a 20 to 30% chance of developing an osteosarcoma
4. Most likely had this lesion in a rib

   A. 1,2,3   B. 1,3   C. 2,4   D. 4 Only   E. All

13. Characteristic features of Ewing's sarcoma include:

1. Origin in epiphyses of long bones
2. Extensive invasion of adjacent soft tissues
3. High degree of cytologic pleomorphism
4. PAS-positive cytoplasmic granules

   A. 1,2,3   B. 1,3   C. 2,4   D. 4 Only   E. All

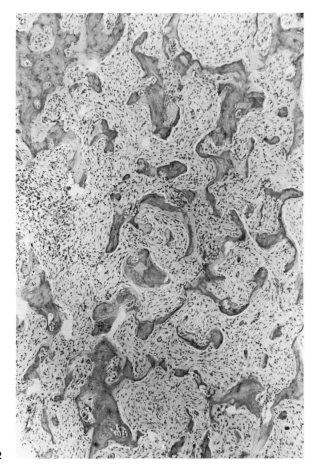

Figure 15–2

DIRECTIONS: For Questions 14 to 32, you are to decide whether EACH choice is TRUE or FALSE.

For each of the following statements about normal skeletal muscle, choose whether it is TRUE or FALSE.

14. A striated muscle cell is known as a myofibril.
15. Muscle cells innervated by a single anterior horn cell constitute a motor unit.
16. Slow twitch (type I) muscle cells usually comprise 30 to 50% of a motor unit.
17. Muscle cells undergo mitosis only when regenerating.
18. During regeneration, new multinucleate muscle cells form from the fusion of mononuclear myoblasts.

For each of the following statements about rheumatoid arthritis (RA), choose whether it is TRUE or FALSE.

19. The process tends to involve the large joints of weight-bearing areas
20. The majority of affected adults have rheumatoid skin nodules
21. The majority of affected adults have antibodies directed against IgG

22. Joint fluid in acute disease typically has normal complement levels
23. The predominant cell type found in the joint fluid in acute disease is the plasma cell
24. In the presence of hypersplenism and leg ulcers, the process is known as Felty's syndrome
25. Amyloidosis develops in over half of cases of long-standing disease

For each of the following statements about gout, choose whether it is TRUE or FALSE.

26. In most cases, an underlying disease process causing excessive breakdown of cells is present
27. In most cases, synthesis of uric acid is increased
28. In most cases, renal excretion of uric acid is relatively reduced
29. At least half of affected individuals develop acute arthritis of the great toe
30. Acute gouty arthritis is the result of urate crystal formation
31. Chronic gouty arthritis is the result of pannus formation
32. Tophi in the central nervous system are one of the most debilitating complications

DIRECTIONS: For Questions 33 to 51, the set of lettered headings is followed by a list of numbered words or phrases. For each numbered word or phrase choose:

A—if the item is associated with (A) only
B—if the item is associated with (B) only
C—if the item is associated with *both* (A) and (B)
D—if the item is associated with neither (A) nor (B)

For each of the features listed below, choose whether it describes desmoid tumors, nodular fasciitis, both, or neither.

    A. Desmoid tumors
    B. Nodular fasciitis
    C. Both
    D. Neither

33. The lesion has a striking female predominance
34. The extremities are often the site of origin
35. Lesions are multifocal in the vast majority of cases
36. The lesion characteristically infiltrates the surrounding soft tissues
37. Histologically, the center of the lesion is often myxoid
38. Incompletely excised lesions tend to recur
39. Malignant transformation occurs in 5 to 10% of cases

For each of the characteristics listed below, choose whether it describes osteochondromatosis, enchondromatosis, both, or neither.

    A. Osteochondromatosis
    B. Enchondromatosis
    C. Both
    D. Neither

40. Has a sex-linked mode of hereditary transmission
41. Characterized by hamartomatous rather than neoplastic lesions
42. Associated with colonic polyps in Gardner's syndrome
43. Associated with cavernous hemangioma in Maffucci's syndrome
44. Associated with an increased risk of developing chondrosarcoma

For each of the characteristics listed below, choose whether it describes osteosarcoma, chondrosarcoma, both, or neither.

    A. Osteosarcoma
    B. Chondrosarcoma
    C. Both
    D. Neither

45. Constitutes the most common form of primary cancer of bones
46. Occurs most frequently in children and adolescents
47. Arises *de novo* as a primary lesion in the majority of cases
48. Tends to arise in pelvic bones
49. Often contains both bone and cartilage
50. Rarely metastasizes to lymph nodes
51. Behaves predictably according to tumor grade

DIRECTIONS: Questions 52 to 70 are matching questions. For each numbered item, choose the most likely associated lettered item from those provided. Each numbered item has ONLY ONE answer. Within each group, each lettered item may be the answer to one, more than one, or none of the numbered items.

For each of the features listed below, choose whether it is characteristic of Duchenne muscular dystrophy, myotonic dystrophy, congenital myopathy, all of these, or none of these.

    A. Duchenne muscular dystrophy
    B. Myotonic dystrophy
    C. Congenital myopathy
    D. All of these
    E. None of these

52. Occurs only in males
53. Rarely associated with mental retardation
54. Incompatible with long survival
55. Characteristically involves extramuscular systems
56. Characteristically produces involvement of a single myofiber type
57. Characterized histologically by "ring fibers"
58. Caused by a myotropic virus

For each of the characteristics listed below, choose whether it describes rhabdosarcoma, synoviosarcoma, malignant fibrous histiocytoma, liposarcoma, or none of these.

    A. Rhabdosarcoma
    B. Synoviosarcoma
    C. Malignant fibrous histiocytoma
    D. Liposarcoma
    E. None of these

59. Constitutes the most common soft tissue malignancy in children
60. Constitutes the most common form of soft tissue malignancy in adults
61. Does *not* have a myxoid histologic variant
62. Characteristically composed of both epithelioid and spindle-shaped cells
63. Typically produces a storiform (pinwheel) histologic pattern of growth
64. Often stains positively for lysozyme by immunohistochemistry

65. Often observed by immunohistochemistry to contain intracytoplasmic keratin proteins

For each of the characteristics listed below, choose whether it describes osteogenesis imperfecta, osteopetrosis, achondroplasia, all of these, or none of these.

    A. Osteogenesis imperfecta
    B. Osteopetrosis
    C. Achondroplasia
    D. All of these
    E. None of these

66. The disorder has a hereditary mode of transmission
67. Affected adults usually enjoy normal longevity
68. The sclerae characteristically appear blue
69. Multiple exostoses are common complications
70. Anemia and hepatosplenomegaly are common complications

15

THE MUSCULOSKELETAL SYSTEM

ANSWERS

1. (A) Morphologic patterns of muscle injury are limited in number and usually lack specificity for any given etiology. Therefore, specific etiologic diagnosis of muscle disease is often impossible from biopsy alone. Clinical features such as the distribution of muscle involvement and the coexistence of other organ involvement must also be considered in order to make a specific diagnosis.

Although it is true that morphologic changes on muscle biopsy are often less than pathognomonic, fairly specific changes are produced by at least some forms of muscle injury. The muscular dystrophies, for example, typically produce a random and irregular variation in myofiber size. It is principally this irregular pattern of individual muscle cell involvement that differentiates muscular dystrophy from denervation—both processes that ultimately produce muscle atrophy. Changes such as proliferation of endomysial and perimysial connective tissue, accumulation of fat cells between myofibers, dislocation and internalization of muscle nuclei, and accumulation of phagocytic macrophages around disintegrating muscle cells are general features of muscular atrophy and do not help to differentiate muscular dystrophy from denervation atrophy. In contrast to the muscle atrophy in the dystrophies, denervation atrophy is not random but is determined by the pattern of innervation of affected motor nerves *(pp. 1306–1308)*.

2. (A) Myasthenia gravis is an autoimmune disorder characterized by antibodies directed against the acetylcholine receptors of the postsynaptic membrane at the motor end-plate. Transmission of neural impulses at neuromuscular junctions is blocked, and muscle weakness is produced. Characteristically, the first manifestation of the disease is weakening of the eye muscles, producing diplopia and drooping of the eyelids. The eye muscles are the first and most consistently affected muscles in the body, whereas proximal muscles and girdle muscles are affected relatively late in the disease. Other distinctive clinical features that set myasthenia gravis apart from other muscular disorders include progression of muscular weakness with persistent use and recovery of strength following a period of rest. Individuals with myasthenia gravis and members of their family have an increased incidence of other autoimmune disorders including diabetes mellitus, thyroid disease, and pernicious anemia. Infants born of myasthenic mothers may manifest a transient motor weakness known as "congenital myasthenia," caused by transplacental passage of maternal IgG antireceptor antibodies *(pp. 1310–1312)*.

3. (E) Osteoblasts are bone-forming cells that synthesize the collagenous component of the osteoid matrix. In addition, they synthesize the calcium-binding proteins that are required for mineralization of the osteoid that they produce. These cells are rich in alkaline phosphatase, which serves as a marker for osteoblastic activity. When osteoblasts become incorporated within the matrix they produce, they become known as osteocytes. It is the osteocyte and not the osteoblast that is thought to be responsible for the rapid mobilization of calcium in such conditions as hyperparathyroidism, osteomalacia, and thyrotoxicosis. The slower remodeling processes involved in normal bone turnover are the province of the osteoclast *(pp. 1317–1319)*.

4. (A) Although osteomyelitis may occasionally arise as an infectious complication in an immunosuppressed individual or as a result of local trauma, metastatic seeding from a distant infection, or local spread of a contiguous soft tissue infection, it most often arises as a primary infection in a previously healthy individual. In this setting, it is believed to be produced by transient bacteremias from such trivial sources as injury to the intestinal mucosa, vigorous chewing of hard foods, or minor injury to the skin *(p. 1323)*.

5. (E) Complications of osteomyelitis in any age group include Brodie's abscesses, skin sinuses, sequestra, and involucra. Brodie's abscesses are chronic niduses of infection that may develop if the initial infection is walled off by inflammatory fibrous tissue. Skin sinuses develop when the spreading infection directly dissects through to the skin surface or follows the evulsion of a sequestrum (fragment of necrotic bone) through the soft tissues to the skin. An involucrum refers to the reactive subperiosteal new bone formation that encloses and envelops the inflammatory focus in a smoldering chronic infection.

Except in infants in the first year of life, osteomyelitis rarely spreads to the adjacent joint space, since the epiphyseal cartilaginous plate is resistant to bacterial invasion. Only in severe disease in which the infection has tracked along the outer surface of the bone and enters the joint space indirectly does suppurative arthritis appear, but this is rare *(pp. 1324–1325)*.

6. (C) The pathognomonic histologic feature of Paget's disease of bone, a mosaic pattern of bone formation, is seen in the accompanying photomicrograph. Paget's disease is an extremely common disorder of bone, but its pathogenesis is still unknown. It is characterized by excessive resorption of normal bone followed by excessive new bone formation in a haphazard arrangement. The newly formed osteons are demarcated by osteoid seams that form the illustrated histologic "mosaic." It is a disorder of adults of middle age or older and virtually never appears in children. Involved bones are characteristically greatly thickened, a feature readily seen on x-ray. The intense osteoblastic activity typically produces high serum alkaline phosphatase levels. In fact, the alkaline phosphatase levels in Paget's disease are generally greater than in any other bone disorder. One of the most ominous complications of Paget's disease is the development of a sarcoma in the pagetic bone, a consequence that occurs in about 1% of patients.

Although involved bones are indeed thickened in this disease, they are, nevertheless, extremely *soft*. Because pagetic bones are composed largely of poorly mineralized osteoid matrix and vascular connective tissue they are usually light, soft, and porous and are prone to pathologic fractures *(pp. 1331–1333)*.

7. (B) Hypertrophic osteoarthropathy is a disorder of unknown etiology characterized by periosteal inflammation at the ends of tubular bones with lifting of the periosteum, subjacent new bone formation, and arthritis of the adjacent joints. Although it may occur in association with a wide variety of neoplastic and inflammatory disorders, the disease with which it most commonly occurs is bronchogenic carcinoma. Pleural mesothelioma, infective endocarditis, and congenital heart disease are among the more common associated disorders, and ulcerative colitis is among the less frequent clinical accompaniments. However, none of these diseases produces hypertrophic osteoarthropathy with as great a frequency (10% of cases) as bronchogenic carcinoma. Hypertrophic osteoarthropathy sometimes precedes clinical manifestations of an underlying disease and can call attention to it. Furthermore, the arthropathy is reversible with the surgical resection or medical correction of the underlying disease process *(p. 1333)*.

8. (E) Giant cell tumors of bone encompass a spectrum of neoplasms that exhibit extremely variable biologic behavior. They are composed of mononuclear fibroblast-like cells admixed with numerous multinucleate giant cells. Most giant cell tumors (70 to 75%) are composed of well-differentiated cells with few, if any, mitoses and minimal atypicality; these lesions behave clinically in a benign fashion. Only about 5 to 15% of giant cell tumors are overtly anaplastic and biologically aggressive. The remainder have an intermediate histologic appearance and a variable and unpredictable clinical course.

Giant cell tumors occur most commonly in young to middle-aged adults and are distinctly uncommon in individuals under the age of 15. Distinctively, the lesions almost always arise in the epiphyses of long bones, most commonly around the knee. Although the tumor is named for its variable complement of osteoclast-like giant cells, it is the mononuclear cells and not the multinucleate giant cells that represent the neoplastic element in this tumor *(pp. 1345–1346)*.

9. (B) Osteoarthritis is the most common form of joint disease. It is a deforming and debilitating destructive process. In adults, it often occurs as a consequence of a variety of congenital, structural, traumatic, metabolic, or inflammatory diseases of joints.

No matter what the pathogenesis, the histologic changes of osteoarthritis are quite constant. Clefts appear in the surface of the articular cartilage and may extend to the underlying subchondral bone, a pathologic feature known as cartilage fibrillation. With progressive erosion of articular cartilage, focal areas of subchondral bone become denuded and sclerotic (eburnation). Bony spurs arise from the margins of the articular cartilage and may project from opposing bone, causing pain and limitation of motion. Osteophytic spurs arising from the base of the terminal phalanges are known as Heberden's nodes and are characteristic of osteoarthritis.

Pannus formation is a process characterized by intense inflammation of the synovial lining; a highly vascularized polypoid mass of inflammatory tissue arises from the synovium and often overgrows the articular surface beginning at the joint margins. Pannus formation is characteristic, although not pathognomonic, of rheumatoid arthritis. Pannus formation may also be seen in association with other inflammatory processes in joints, including the arthritis associated with psoriasis or gout. However, pannus formation is not a feature of osteoarthritis *(pp. 1349–1350, 1352, 1359, 1362)*.

10. (E) Granular cell tumors are soft tissue neoplasms that are almost always benign and arise from the precursors of Schwann cells. In the past, because they were thought to arise from myoblastic cells, these tumors were called myoblastomas. They arise most commonly in the tongue and in the dermal tissues of the trunk and upper extremities. In their subepithelial locations, granular cell tumors induce pseudoepitheliomatous hyperplasia of the overlying epithelium that can be mistaken for a squamous cell carcinoma *(pp. 1316–1317)*.

11. (D) Osteoporosis is a condition characterized by reduction in both the mineral and matrix phases of structurally normal bone. It is a ubiquitous but asymptomatic condition seen in women over the age of 45 and in men between the ages of 50 and 60. The condition is believed to be caused by accelerated bone loss, the reasons for which are as yet unclear. The bone loss is greater in trabecular than in cortical bone. Therefore, fractures of bone composed predominantly of trabecular bone such as vertebral bodies and the femoral necks are common.

Impaired osteoid mineralization is the characteristic defect in a different systemic bone disorder known as osteomalacia (pp. 1327–1328).

12. (D) The bony lesion pictured in the photomicrograph is composed of haphazardly arranged trabeculae of woven bone within a background of cellular connective tissue and is known as fibrous dysplasia. In about 70 to 75% of cases the lesion is limited to a single bone, and the condition is referred to as monostotic fibrous dysplasia. As in the case described, the condition typically becomes manifest in childhood. The lesion is usually asymptomatic and is therefore often discovered as an incidental finding on x-ray. The rib is the most common location of monostotic fibrous dysplasia, followed by the femur, tibia, maxilla, mandible, calvarium, and humerus.

In about 30% of cases of fibrous dysplasia, multiple bones are involved. The polyostotic form of the disease usually appears at a slightly earlier age, is more likely to involve the craniofacial bones, and is less likely to involve the ribs than the monostotic form. In about 3% of cases of polyostotic fibrous dysplasia, the condition is accompanied by skin pigmentation and a variety of endocrine disorders, including precocious sexual development (Albright's syndrome), hyperthyroidism, Cushing's syndrome, hyperparathyroidism, and others.

There is no known association between the monostotic and polyostotic forms of fibrous dysplasia; transition from the monostotic to the polyostotic form has never been reported. Therefore, a patient with a single lesion such as the one described is not at increased risk of developing multiple lesions.

Only about 0.5% of the lesions of fibrous dysplasia undergo sarcomatous change. Therefore, the risk of malignant transformation is low in the monostotic form of the disease (pp. 1333–1334).

13. (C) Ewing's sarcoma is a highly malignant form of primary bone tumor that is believed to originate from a primitive mesenchymal cell having no tendency to differentiate into a specific bone or marrow cell type. It typically arises in the metaphyses of long tubular bones and virtually never originates in epiphyseal regions. It tends to perforate the bony cortex and penetrate adjacent soft tissues, often producing larger extraosseous than intraosseous masses. Histologically, the tumor is composed of masses of small uniform cells with little cytologic pleomorphism. A helpful diagnostic feature of Ewing's sarcoma is the finding of characteristic PAS-positive granules in the cytoplasm of the tumor cells (pp. 1343–1345).

14. (False); 15. (True); 16. (False); 17. (False); 18. (True)

(14) Normal skeletal muscle is a marvel of structural organization from the gross to the ultrastructural level. Each muscle is composed of numerous fascicles that represent groups of muscle cells enclosed in perimesial connective tissue. Individual muscle cells within a fascicle are known as myofibers; each contains numerous myofibrils within its cytoplasm. Myofibrils are the submicroscopic structures that constitute the contractile elements of the cell and are composed of a highly ordered array of interdigitating actin and myosin myofilaments.

(15) The functional organization of groups of muscle cells does not always correspond precisely to the architectural organization described above. Functional groupings of myofibers are known as motor units and are determined by innervation rather than by spacial contiguity or fascicular grouping. A motor unit, therefore, is composed of all myofibers innervated by a single anterior horn cell. **(16)** Since it is innervation that determines myofiber type, all of the myofibers within a motor unit are of the same type.

(17) Skeletal muscle cells, along with cardiac muscle and nerve cells, are classified as "permanent" cells since they lack the capacity to undergo mitotic division in postnatal life. **(18)** Nevertheless, skeletal muscle is capable of regeneration in many forms of muscular disease. Many of the means by which it reconstitutes itself are unique to this tissue type and include fusion of myoblasts normally present between myofibers as "satellite cells" and the process known as "budding" of old myofibers (pp. 71, 1305).

19. (False); 20. (False); 21. (True); 22. (False); 23. (False); 24. (True); 25. (False)

Rheumatoid arthritis (RA) is a chronic systemic inflammatory disease that is autoimmune in nature and produces a progressive deforming arthritis as one of its primary manifestations.

(19) In contrast to osteoarthritis, which tends to involve weight-bearing joints, RA typically affects the small joints of the hands and feet in a symmetrical distribution. **(20)** Rheumatoid skin nodules are a particularly distinctive but variable feature of RA and are present only in about 20% of patients. **(21)** Nearly all adult patients with RA have antibodies against the Fc fragment of autologous IgG. These autoantibodies, called rheumatoid factor (RF), are present only infrequently in the juvenile form of rheumatoid arthritis occurring in individuals under the age of 16. **(22)** In the adult form of the disease, most of the rheumatoid factor is formed locally by the lymphoplasmacytic inflammatory infiltrate in the joints. The IgG-RF immune complexes that are formed bind and activate complement and initiate an inflammatory response.

Thus, complement levels are characteristically low in the acute rheumatoid synovial effusions. (23) The neutrophil, attracted by the chemotactic fragments from C3 and C5, is the predominant cell type present.

(24) Felty's syndrome is one of the variant forms of rheumatoid arthritis; it refers to the combination of splenomegaly with hyperplenism and leg ulcers in association with the characteristic rheumatoid polyarthritis. Other variant forms of the disease include juvenile rheumatoid arthritis (see Question 21), ankylosing spondylitis, and arthritis associated with ulcerative colitis.

(25) Although rheumatoid arthritis is the second most common cause of secondary amyloidosis, only about 15 to 25% of cases of long-standing RA are complicated by this disorder. Thus, the likelihood of developing secondary amyloidosis is less for patients with RA than for those with tuberculosis or leprosy, diseases in which the prevalence of amyloidosis approaches 50% (*pp. 1351–1354*).

26. (False); 27. (True); 28. (True); 29. (True); 30. (True); 31. (True); 32. (False)

Gout is a chronic disabling disease caused by the precipitation of monosodium urate crystals from supersaturated body fluids in patients with hyperuricemia. (26) Although gout may occur as a secondary phenomenon in any disease process causing hyperuricemia, the vast majority of cases (approximately 90%) occur in the absence of a known metabolic defect and are referred to as "primary idiopathic gout." (27) Metabolic studies have shown that in most cases the cause of the hyperuricemia is increased synthesis of uric acid rather than impaired excretion. (28) However, it is also clear that in the majority of patients a *relative* underexcretion of uric acid coexists with increased urate synthesis but is not the primary abnormality. In about 30% of cases, no increased synthesis of uric acid can be detected. In these individuals the primary pathogenesis of gout is believed to be renal in origin, and a tubular defect in the excretion of urates can be detected in many of these patients.

(29) Acute gouty arthritis of the metatarsal phalangeal joint of the great toe is the most common presentation of the disease. At least half of the initial attacks involve this joint. (30) As alluded to above, *acute* attacks of arthritis are evoked by the precipitation of urate crystals into the joint fluid. (31) *Chronic* gouty arthritis is the result of multiple recurrent attacks of acute arthritis that induce inflammatory synovial pannus formation. The pannus, in turn, destroys the underlying articular cartilage and ultimately causes chronic disabling disease. (32) Tophi, the pathognomonic lesions of gout, are composed of a mass of crystalline or amorphous urates surrounded by an intense inflammatory and foreign body giant cell reaction. Because urates do not penetrate

the blood-brain barrier, tophi do not develop in the central nervous system (*pp. 1356–1361*).

33. (A); 34. (B); 35. (D); 36. (C); 37. (B); 38. (A); 39. (D)

Desmoid tumors and nodular fasciitis are both considered to be forms of fibromatosis. These entities are both misnomers of a sort, since neither is neoplastic or clearly inflammatory as their names would imply. Furthermore, nodular fasciitis does not primarily arise in the fascia but rather in subcutaneous tissues.

(33) Desmoid tumors appear to be hormonally responsive lesions. They have a striking female predominance and have been found to contain estrogen receptors. Furthermore, desmoid-like tumors have been produced in guinea pigs by the injection of estrogens. (34) In contrast to desmoids, which arise predominantly in the anterior abdominal wall of females, nodular fasciitis has a predilection for the extremities (forearm, leg, and arm) and face of either sex. (35) Both desmoids and nodular fasciitis tend to be unifocal lesions (36) that have irregular borders and characteristically infiltrate the surrounding soft tissues. (37) Histologically, desmoid tumors are characteristically heavily collagenized in their central regions, whereas nodular fasciitis is most frequently myxoid in the center and increases in cellularity toward the periphery of the lesion. (38) Both desmoid tumors and nodular fasciitis can be cured by surgical resection. However, incompletely excised desmoid tumors tend to recur locally, whereas even incompletely resected lesions of nodular fasciitis do not recur. (39) Neither of these lesions has a propensity for neoplastic transformation. The rare reports of metastatic dissemination of a desmoid tumor are believed to represent misdiagnoses of low grade fibrosarcomas (*pp. 1312–1314*).

40. (D); 41. (C); 42. (A); 43. (B); 44. (C)

(40 and 41) Osteochondromatosis and enchondromatosis are diseases characterized by hamartomatous overgrowths of cartilaginous and bony tissue growing from the lateral contours or within the medullary cavities of endochondral bones respectively. Although osteochondromatosis is a hereditary disorder, its mode of transmission is uncertain. However, it is believed to be an autosomal dominant condition affecting both males and females. Enchondromatosis usually develops at a younger age than osteochondromatosis and is typically discovered early in childhood, but there is no clear evidence of hereditary or familial influences in this disease. (42) Furthermore, osteochondromas may occur as a part of another hereditary disorder known as Gardner's syndrome, which also includes desmoid tumors, sebaceous cysts, and adenomatous polyps of the colon. The latter pose a significantly increased risk of colonic adenocarcinoma.

(43) Although, as stated above, enchondromatosis

alone does not appear to have a clear-cut familial mode of transmission, it may occur as part of a familial syndrome that includes multiple cavernous hemangiomas and is known as Maffucci's syndrome.

(44) Although both osteochondromatosis and enchondromatosis are associated with an increased incidence of chondrosarcoma, the rate of malignant transformation appears to be lower for osteochondromatosis (3 to 5% of hereditary cases) than enchondromatosis (5 to 50% of cases). Nearly half of all chondrosarcomas arise from enchondromas. Therefore, patients with enchondromatosis (Ollier's disease) are at particular risk of developing this malignancy (pp. 1321–1323).

45. (A); 46. (A); 47. (C); 48. (B); 49. (C); 50. (C); 51. (B)

Malignancies arising from the cell types found in bone are much less common than those arising from marrow elements (myeloma and leukemia). Although infrequent, primary bone tumors are among the most biologically aggressive neoplasms in humans. (45) Osteosarcoma is the most common cancer of bone, followed by Ewing's sarcoma, chondrosarcoma, and malignant giant cell tumor of bone, in descending order of frequency. (46) Osteosarcoma constitutes the most common form of primary bone cancer in children and young adults. (47) Like chondrosarcomas, osteosarcomas tend to arise as primary lesions in the majority of cases, although they do occur occasionally in the background of preexisting bone disease such as Paget's disease, multiple enchondromas, multiple osteochondromas, chronic osteomyelitis, fibrous dysplasia, infarcts, or fractures of bone.

(48) Unlike osteosarcoma, which tends to arise about the knee, chondrosarcomas originate most frequently in the pelvic bones. (49) Histologically, both osteosarcomas and chondrosarcomas often contain both bony and cartilaginous elements. Their diagnosis depends on the identification of frankly malignant, anaplastic cells in association with osteoid matrix in the case of osteosarcoma or chondroid matrix in the case of chondrosarcoma. In chondrosarcomas with ossification, the bone formation occurs within cartilage, whereas in osteosarcomas, the neo-osteogenesis arises out of the background of anaplastic, osteoblastic cells. (50) It is rare for either osteosarcoma or chondrosarcoma to metastasize to lymph nodes. Hematogenous dissemination is the major mode of metastasis of both of these tumors. (51) In contrast to the experience with osteosarcoma in which there is little correlation between histologic grade and patient survival, there is an excellent correlation between the histopathology of chondrosarcomas and tumor behavior. Obviously, then, histologic grading of chondrosarcoma is of much greater clinical significance than grading of osteosarcomas. Stage is a much better predictor of the prognosis of osteosarcoma: tumor size and the presence or absence of metastatic disease

correlate best with the overall survival rate (pp. 1335–1340, 1342–1343).

52. (A); 53. (C); 54. (A); 55. (B); 56. (E); 57. (B); 58. (E)

Muscular dystrophies and congenital myopathies are inherited primary disorders of muscle fibers that produce muscle weakness, atrophy, and loss of tendon reflexes. Although the muscular dystrophies tend to manifest distinctive clinical patterns, they produce the same basic morphologic changes in the involved muscles. Congenital myopathies, in contrast, are not clinically distinctive but produce fairly specific morphologic changes.

(52) Among the hereditary dystrophies and myopathies, the Duchenne type and Becker type muscular dystrophies are the two that are inherited as sex-linked conditions and occur only in males. (53) Both Duchenne muscular dystrophy and myotonic dystrophy, the most severe and the most prevalent dystrophies respectively, are associated with decreased intelligence. Although mild reduction in intelligence is common among individuals with Duchenne muscular dystrophy, frank mental retardation is present only in about 30%. The majority of individuals with myotonic dystrophy, however, manifest frank mental retardation or even dementia. Congenital myopathies, in contrast, are rarely associated with mental retardation.

(54) The Duchenne muscular dystrophy is incompatible with long survival; it is a progressive disease that usually leads to death by age 20. Although myotonic dystrophy is also a progressive disease, muscle involvement generally proceeds far more slowly and is not totally incapacitating nor incompatible with long survival. In contrast to the muscular dystrophies, the congenital myopathies are not progressive and are compatible with a normal life span and a useful existence.

(55) Unlike the other forms of muscular dystrophy and the congenital myopathies, myotonic dystrophy characteristically involves many extramuscular systems. Thus, in addition to weakness and myotonia of the distal muscles, frontal baldness, cataracts, and testicular atrophy are major clinical features.

(56) In all forms of muscular dystrophy, there is a loss of histochemical differentiation between type I and type II myofibers, but neither fiber type is spared. Several of the congenital myopathies tend to involve one fiber type more than the other, but in no case is the damage limited to a single fiber type. (57) "Ring fibers" represent single myofibers transversely encircling other myofibers in the same bundle. They are a distinctive histologic feature of myotonic dystrophy and when present provide the opportunity to identify this form of dystrophy morphologically. (58) As stated above, the muscular dystrophies and congenital myopathies are hereditary disorders of muscle fibers and are not known to be

related to any acquired disease such as viral infection (*pp. 1308–1310*).

59. (A); 60. (D); 61. (B); 62. (B); 63. (C); 64. (C); 65. (B)

(**59**) Among the soft tissue sarcomas, rhabdosarcoma is the most common form in children, and (**60**) liposarcoma is the most common form in adults. (**61**) Regardless of their cell of origin, most soft tissue sarcomas manifest a variety of histologic growth patterns. Unfortunately, many of these histologic variants overlap, making specific diagnosis of soft tissue sarcomas a challenging endeavor. For example, rhabdosarcoma, malignant fibrous histiocytoma, and liposarcoma are all capable of producing myxoid histologic variants. Only synoviosarcoma fails to produce a myxoid variant. (**62**) Instead, synoviosarcoma is characterized by biphasic histology; it is composed of both epithelioid and spindle-shaped cells recapitulating the derivation of cuboidal synovial lining cells from primitive mesenchymal cells.

(**63**) Storiform or pinwheel patterns of growth characterize malignant fibrous histiocytomas. (**64**) These tumors are composed of spindle-shaped fibroblasts and histiocytes. The latter can be identified by immunohistochemical stains for lysozyme or chymotrypsin, enzymes that are typically present in normal histocytes. (**65**) Immunoperoxidase staining for keratin, on the other hand, is unusual for sarcomas but can often be seen in the epithelium-like components of synoviosarcomas (*pp. 270, 1314–1316, 1362–1365*).

66. (D); 67. (C); 68. (A); 69. (E); 70. (B)

(**66**) Osteogenesis imperfecta, osteopetrosis, and achondroplasia are hereditary disorders of bone with varying morbidity and mortality. (**67**) Only the heterozygotic form of achondroplasia is compatible with normal longevity, although homozygotes with this disease die *in utero* or soon after birth. Osteogenesis imperfecta can be divided clinically into two categories: a highly lethal "congenita" category marked by clinical manifestations from birth and a more common "tarda" variety that usually manifests itself later (in early childhood) but is not compatible with long survival. Osteopetrosis also has two modes of transmission and two correspondingly different clinical subsets. The autosomal recessive disease appears in infancy and results in an early death, whereas the autosomal dominant disease is relatively benign and is compatible with a *nearly* normal life span, although affected individuals are at high risk of developing fractures (even with mild trauma) and infections (particularly osteomyelitis), which are a threat to life. (**68**) One of the most distinctive clinical features of osteogenesis imperfecta is the appearance of the sclerae, which are translucent and look blue because of the visualization of the underlying choroid plexus.

(**69**) Exostoses are not associated with any of these three hereditary conditions but rather constitute a separate and unrelated hereditary condition of bone known as osteochondromatosis.

(**70**) Anemia and hepatosplenomegaly are common complications of osteopetrosis. In this condition, the marked overgrowth of bone narrows the marrow cavity and in advanced cases may obliterate it altogether. In such cases, hepatosplenomegaly results from extramedullary hematopoiesis (*pp. 1320–1321*).

16

THE NERVOUS SYSTEM

DIRECTIONS: For Questions 1 to 7, choose the ONE BEST answer to each question.

1. All of the following conditions cause increased intracranial pressure EXCEPT:

   A. Alzheimer's disease
   B. Metastatic tumor
   C. Lead encephalopathy
   D. Water intoxication
   E. Contusions

2. Diseases of the CNS that are primarily iatrogenic include all of the following EXCEPT:

   A. Progressive multifocal leukoencephalopathy
   B. Citrobacter meningitis
   C. Cerebral toxoplasmosis
   D. Central pontine myelinolysis
   E. Metachromatic leukodystrophy

3. All of the following features describe subacute sclerosing panencephalitis (SSPE) EXCEPT:

   A. Occurs as a complication of rubeola infection
   B. Has a long latent period
   C. Has a protracted course
   D. Has a high mortality rate
   E. Causes primary demyelinization in the CNS

4. Which of the following statements about subacute spongiform encephalopathy (Creutzfeldt-Jakob disease) is correct?

   A. The causative agent is visible only with the electron microscope
   B. The causative agent is typically inactivated by ionizing radiation
   C. The usual mode of transmission is man-to-man via aerosolized droplet exposure

   D. A brisk cellular immune response without granuloma formation is characteristic
   E. The disease typically causes a rapidly progressive dementia

5. Which of the following statements about epidural hematoma is correct?

   A. It is almost always accompanied by a skull fracture
   B. The bleeding is usually of venous origin
   C. The onset of symptoms is typically delayed for several hours after the vascular rupture
   D. The major symptom is a fluctuating level of consciousness
   E. It occasionally occurs as a result of rupture of a mycotic aneurysm

6. The most common cause of spinal cord compression is:

   A. Penetrating wounds with hemorrhage into the cord
   B. Spinal meningioma
   C. Traumatic vertebral fracture
   D. Epidural hematoma
   E. Metastatic tumor

7. All of the following pathologic features are characteristic of Alzheimer's disease EXCEPT:

   A. Hirano bodies in proximal dendrites
   B. Senile plaques
   C. Neurofibrillary tangles
   D. Iron-containing pigment in the globus pallidus
   E. Granulovacuolar degeneration of neurons

DIRECTIONS: For Questions 8 to 16, ONE or MORE of the completions given correctly finishes the incomplete statement. Choose:

A—if only *1,2, and 3* are correct
B—if only *1 and 3* are correct
C—if only *2 and 4* are correct
D—if only *4* is correct
E—if all are correct

8. Subdural empyema is associated with:

1. Bacterial meningitis
2. Skull fracture
3. Brain abscess
4. Sinusitis

A. 1,2,3   B. 1,3   C. 2,4   D. 4 Only   E. All

9. Herpes simplex causes:

1. Neonatal panencephalitis
2. Cold sores
3. Benign recurrent (Mollaret) meningitis
4. Postherpetic neuralgia

A. 1,2,3   B. 1,3   C. 2,4   D. 4 Only   E. All

10. Berry aneurysms are:

1. Usually atherosclerotic in origin
2. Nearly always solitary
3. Most commonly located in the vertebrobasilar artery circulation
4. The most common cause of ruptured intracranial aneurysm

A. 1,2,3   B. 1,3   C. 2,4   D. 4 Only   E. All

11. In the CNS, the middle cerebral artery is the most common site of:

1. Embolic obstruction
2. Bleeding from arteriovenous malformations
3. Arterial tears producing epidural hematoma
4. Atherosclerotic thrombosis

A. 1,2,3   B. 1,3   C. 2,4   D. 4 Only   E. All

12. Carcinomatous meningitis is associated with which of the following tumors?

1. Pineal tumors
2. Metastatic lung cancer
3. Medulloblastomas
4. Metastatic breast cancer

A. 1,2,3   B. 1,3   C. 2,4   D. 4 Only   E. All

13. Meningiomas are commonly associated with:

1. Infiltrative, irregular borders
2. Penetration of the adjacent bone
3. A poor prognosis
4. Psammoma bodies

A. 1,2,3   B. 1,3   C. 2,4   D. 4 Only   E. All

14. Typical histologic features of idiopathic parkinsonism include:

1. Neurofibrillary tangles
2. Lewy bodies
3. Severe neuronal loss in the putamen
4. Depigmentation of the substantia nigra

A. 1,2,3   B. 1,3   C. 2,4   D. 4 Only   E. All

15. Typical features of amyotrophic lateral sclerosis (ALS) include:

1. Degeneration of the upper motor neurons
2. Degeneration of the lower motor neurons
3. An inevitably fatal course
4. Infection with an enterovirus

A. 1,2,3   B. 1,3   C. 2,4   D. 4 Only   E. All

16. Neurofibromata:

1. Are derived from Schwann cells
2. Contain Verocay bodies
3. Are often multiple
4. Are eccentrically located on distal nerves

A. 1,2,3   B. 1,3   C. 2,4   D. 4 Only   E. All

DIRECTIONS: For Questions 17 to 32, you are to decide whether EACH choice is TRUE or FALSE.

For each of the following statements about vascular disease of the CNS, choose whether it is TRUE or FALSE.

17. Pure hypoxia irreversibly damages neurons within a few minutes

18. Ischemic encephalopathy is most commonly associated with inadequate cardiopulmonary resuscitation following cardiac arrest

19. A hemorrhagic infarct often overlaps arterial supplies

20. Cerebral hemorrhage is most often caused by hypertensive vascular disease

21. Supratentorial hemorrhage often presents clinically as intractable vomiting

22. Emboli are the most common cause of cerebral infarction

23. Lacunar infarcts in the internal capsule are characteristic of hypertensive vascular disease

24. Pure motor hemiparesis without sensory deficit is characteristic of lacunar strokes

25. The most common cause of vascular injury in the spinal cord is hypertensive vascular disease

For each of the following statements about multiple sclerosis, choose whether it is TRUE or FALSE.

26. Most cases occur in children

27. The primary pathologic process is generalized CNS demyelinization

28. Intellectual deterioration is an early manifestation of the disease

29. The cerebrospinal fluid typically contains increased immunoglobulins

30. Onset usually occurs shortly after a viral infection

31. Dense "plaques" of gliosis are a characteristic histologic feature

32. Long-term corticosteroid treatment prevents progression of the disease

DIRECTIONS: For Questions 33 to 49, the set of lettered headings is followed by a list of numbered words or phrases. For each numbered word or phrase choose:

A—if the item is associated with (A) only
B—if the item is associated with (B) only
C—if the item is associated with *both* (A) and (B)
D—if the item is associated with *neither* (A) nor (B)

For each of the features listed below, choose whether it describes communicating hydrocephalus, noncommunicating hydrocephalus, both of these, or neither of these.

A. Communicating hydrocephalus
B. Noncommunicating hydrocephalus
C. Both of these
D. Neither of these

33. Often fails to produce ventricular distention
34. Associated with postmeningitic states
35. Associated with neoplasms
36. Associated with thrombosis of the dural sinuses
37. Associated with the Dandy-Walker syndrome

For each of the features listed below, choose whether it describes rabies, poliomyelitis, both of these, or neither of these.

A. Rabies
B. Poliomyelitis
C. Both of these
D. Neither of these

38. A primary infection elsewhere precedes nervous system disease
39. Diagnostic inclusions are seen in infected cells

40. The causative viral agent affects only dorsal root ganglion cells

41. Lower motor neuron paralysis is produced

42. The most common cause of death is respiratory center failure

For each of the features listed below, choose whether it describes acute disseminated encephalomyelitis, acute hemorrhagic leukoencephalopathy, both of these, or neither of these.

A. Acute disseminated encephalomyelitis
B. Acute hemorrhagic leukoencephalitis
C. Both of these
D. Neither of these

43. The disorder is a common disease of white matter in children

44. Development of the disease is usually preceded by a nonspecific respiratory infection

45. Lymphocytes from patients with the disease are sensitized to myelin basic protein

46. Circulating antibodies to myelin basic protein are a characteristic feature

47. Recovery without neurologic impairment is the rule

48. On gross examination, the brain is usually normal

49. Vasculitis is characteristically present on histologic examination

DIRECTIONS: Questions 50 to 81 are matching questions. For each numbered item, choose the most likely associated lettered item from those provided. Each numbered item has ONLY ONE answer. Within each group, each lettered item may be the answer to one, more than one, or none of the numbered items.

For each of the characteristics of central nervous system (CNS) cells listed below, choose whether it describes astrocytes, oligodendrocytes, ependymal cells, all of these, or none of these.

    A. Astrocyte
    B. Oligodendrocyte
    C. Ependymal cells
    D. All of these
    E. None of these

50. Defined as a neuroglial cell
51. Functions as a macrophage
52. Forms glial scars following CNS injury
53. Provides physical (structural) support for neurons
54. Maintains CNS myelin
55. Produces cerebrospinal fluid
56. Resorbs cerebrospinal fluid

For each of the features listed below, choose whether it describes meningococcal meningitis, mumps meningitis, tuberculous meningitis, all of these, or none of these.

    A. Meningococcal meningitis
    B. Mumps meningitis
    C. Tuberculous meningitis
    D. All of these
    E. None of these

57. The cerebrospinal fluid (CSF) sugar content is usually normal
58. The CSF protein content is usually elevated
59. Neutrophils are characteristically found in the CSF
60. Photophobia and stiff neck are *not* commonly present
61. Obliterative endarteritis of subarachnoid vessels is an associated complication

For each of the features listed below, choose whether it is characteristic of astrocytoma, oligodendroglioma, ependymoma, or none of these.

    A. Astrocytoma
    B. Oligodendroglioma
    C. Ependymoma
    D. None of these

62. Constitutes the most common brain tumor in children
63. Constitutes the most common brain tumor in adults

64. Constitutes the most common type of intraspinal glioma
65. Gives rise to glioblastoma multiforme
66. Characteristically tends to calcify markedly
67. Forms tumor cell rosettes as a typical histologic feature
68. Forms tumor cell pseudorosettes as a typical histologic feature
69. Typically metastasizes to bone
70. Frequently responds dramatically to chemotherapy

For each of the features listed below, choose whether it describes metachromatic leukodystrophy, Krabbe's disease (globoid cell leukodystrophy), adrenoleukodystrophy, or none of these.

    A. Metachromatic leukodystrophy
    B. Krabbe's disease (globoid cell leukodystrophy)
    C. Adrenoleukodystrophy
    D. None of these

71. Usually becomes clinically manifest after age 10
72. Produced by a deficiency of cerebroside sulfatase
73. Produced by a deficiency of galactocerebroside β-galactosidase
74. Characterized histologically by multinucleate histiocytic cells in the white matter
75. Characterized histologically by diagnostic inclusion bodies in Schwann cells

For each of the causes of peripheral neuropathies listed below, decide whether it is usually associated with a pattern of acute ascending motor paralysis, subacute symmetrical sensorimotor polyneuropathy, subacute asymmetrical sensorimotor polyneuropathy, or none of these.

    A. Acute ascending motor paralysis
    B. Subacute symmetrical sensorimotor polyneuropathy
    C. Subacute asymmetrical sensorimotor polyneuropathy
    D. None of these

76. Diabetic neuropathy
77. Alcoholic neuropathy
78. Landry-Guillain-Barré syndrome
79. Diphtheritic neuropathy
80. Polyarteritis nodosa neuropathy
81. Sarcoidosis neuropathy

16

THE NERVOUS SYSTEM

ANSWERS

1. (A) Increased intracranial pressure is the end result of myriad pathological processes that expand the volume of the intracranial contents beyond the limits set by its bony confines. Thus, processes that are characterized by cellular swelling, interstitial edema, space-occupying lesions (e.g., tumors, hemorrhage, increased amounts of cerebrospinal fluid), or a combination of these lead to increased intracranial pressure. Metastatic tumor, in addition to constituting a space-occupying lesion, causes local damage to capillary endothelial cells and/or induces new capillary formation, which contributes to vasogenic cerebral edema. Similar mechanisms of vascular injury producing vasogenic edema occur in association with lead encephalopathy and contusions. Water intoxication leads to cytotoxic edema by producing an acute hypo-osmolar state in the plasma with a resultant shift of water into the cerebral cells to maintain osmotic equilibrium.

Alzheimer's disease is not associated with increased intracranial pressure. On the contrary, brain volume is reduced as a result of severe atrophy. The compensatory enlargement of the ventricular system is known as hydrocephalus *ex vacuo*, not to be confused with other forms of obstructive or communicating hydrocephalus that are well-known causes of increased intracranial pressure (*pp. 1375–1376*).

2. (E) It is clear that many forms of CNS disease arise primarily as a consequence of modern forms of treatment. Principal among these are the infectious diseases of the CNS that occur almost exclusively in iatrogenically immunosuppressed patients; these include progressive multifocal leukoencephalopathy (a viral disease of oligodendrocytes), infection by unusual organisms such as Citrobacter meningitis, and cerebral toxoplasmosis. Another iatrogenic disease, central pontine myelinolysis, is produced by rapid rises in serum sodium concentrations most frequently associated with intravenous administration of sodium-containing solutions. This disease leads to demyelination in the mid portion of the pons.

Metachromatic leukodystrophy is a genetic autosomal recessive disorder of sphingomyelin metabolism that produces demyelination in both the central and peripheral nervous system and has no iatrogenic component (*pp. 1377–1378, 1386, 1424*).

3. (E) Subacute sclerosing panencephalitis (SSPE) is a slow viral infection of the central nervous system. It is caused by the measles virus and therefore usually follows either active infection or immunization against rubeola. The disease has a long latent period and a protracted course that usually leads to death. Pathologically, the disease is characterized by inclusion bodies in neurons and oligodendroglia, extensive neuronal loss, and perivascular mononuclear cell infiltrates. Most of the injury in SSPE is sustained by the neurons, and primary demyelinization is not a feature. Rather, primary demyelinization is the characteristic feature of progressive multifocal leukoencephalopathy, a viral infection of oligodendrocytes (*p. 1385*).

4. (E) Subacute spongiform encephalopathy (Creutzfeldt-Jakob disease) is a rapidly progressive dementia caused by a poorly defined transmissible agent with some unusual features. The agent is *not* visible with the electron microscope and has an atypical *resistance* to standard methods for viral inactivation such as exposure to ionizing radiation, ultraviolet light, or formalin. Unfortunately, the mode of transmission is unknown at present, although the disease does not appear to be highly contagious. Documented cases of man-to-man transmission have occurred via a *parenteral* route. The disease is characterized pathologically by neuronal loss and marked gliosis in the *absence* of inflammation. Clinically, a rapidly progressive dementia is the rule, and death usually ensues following an average survival of seven months (*p. 1387*).

5. (A) An epidural hematoma results from bleeding into the potential space between the skull and the dura mater. Unlike subdural hematomas, which often result from blunt trauma without skull fractures, epidural hematomas almost always occur in association with an overlying skull fracture. Since the bleeding is usually of arterial origin, the rise in intracranial pressure and the onset of symptoms are typically rapid, usually developing within minutes to a few hours of the trauma. The major symptom is a progressively deepening coma. A fluctuating level of consciousness is suggestive instead of a subdural hematoma. Epidural hematomas are almost always due to trauma; other causes are distinctly uncommon. Although they are rarely a cause of intracranial hemorrhage, ruptured mycotic aneurysms usually produce subarachnoid hemorrhage rather than epidural hematoma *(pp. 1396–1397)*.

6. (E) Mechanical injury to the spinal cord occurs by two mechanisms: penetration and/or compression injuries. Compression injuries produce contusions of the cord and are most frequently caused by metastatic tumor causing pathologic fractures in the spinal canal and within the vertebral bodies. Although penetrating wounds usually produce lacerations of the spinal cord, an element of compression may be introduced when concomitant hemorrhage into the cord parenchyma occurs (hematomyelia) *(p. 1399)*.

7. (D) Alzheimer's disease is a degenerative disease of the cerebral cortex that ultimately leads to dementia. Although the pathogenesis of the disease is unknown, several distinctive pathologic features are produced. Hirano bodies, glassy eosinophilic inclusions composed principally of actin filaments, are seen in proximal dendrites. Senile plaques, which are composed of dilated, tortuous, presynaptic axon terminals, are typically found in the cerebral cortex. Neurofibrillary tangles, which are neurofilaments in the cytoplasm of neurons that typically encircle the nucleus and denote neuronal degeneration, are most notably, but not exclusively, associated with Alzheimer's disease. Granulovacuolar degeneration of neurons refers to clear intraneuronal cytoplasmic vacuoles, each of which contains an argyrophilic granule of unknown composition. This form of neuronal degeneration is particularly characteristic of Alzheimer's disease.

Iron-containing pigment in the globus pallidus is a feature of Hallervorden-Spatz disease, an autosomal recessive disorder that affects the globus pallidus and the substantia nigra *(pp. 1414–1417)*.

8. (D) A subdural empyema is an infection (most frequently bacterial) of the skull bones or air sinuses that has penetrated into the subdural space. Thus, most patients with a subdural empyema also have sinusitis and fever. Usually, the process remains localized, and the underlying arachnoid mater and subarachnoid space are uninvolved. Injury to the brain may occur by indirect means such as secondary thrombophlebitis of central veins crossing the subdural space with venous infarction of the brain, but brain abscesses are not produced *(p. 1380)*.

9. (A) Herpes simplex virus (HSV I) infections take many forms in man. In addition to causing the common cold sore, HSV I produces both a neonatal and an adult form of encephalitis. In contrast to the adult form, which typically involves the inferior and medial regions of the temporal lobes and the orbital gyri of the frontal lobes, the neonatal form affects the entire brain. This virus is also a known cause of benign recurrent (Mollaret) meningitis, a rare self-limited recurrent meningitis. Postherpetic neuralgia, however, is a product of latent herpes zoster infection and refers to a lingering pain following a case of "shingles" (see Question 40) *(pp. 1383–1384)*.

10. (D) Berry aneurysms are developmental (congenital) arterial defects that are the most common cause of aneurysmal rupture in the CNS. Only 6% are located in the vertebrobasilar artery circulation; the vast majority occur in the internal carotid artery circulation. Although they are often solitary, more than one aneurysm is found in up to 30% of cases *(p. 1393)*.

11. (B) The middle cerebral artery is the vessel most commonly involved by several different types of CNS vascular disorders. It is the most common site of bleeding from arteriovenous malformations and embolic obstruction. Arterial tears producing epidural hematomas are most common in the middle meningeal artery. Atherosclerotic thrombosis usually occurs in the larger arteries of the brain and most often involves the internal carotid, vertebral, and lower basilar arteries *(pp. 1394, 1396)*.

12. (E) Carcinomatous meningitis refers to metastatic spread of tumor via the cerebrospinal fluid to the meningeal surfaces of the brain, spinal cord, and nerve roots. This mode of dissemination is frequently associated with two primary brain tumors—medulloblastomas and pineal tumors. Tumors metastatic to the brain may also spread in this manner, and the two that do so most frequently are lung and breast cancers *(p. 1400)*.

13. (C) Meningiomas are primary tumors of the meninges that are most frequently slow-growing, well-circumscribed, benign tumors associated with a good prognosis. Only rarely do the anaplastic and papillary variants of this tumor behave in a malignant fashion. Despite their benign behavior, penetration of the tumor into the adjacent bone is common. A characteristic histologic feature is the presence of psammoma bodies, concentrically laminated spheroids of calcium salts that give the tumor a gritty appearance and may appear as stippling on x-ray examination *(pp. 1407–1409)*.

14. (C) Idiopathic parkinsonism is a progressive disorder of motor function characterized by damage to the striatonigral dopaminergic system. Histologically, the disease is characterized by the presence of Lewy bodies, eosinophilic intracytoplasmic inclusion bodies, in the neurons of the substantia nigra and locus ceruleus. In addition, the melanin-containing neurons in these regions of the brain are typically depigmented.

Neurofibrillary tangles are seen in the affected neurons of postencephalitic parkinsonism (not Lewy bodies). They are not associated with idiopathic parkinsonism, however. Neuronal loss in the putamen is a characteristic of striatonigral degeneration, another degenerative disease of the basal ganglia that is clinically similar to idiopathic parkinsonism but is pathologically different *(p. 1417)*.

15. (A) Amyotrophic lateral sclerosis (ALS) is a degenerative disease of the pyramidal motor system. Although there are four clinical variants, the most frequent produces degeneration of both the upper motor neurons in the motor cortex and the lower motor neurons in the cranial motor nuclei or in the anterior horns of the spinal cord. The disease has an invariably fatal outcome after a variable two- to six-year course. Unlike poliomyelitis, a disease of lower motor neurons caused by an enterovirus, ALS is not known to be associated with a viral agent *(p. 1419)*.

16. (B) Neurofibromata are peripheral nerve tumors derived from Schwann cells. They are often multiple and are composed of interlacing bands of delicate spindle cells with slender, wavy nuclei. In neurofibromata, nerve fibers are found scattered throughout the tumor mass, which appears as a bulbous expansion of the entire nerve fascicle. In contrast to schwannomas, which are eccentrically located on the side of the nerve and can be surgically excised, neurofibromas cannot be resected without removing the involved nerve. Verocay bodies are a histologic feature of schwannomas and consist of palisaded nuclei in the areas of high cellularity known as Antoni A tissue *(pp. 1432–1433)*.

17. (False); 18. (True); 19. (False); 20. (True); 21. (False); 22. (False); 23. (True); 24. (True); 25. (False

As a group, vascular disorders are the most common cause (about 50% of cases) of neurologic problems encountered in general hospitals. **(17)** The separate contributions of hypoxia and reduced blood flow to neurologic dysfunction are important to differentiate. Pure hypoxia (deprivation of oxygen) with maintenance of normal blood flow, as might occur on exposure to reduced atmospheric pressures, is tolerable to neurons for much longer periods of time than ischemia (reduced or interrupted blood flow). Evidence from experimental studies suggests that neurons can tolerate pure hypoxia for as long as 25 minutes, whereas ischemia produces permanent neuronal damage after about 4 minutes. **(18)** Encephalopathic changes induced by ischemia are most commonly the result of less than effective cardiopulmonary resuscitation following cardiac arrest, not surprising in these resuscitation-conscious times.

(19) Prolonged ischemia from a localized vascular obstruction, either from thrombus, embolus, or external compression, produces cerebral infarction in the distribution of the affected vessel. The infarction does *not* overlap arterial territories. Thus, a hemorrhagic infarct can often be differentiated from a cerebral *hemorrhage* that does not necessarily cause a pattern of involvement corresponding to a given vascular distribution. **(20)** Cerebral hemorrhage (bleeding into the brain substance) is more commonly caused by hypertensive vascular disease. In this disorder, bleeding is caused by rupture of blood vessels within the CNS, most commonly in the putamen (55%). **(21)** Supratentorial cerebral hemorrhages tend to present as hemiplegias, frequently with an eye movement disorder. Intractable vomiting is a symptom associated with hemorrhage in the posterior fossa (a cerebellar hematoma, for example). **(22)** Although emboli are the most common cause of cerebral infarction in the distribution of the middle cerebral artery, the most common cause of cerebral infarction *overall* is large vessel thrombosis, usually atherosclerotic in origin.

(23) Lacunar infarcts are small infarcts in the deep portions of the brain (especially the thalamus, putamen, and internal capsule) that are characteristic of hypertensive vascular disease. **(24)** Owing to their small size and variable location, lacunar infarcts can produce a variety of ischemic syndromes or may even be asymptomatic. A pure motor hemiparesis or a pure sensory deficit are two of the recognized lacunar syndromes. They can occur from a small infarct in the internal capsule where the major tracts are compressed into a small volume.

(25) In contrast to the brain, the spinal cord most often sustains vascular injury from disruption of the spinal arteries secondary to dissecting aortic aneurysms *(pp. 1388–1395)*.

26. (False); 27. (True); 28. (False); 29. (True); 30. (False); 31. (False); 32. (False)

(26 and 27) Multiple sclerosis (MS) is a disease of undetermined etiology that causes diffuse primary demyelinization in the central nervous system. Although it may occur in children, it usually affects adults between 20 and 40 years of age and is rare after age 50. **(28)** The disease typically begins with paresthesias, diplopia, or cerebellar incoordination, but intellectual deterioration is not an early manifestation. **(29)** The cerebrospinal fluid typically contains an increased immunoglobulin content, and immunoelectrophoretic analysis demonstrates oligoclonal bands that are not present in the serum. In contrast to the CSF immunoglobulins found in subacute sclerosing panencephalitis (SSPE; see Question 3), which are directed against measles viral antigen, the antigen against which the CSF immunoglobulin is directed in MS patients is as yet unknown. **(30)** In further contrast to SSPE, which typically occurs after a case of measles, MS is not associated with a preceding viral infection. **(31)** The characteristic brain and spinal cord plaques that occur in MS are not produced by gliosis. Rather, they consist of multiple small foci of demyelination and perivascular inflammation that have coalesced to form macroscopically visual lesions. (32) Although clinical trials have shown that high levels of immunosuppression can temporarily arrest the progression of MS in children, there is at present no truly effective treatment for this disease. During relapses, however, patients are often treated with ACTH with some temporary benefit *(pp. 1410–1412)*.

33. (D); 34. (C); 35. (B); 36. (A); 37. (B)

Distention of the ventricles by an increased volume of cerebrospinal fluid (CSF) is known as hydrocephalus. Although it can be caused by overproduction of fluid, decreased absorption of CSF is the most common cause. Decreased CSF absorption may, in turn, result either from decreased transfer of CSF to the venous system by the arachnoid villi (communicating hydrocephalus) or from decreased flow through the CSF pathway to the villi due to obstruction (noncommunicating hydrocephalus). (33) Both types produce ventricular distention. (34) Either type may occur in a postmeningitis state, depending upon the nature and extent of the injury and the location of the subsequent fibrosis. For example, severe pneumococcal meningitis may lead to communicating hydrocephalus from arachnoid fibrosis induced by large quantities of pneumococcal capsular polysaccharides in the subarachnoid space. In fact, acute pyogenic meningitis of any cause may produce fibrotic adhesions between the meninges and the brain. Basal adhesive arachnoiditis obliterating the subarachnoid space around the brainstem may occlude the foramina of Magendie and Luschka, producing noncommunicating hydrocephalus. (35) Obstructive (noncommunicating) hydrocephalus is characteristically seen in association with neoplasms that invade or compress the foramina in the CSF pathway. (36) Thrombosis of the dural sinuses inteferes with transport of CSF into the venous system and typically produces communicating hydrocephalus. (37) The Dandy-Walker syndrome is a congenital malformation of the cerebellum in which the cerebellar vermis fails to develop. Consequently, occlusion or obliteration of the foramina of Magendie and Luschka occurs and noncommunicating hydrocephalus is produced *(pp. 1376–1377)*.

38. (B); 39. (A); 40. (D); 41. (B); 42. (A)

Rabies and poliomyelitis are viral diseases of the CNS that end in paralysis. (38) As typically occurs with most viral diseases of the CNS, poliomyelitis is preceded by a primary infection elsewhere, in this case the gastrointestinal tract. Rabies is a noteworthy exception to this rule since the virus is inoculated directly into the peripheral nerves and ascends promptly to the brain. (39) Although other forms of viral encephalitis may be associated with inclusion bodies, the only diagnostic inclusion is the intracytoplasmic Negri body of rabies. It is an eosinophilic cytoplasmic inclusion, usually round, oval, or bullet-shaped and often multiple. (40) Although rabies virus does affect the dorsal root ganglia, it also typically involves the neurons of Ammon's horn in the temporal lobe as well as the Purkinje cells of the cerebellum and the spinal cord. The principal target of poliovirus is the anterior horn cell of the spinal cord, although the posterior horn may be affected in very fulminant cases. The viral agent that shows specific and exclusive tropism for the dorsal root ganglion cells is herpes zoster. Following acute infection by herpes zoster (chickenpox), the virus remains latent for long periods of time within the dorsal root ganglia. Recrudescence of the viral infection ("shingles") may occur with immunosuppression or advancing age. (41) In contrast to rabies, which produces a characteristic severe encephalitis with flaccid paralysis occurring only in the late stage of the disease, poliomyelitis with its specifically targeted injury characteristically causes a lower motor neuron paralysis. (42) Although the most common cause of death in both these diseases is respiratory failure, it occurs on the basis of respiratory center failure in rabies and from paralysis of the respiratory muscles in polio *(pp. 1383–1385)*.

43. (D); 44. (B); 45. (C); 46. (D); 47. (D); 48. (A); 49. (B)

Acute disseminated encephalomyelitis and acute hemorrhagic leukoencephalitis are two disorders with impossibly long names that fall into the category of perivenous encephalomyelitis. They are characterized by perivenular demyelinization and a pronounced mononuclear inflammatory infiltrate. (43) Although they may occur in either children or adults, both of these diseases are extremely *rare*. (44) In contrast to acute disseminated encephalomyelitis, which typically occurs after a well-defined viral infection such as measles, mumps or chickenpox, acute hemorrhagic leukoencephalitis is usually preceded only by a nonspecific respiratory infection. (45) Both diseases, however, are believed to be autoimmune in origin, since lymphocytes from patients with these diseases are sensitized to myelin basic protein. (46) In both diseases, the autoimmune response appears to be largely cellular rather than humoral, since antibodies to myelin proteins are not found.

(47) Unfortunately, both diseases have an extremely poor prognosis. About half of the patients with acute disseminated encephalomyelitis die in the acute phase of the disease, and those who survive usually have severe neurologic impairment. Acute hemorrhagic leukoencephalitis is typically a rapidly fatal disorder with only rare survivors. (48) The pathologic findings in these diseases reflect their differing severity. In acute disseminated encephalomyelitis, the brain usually appears normal on gross examination, whereas in acute hemorrhagic leukoencephalitis (a necrotizing process), the brain is soft,

sometimes liquefied, and flecked with tiny hemorrhages. (49) On histologic examination, necrotizing vasculitis is seen in acute hemorrhagic leukoencephalitis and corresponds to the hemorrhagic areas seen grossly. Although perivascular inflammation is seen in acute disseminated encephalomyelitis, vasculitis does not occur (pp. 1412–1413).

50. (D); 51. (E); 52. (A); 53. (A); 54. (B); 55. (E); 56. (E)

Although the neuron is the basic parenchymal element of the central nervous system, numerous specialized supportive and protective interstitial cells are necessary for normal neuronal functioning. (50) These supportive elements, called neuroglial cells, consist of astrocytes, oligodendrocytes, ependymal cells, and microglial cells. (51) It is the *microglial* cells (not presented as a choice above) that represent the CNS component of the monocyte-macrophage system. When activated, these cells resemble macrophages in both their cytoplasmic histochemical profiles and their phagocytic activity.

(52 and 53) Astrocytes form an extensive cellular plexus that serves as the structural framework for the all-important neurons. They are also thought to provide biochemical support and insulation to neighboring neurons. Following injury, astrocytes are responsible for the CNS equivalent of scar formation, a process known as gliosis. In contrast to fibrosis, gliosis does not lead to the production of collagen. Rather, defects are filled by "glial fibers," which are actually cellular processes of astrocytes containing abundant intermediate filaments made up of vimentin and glial fibrillary acidic protein (GFAP).

(54) Oligodendrocytes, so called because they have fewer and shorter dendrites than astrocytes, are responsible for the production and maintenance of CNS myelin. In contrast to the Schwann cell, the myelin-forming cell of the peripheral nervous system, each oligodendrocyte contributes segments of myelin sheaths to multiple axons. In demyelinating diseases of the CNS, oligodendrocytes sustain most of the injury.

(55 and 56) Although ependymal cells line the ventricles of the brain, they are not responsible for the production of the cerebrospinal fluid contained within, nor are they responsible for its resorption. The cells of the choroid plexus produce cerebrospinal fluid, which, after traversing the ventricles and entering the subarachnoid space, is resorbed by the cells of the arachnoid villi (pp. 1373–1374).

57. (B); 58. (D); 59. (A); 60. (C); 61. (C)

Meningitis refers to inflammation limited to the leptomeninges in the subarachnoid space and is most often caused by infection. The nature of the inflammatory process is largely determined by the causal organism. Acute pyogenic meningitis is usually bacterial in origin; meningococcal meningitis is a com-

mon example. Acute lymphocytic meningitis, usually virally induced, is exemplified by mumps meningitis. Chronic meningitis, a more slowly evolving process, is associated with infection by bacteria or fungi; tuberculous meningitis is a prototypic example. (57) Only in acute lymphocytic meningitis is the sugar content of the CSF almost invariably normal. Pyogenic meningitis causes a strikingly reduced CSF sugar content, whereas chronic meningitis is associated with a variably reduced sugar content. (58) In contrast, all forms of meningitis usually produce elevations in the protein content of the CSF. These vary only in magnitude.

(59) Large numbers of neutrophils in the CSF are characteristic of acute pyogenic meningitis such as that of meningococcal origin. In mumps meningitis, the CSF pleocytosis consists mainly of lymphocytes and in tuberculous meningitis is composed largely of mononuclear cells. (60) Only the acute forms of meningitis, either pyogenic or lymphocytic, are associated clinically with signs of meningeal irritation: a stiff neck, headache, photophobia, irritability, and clouding of consciousness. Chronic meningitis, such as tuberculous meningitis, presents with more generalized neurologic symptoms including headache, malaise, mental confusion, and vomiting rather than a stiff neck. (61) Obliterative endarteritis is a complication of chronic meningitis caused by the continuing inflammatory reaction around the vessels of the subarachnoid space. Since infarctions in the underlying brain may result, obliterative endarteritis is one of the most feared complications of this type of meningitis (pp. 1378–1380).

62. (A); 63. (D); 64. (C); 65. (A); 66. (B); 67. (C); 68. (C); 69. (D); 70. (D)

Astrocytomas, oligodendrogliomas, and ependymomas are all neuroglial tumors with distinctive characteristics. (62) Astrocytomas are the most common type of primary brain tumor in children. In contrast to adult astrocytomas, most of which occur in the cerebral hemispheres, the majority of astrocytomas in children occur in the cerebellum. (63) The most common primary brain tumor in adults is glioblastoma multiforme, constituting 25 to 30% of cases. (64) In the spinal cord, the most common type of glial tumor is the ependymoma. Ependymomas constitute about 63% of intraspinal gliomas but only 5 to 6% of all intracranial gliomas. (65) The astrocytoma is the tumor type that gives rise to glioblastoma multiforme, the most anaplastic of all the gliomas. Although they may arise *de novo*, most glioblastomas develop in preexisting astrocytomas by progressive dedifferentiation.

(66) One of the most distinctive pathologic features of oligodendroglioma is its tendency to calcify. This feature is actually a diagnostic aid, since the tumor characteristically appears strippled with calcifications on x-ray examination and CT scan.

(**67 and 68**) Histologic features that are particularly characteristic of ependymomas are rosette and pseudorosette formation. A rosette is a small circle of tumor cells arranged around a central space that may contain neuroglial fibers. The tumor cells in pseudorosettes, on the other hand, are arranged around a blood vessel.

(**69 and 70**) Extraneural metastases from any primary intracranial tumor are distinctly uncommon, and when they occur, they are most likely to be from a glioblastoma or medulloblastoma. Another characteristic shared by all neuroglial tumors is their resistance to chemotherapy. Depending on the feasibility of surgical resection, excision and radiotherapy have thus far provided the most successful therapeutic approaches to neuroglial tumors (*pp. 1401–1405*).

71. (D); 72. (A); 73. (B); 74. (B); 75. (C)
The leukodystrophies are diseases of the white matter resulting from biochemical defects in the pathway of myelin metabolism. (**71**) All of these diseases become manifest in early childhood as symmetrical, global disorders of myelinization. (**72**) Metachromatic leukodystrophy is an autosomal recessive disorder of sphinogomyelin metabolism produced by a deficiency of aryl-sulfatase A (cerebroside sulfatase). It usually presents as a progressive motor impairment with mental deterioration and can be diagnosed by measuring urinary aryl-sulfatase A. (**73 and 74**) Another autosomal recessive disorder, Krabbe's disease, results from a deficiency of galactocerebroside β-galactosidase. This disease usually begins within the first six months of life and leads to death within a year. In addition to demyelinization, a characteristic histologic feature is the presence of multinucleate, histiocytic cells called globoid cells. (**75**) Adrenoleukodystrophy, a familial sex-linked disease producing symmetrical demyelinization in the cerebral hemispheres and adrenal failure, has a diagnostic ultrastructural feature. By electron microscopy, specific cytoplasmic inclusions composed of dense, long, thin leaflets enclosing an electron-lucent space are seen in the cerebral macrophages, adrenocortical cells, testicular Leydig cells, and Schwann cells of patients with this disease (*pp. 1424–1425*).

76. (C); 77. (B); 78. (A); 79. (A); 80. (C); 81. (C)
Peripheral neuropathies develop whenever axonal degeneration, demyelinization, or a combination of these occurs in the peripheral nervous system. They may occur in association with a large number of diseases and produce varied clinical syndromes, depending upon the size and the type (sensory, motor, or autonomic) of the axons principally involved. Most major causes of peripheral neuropathy tend to produce a specific pattern of injury and corresponding clinical syndrome with variable predictability. (**76, 80, 81**) Diseases that produce focal lesions rather than generalized injury tend to affect only individual nerves and produce a mononeuritis or, if more than one nerve is affected, a mononeuritis multiplex. If the disease is severe and widespread, however, a polyneuritis may be produced that is often symmetrical. Diabetes mellitus, polyarteritis nodosa, and sarcoidosis are examples of processes that typically produce focal lesions and cause focal and/or diffuse sensorimotor axonal neuropathies that are usually asymmetrical. (**77**) Alcohol has diffuse systemic effects and is therefore associated with diffuse demyelinization and axonal degeneration manifested as a symmetrical sensorimotor polyneuropathy.

(**78 and 79**) Diseases that cause acute demyelinization without significant axonal injury and an acute ascending motor paralysis include the Landry-Guillain-Barré syndrome (acute idiopathic polyneuritis) and diphtheria. The cause of the acute demyelinization in the Landry-Guillain-Barré syndrome is as yet unknown, although immunologic mechanisms have been implicated. Diphtheritic peripheral neuritis is the direct result of the action of diphtheria toxin on the peripheral nerve. In diphtheria, demyelinization is limited to the dorsal root ganglia and the adjacent motor and sensory roots, since there is a naturally occurring defect in the blood barrier at these points, allowing penetration of the toxin (*pp. 1429–1431*).